Essentials of Radiotherapy in Uro-Genital Malignancies

Renu Madan • Shikha Goyal
Editors

Essentials of Radiotherapy in Uro-Genital Malignancies

Springer

Editors
Renu Madan
Department of Radiotherapy and Oncology
Post Graduate Institute of Medical
Education and Research
Chandigarh, India

Shikha Goyal
Department of Radiotherapy and Oncology
Post Graduate Institute of Medical
Education and Research
Chandigarh, India

ISBN 978-981-95-5944-2 ISBN 978-981-95-5945-9 (eBook)
https://doi.org/10.1007/978-981-95-5945-9

This Springer imprint is published by the registered company Springer Nature Singapore Pte Ltd.
The registered company address is: 152 Beach Road, #21-01/04 Gateway East, Singapore 189721, Singapore

Foreword

The editors of *Essentials of Radiotherapy in Uro-Genital Malignancies* are to be commended for their meticulous effort in compiling a succinct and informative textbook which brings together the expert insights and knowledge from radiation oncology, medical oncology, and uro-oncology. The textbook presents a practical approach to urogenital cancers, including radiology, pathology, and clinical expertise for optimum patient care.

Multidisciplinary management is crucial for achieving better outcome, and radiotherapy has emerged as a crucial component in the treatment of most urogenital cancers. This textbook offers comprehensive and multidisciplinary approach for managing urogenital cancers and covering topics such as prostate, bladder, testicular, kidney, and penile cancer. Additionally, it explores crucial areas such as epidemiology, cancer genetics, role of brachytherapy, and survivorship concerns.

The field of uro-oncology continues to evolve with significant developments and breakthroughs over the past decade. As a comprehensive guide designed for oncologists, students, and healthcare professionals dedicated to the care of patients with urogenital malignancies, this book skillfully consolidates the latest evidence, expert opinions, and clinical practices.

We hope that this comprehensive guide will contribute to improved outcomes, and increased hope for patients and families affected by urogenital cancers.

It's an honor to write the foreword for this book. I'm confident that this will prove to be a valuable resource for oncologists in their clinical practice.

Department of Radiation Oncology,
Ex Chief DR.B.R.A.I.R.C.H, AIIMS
New Delhi, India

Ex-head National Cancer Institute
(2nd Campus AIIMS), Jhajjar,
Haryana, India

G. K. Rath

October 3, 2025

Preface

We are pleased to introduce *Essentials of Radiotherapy in Uro-Genital Malignancies*, a comprehensive textbook that synthesizes the latest evidence and best practices for managing urogenital malignancies. After a two-year journey that began in 2023, this textbook represents a significant milestone, made possible by the dedication and hard work of our expert authors.

As a field that is constantly evolving, radiation oncology necessitates a deep understanding of the complexities involved in treating urogenital malignancies. The textbook is organized into 17 chapters, providing an in-depth exploration of the management of various urogenital cancers, including genetics, brachytherapy, and survivorship issues. We trust that this textbook will serve as a valuable resource for healthcare professionals dedicated to the care of patients with urogenital cancers.

We are deeply grateful for the inspiration provided by patients and families battling urogenital cancers, who drive us to improve care and treatment.

This book has been prepared to the best of our ability, and while we strive for accuracy, we acknowledge the possibility of errors. We welcome constructive feedback from readers to help us improve future editions.

Chandigarh, India Renu Madan
Chandigarh, India Shikha Goyal

Contents

1 Introduction to Urogenital Cancers

Arun Kumar Yadav, Renu Madan, Arnav Tiwari,
Shikha Goyal, and Narendra Kumar

1.1 Introduction

Genitourinary (GU) cancers comprise of distinct neoplasm of prostate, bladder, kidney, testis, and penis. With population aging, the incidence of these cancers is increasing [1]. According to the data from International agency for Research on Cancer, kidney, bladder, and prostate cancers are the ninth, sixth, and third most common causes of cancer in males, respectively. [2]. From 1971 to 2019, mortality rate from prostate, Kidney, and bladder cancers is declining due to early detection and improvement in the therapeutic strategies [3]. However, the testicular cancer survival rate remained stable at >90%. Outcome in penile cancer patients still remains poor. Over the last few decades, understanding of tumor biology has shown that some patients require aggrevise treatment, while others may not require any treatment at all.

Multi-disciplinary care is the key to the cancer management. The first structured fellowship in uro-oncology was started in 1971, under the vision of the then chief Willet F. Whitmore, Jr., at Memorial Sloan Kettering Cancer Centre (MSKCC), New York [4]. Prestigious Society of Urology Oncology was founded in 1984.

A. K. Yadav
Department of Radiotherapy and Radiation Medicine, Banaras Hindu University, Varanasi, India

R. Madan (✉) · A. Tiwari · S. Goyal · N. Kumar
Department of Radiotherapy and Oncology, Postgraduate Institute of Medical Education and Research (PGIMER), Chandigarh, India

R. Madan, S. Goyal (eds.), *Essentials of Radiotherapy in Uro-Genital Malignancies*, https://doi.org/10.1007/978-981-95-5945-9_1

1.2 Prostate Cancer

Since the approval of the prostate cancer–specific antigen (PSA) for screening by the Food and Drug Administration (FDA) in 1984, and better imaging techniques, majority of the prostate cancers are now diagnosed at early stage of the disease. Advanced imaging modalities such as prostate specific–membrane antigen (PSMA) PET help in personalized treatment and treatment individualization [5].

The ideal approach for an individual with prostate cancer is a complex decision process. Various treatment options include active surveillance (AS) or watchful waiting, surgery, radiotherapy (RT), androgen deprivation therapy (ADT), and chemotherapy depending on the stage, risk, symptomatology, and patient preference. Normograms, first developed for prostate cancers, can be used to detect recurrence and help in personalized treatment. The concept of AS for indolent prostate cancer patients arose in 1970s and avoids overtreatment in a significant number of the patients [6]. Laparoscopic radical prostatectomy (RP) replaced the open retropubic approach in 1998, which was soon replaced by robot-assisted RP [4]. Minimally invasive surgeries have allowed the complex oncological procedures to be performed in an ambulatory setting. An ambulatory recovery model was established to permit same-day surgery and discharge [7].

Radiotherapy (RT) is an equally effective therapeutic option in prostate cancer patients. Newer RT techniques such as intensity-modulated radiation therapy (IMRT), volumetric-modulated arc therapy (VMAT), and image-guided radiation therapy (IGRT) help in optimizing the dose delivered to the target while minimizing exposure to surrounding healthy tissues, which in turn lead to dose escalation and improved outcome. The role of RT is evolving particularly in those with oligo-metastatic disease. Prostate cancer shows RT dose–response relationship and, unlike majority of the cancer, the α/β ratio for prostate cancer is low, compared to the surrounding normal tissue; hence, hypofractionated RT improves outcome. Both moderate hypofractionated RT (2.4–3.4 Gy/#) and stereotactic body radiotherapy (SBRT) or ultra-hypofractionated RT (>5 Gy/#) are acceptable regimens [8–10]. Another method of dose escalation, i.e. boost to the visible tumor, improves biochemical disease-free survival in intermediate- and high-risk prostate cancer, without increasing toxicities and quality of life [11]. Proton beam therapy (PBT) is the most advanced technique of RT; however, till date, none of the trial has demonstrated clear benefit of PBT. One trial showed that PBT reduces the acute toxicity with no impact on late toxicity compared to photon beam therapy [12]. RT to primary in those with oligometastatic disease has shown encouraging results [13, 14]. Aggressive metastasis-directed therapy improves ADT-free and biochemical relapse-free survival [15, 16]. However, further studies are required to understand the impact of metastatis-directed therapy (MDT) and RT to the primary site in the setting of metastatic disease. Interstitial brachytherapy can also be used in selected patients [17].

Eventual failure to conventional ADT leads to castration-resistant prostate cancer (CRPC). Understanding the mechanism of resistance to ADT has led to the development of second-generation ADT (Abiraterone, Enzalutamide, Apalutamide, Darolutamide), which prolong the survival in advanced prostate cancer [18].

Besides, PSMA-targeted therapy is widely used in the metastatic CRPC [19]. More recent trials have shown the efficacy of PARP inhibitors in advanced prostate cancer patients with alteration in gene involving homologous recombination repair [20].

1.3 Bladder Cancer

Bladder cancer is classified into non-muscle-invasive and muscle-invasive tumors and low- and high-grade tumors. Cystoscopy and trans-urethral resection of bladder tumor (TURBT) aim to remove all visible tumor and determine the histological types and depth of the invasion. Restage TURBT improves staging, disease control, and response to intravesical treatment [21]. Intravesical Bacillus-Calmette-Guerin (BCG) was approved by the FDA in 1990s and is still considered as a standard of care in non muscle invasive bladder cancer (NMIBC). Despite an early response to intravesical therapy, patients are at increased risk of recurrence which mandates long-term surveillance. This led to a paradigm shift in 1990s toward early cystectomy in those who failed to intravesical BCG [22]. Further studies showed that about 25% of the patients resistant to BCG respond to intravesical chemotherapy and immunotherapy [23, 24].

The main therapeutic modalities for muscle invasive bladder cancer (MIBC) include radical cystectomy (RC) or bladder preservation therapy or trimodality therapy (TMT) that includes maximum TURBT and chemoradiation. Despite the success of bladder-preserving treatment protocol in MIBC, a major proportion of patients undergo radical cystectomy and pelvic lymph node dissection (PLND). Orthotropic neo-bladder was introduced four decades back as a substitute for conventional ileal conduit. Randomized trials of open RC and robot-assisted RC did not show any difference in recovery time and outcome [25].

Advances in RT techniques have helped in dose escalation, hypofractionation, and adaptive RT planning in bladder cancer patients. There is no standard of care for radiotherapy dose and fractionation. After the results of a meta-analysis comparing two fractionation schedule—55 Gy/20# and 64 Gy/32#—hypofractionated RT is being increasingly used and preferred by many physicians [26]. Trials are exploring the role of adaptive RT for tumor-directed dose escalation [27].

Chemotherapy remains an important component of treatment in MIBC and advanced bladder cancer. The first effective chemotherapy regimen in bladder cancer—methotrexate, vinblastine, adriamycin, and cisplatin (MVAC)—was developed in 1980s [28]. Gemcitabine- and cisplatin-based chemotherapy is considered as equally effective and less toxic to dose-dense MVAC (ddMVAC) chemotherapy. BCON trial showed that the addition of carbogen and nicotinamide can be used to modify hypoxia and improved survival in patients not suitable for concurrent chemotherapy [29].

The treatment options for metastatic disease include chemotherapy, immune check-point inhibitors (ICIs), and antibody-drug conjugates.

ICIs have the potential to improve outcome when given synergistically with RT. Ongoing trials are exploring the role Atezolizumab (NCT03775265),

Pembrolizumab (NCT04241185), and Durvalumab (NCT04216290) with TMT. However, there is a concern of increase in grade 3 gastrointestinal toxicity particularly with hypofractionated RT.

Epidermal growth factor receptor (EGFR) overexpression assessed by IHC is associated with improved outcome, whereas HER2 overexpression is associated with poor outcome and reduced response to chemoradiation [30, 31]. RTOG0524 trial found that addition of trastuzumab can mitigate the worse outcome in HER 2 PLUS_SPI or 3 PLUS_SPI bladder cancer patients.

1.4 Kidney Cancer

Radical nephrectomy (RN) was the standard of care for all renal cell carcinoma (RCC) patients until 1990s, when partial nephrectomy (PN) yielded comparable outcome to RN for localized RCC [32]. The number of PN is increasing due to wide availability of advanced imaging and detection of small localized RCC. In the last two decades, several new tyrosine kinase inhibitors (TKI) and immune-oncology (I/O) drugs became available which have significantly improved the outcome and are the current standard of care for advanced or metastatic RCC [33, 34].

Traditionally RCC was considered as a radio-resistant tumor, and the role of RT was limited to only palliation. However, with the availability of image guidance and advanced techniques of radiation, it is now possible to deliver high dose of radiation or stereotactic body radiotherapy (SBRT) to the tumor, which reduces radio-resistance. [35]. Several studies have demonstrated the benefit of SBRT in oligo-metastatic or oligo-progressive RCC. There is increasing interest in combining SBRT and immunotherapy due to the abscopal effect [36].

1.5 Testicular Cancer

Germ cell tumors (GCT) are the most common type of testicular cancer. These are classified into seminoma and non-seminomatous germ cell tumors (NSGCT) and have a predictable pattern of spread, first to retroperitoneal lymph nodes followed by lungs and other visceral organs. Germ cell tumors are extremely chemo-sensitive and radio-sensitive leading to a cure rate of more than 90%, even in advanced stage of the disease. Orchiectomy is the initial treatment for majority of the adults with GCT [37].

Traditionally, RT was the preferred adjuvant treatment for these patients. However, the treatment landscape has changed in the last few decades. For advanced stage of the disease, 3–4 cycles of chemotherapy with bleomycin, cisplatin, and etoposide are preferred over radiotherapy. Wherever RT is indicated, efforts are being made to reduce the total dose and field size in this group of young patients. Data on PBT is limited. A recent study comparing proton and photon therapy has shown excellent outcome with no in-field recurrence and better sparing of organs at risks (OARs) with PBT [38]. With the advent of chemotherapy, retro-peritoneal lymph node dissection (RPLND) is not routinely performed. The current indications of RPLND are measurable residual disease after chemotherapy, particularly in NSGCT.

1.6 Penile Cancer

Penile cancer is a rare malignancy and is more prevalent in developing countries. Despite medical advancement, the outcome in these patients remained stable over the last few years. Organ preservation surgery or brachytherapy provide durable response in early-stage cancer. In advanced disease, the outcome is poor despite multi-modality treatment including penile amputation with lymph node dissection, chemotherapy, and radiotherapy. The data on immune check-point inhibitors is limited [39]. Ongoing InPACT trial will determine the optimal sequencing of surgery and chemoradiotherapy in advanced penile cancer [40].

1.7 Role of CAR-T Cell Therapy

The role of chimeric antigen receptor T-cell (CAR-T) therapy in GU cancers is evolving. These tumors often express tumor-associated antigens (TAAs) like PSMA, PSCA, CAIX, and EGFR, making them promising candidates for targeted cellular immunotherapy [41, 42]. Prostate cancer is the most extensively explored GU cancer for CAR-T therapy. Key targets include prostate-specific membrane antigen (PSMA) and prostate stem cell antigen (PSCA) [43]. One study of 14 patients with metastatic castration-resistant prostate cancer (mCRPC) received PSCA CAR-T cells. The study demonstrated safety with grade 1–2 cytokine release syndrome in 5 patients, and PSA decline >30% in 4 of 14 patients [43]. Target antigens for RCC include carbonic anhydrase IX (CAIX), ROR1, and CD70. Preclinical studies using CAIX-directed CARs have demonstrated antitumor activity but raised concerns for toxicity to normal tissues expressing CAIX, especially in bile ducts [44]. Pantuck et al. emphasized that RCC's slow progression provides a potential therapeutic window, and combining CAR-Ts with tyrosine kinase inhibitors (TKIs) or checkpoint inhibitors may overcome stromal resistance [45]. Targets for CAR-T cell therapy in bladder cancer include epidermal growth factor receptor (EGFR), MUC1, HER2, and integrins. Although no CAR-T product is clinically approved for bladder cancer, experimental models show cytolytic efficacy of anti-EGFR and anti-HER2 CAR-Ts [46]. Combining CAR-T therapy with BCG or ICIs is being explored to improve immune activation and tumor recognition [44, 46].

1.8 Quality of Life Issues

Cancer itself and its treatment can have a significant impact on the quality of life (QOL). These patients often encounter with recurrent urinary tract infection, urinary retention, hematuria, pelvic pain, erectile dysfunction and sexual health issues, urinary incontinence, fistula, fatigue, and psychological and financial burden. It is important to discuss the treatment options and patient preferences considering the risk, benefits, and outcomes since many patients with terminal illnesses preferring a less aggressive approach. Early initiation and timely referral for palliative care is important.

1.9 Summary

Advanced surgical and radiotherapy techniques and availability of newer chemo-immunotherapeutic agents have led to the improved outcome in urogenital cancers. However, the outcome still remains poor in a significant proportion of the patients necessitating the need for further research. It is important to incorporate the molecular information in the treatment protocol for personalized care.

References

1. Dy GW, Gore JL, Forouzanfar MH, Naghavi M, Fitzmaurice C. Global burden of urologic cancers, 1990–2013. Eur Urol. 2017;71(3):437–46.
2. Sung H, Ferlay J, Siegel RL, Laversanne M, Soerjomataram I, Jemal A, et al. Global cancer statistics 2020: GLOBOCAN estimates of incidence and mortality worldwide for 36 cancers in 185 countries. CA Cancer J Clin. 2021;71(3):209–49.
3. Kratzer TB, Siegel RL, Miller KD, Sung H, Islami F, Jemal A. Progress against cancer mortality 50 years after passage of the National Cancer Act. JAMA Oncol. 2022;8(1):156–9.
4. Herr H, Sogani P, Eastham J. Genitourinary tumors. J Surg Oncol. 2022;126(5):926–32.
5. Petit C, Delouya G, Taussky D, Barkati M, Lambert C, Beauchemin MC, et al. PSMA-PET/CT-guided intensification of radiation therapy for prostate cancer (PSMAgRT): findings of detection rate, effect on cancer management, and early toxicity from a phase 2 randomized controlled trial. Int J Radiat Oncol Biol Phys. 2023;116(4):779–87.
6. Whitmore WF. Proceedings: the natural history of prostatic cancer. Cancer. 1973;32(5):1104–12.
7. Tokita H, Twersky R, Laudone V, Levine M, Stein D, Scardino P, et al. Complex cancer surgery in the outpatient setting: the Josie Robertson surgery Center. Anesth Analg. 2020;131(3):699–707.
8. Widmark A, Gunnlaugsson A, Beckman L, Thellenberg-Karlsson C, Hoyer M, Lagerlund M, et al. Ultra-hypofractionated versus conventionally fractionated radiotherapy for prostate cancer: 5-year outcomes of the HYPO-RT-PC randomised, non-inferiority, phase 3 trial. Lancet Lond Engl. 2019;394(10196):385–95.
9. Dearnaley D, Syndikus I, Mossop H, Khoo V, Birtle A, Bloomfield D, et al. Conventional versus hypofractionated high-dose intensity-modulated radiotherapy for prostate cancer: 5-year outcomes of the randomised, non-inferiority, phase 3 CHHiP trial. Lancet Oncol. 2016;17(8):1047–60.
10. Catton CN, Lukka H, Gu CS, Martin JM, Supiot S, Chung PWM, et al. Randomized trial of a hypofractionated radiation regimen for the treatment of localized prostate cancer. J Clin Oncol Off J Am Soc Clin Oncol. 2017;35(17):1884–90.
11. Kerkmeijer LGW, Groen VH, Pos FJ, Haustermans K, Monninkhof EM, Smeenk RJ, et al. Focal boost to the intraprostatic tumor in external beam radiotherapy for patients with localized prostate cancer: results from the FLAME randomized phase III trial. J Clin Oncol Off J Am Soc Clin Oncol. 2021;39(7):787–96.

12. Vapiwala N, Wong JK, Handorf E, Paly J, Grewal A, Tendulkar R, et al. A pooled toxicity analysis of moderately hypofractionated proton beam therapy and intensity modulated radiation therapy in early-stage prostate cancer patients. Int J Radiat Oncol Biol Phys. 2021;110(4):1082–9.
13. Ali A, Hoyle A, Haran ÁM, Brawley CD, Cook A, Amos C, et al. Association of bone metastatic burden with survival benefit from prostate radiotherapy in patients with newly diagnosed metastatic prostate cancer: a secondary analysis of a randomized clinical trial. JAMA Oncol. 2021;7(4):555–63.
14. Parker CC, James ND, Brawley CD, Clarke NW, Hoyle AP, Ali A, et al. Radiotherapy to the primary tumour for newly diagnosed, metastatic prostate cancer (STAMPEDE): a randomised controlled phase 3 trial. Lancet Lond Engl. 2018;392(10162):2353–66.
15. Phillips R, Shi WY, Deek M, Radwan N, Lim SJ, Antonarakis ES, et al. Outcomes of observation vs stereotactic ablative radiation for oligometastatic prostate cancer: the ORIOLE phase 2 randomized clinical trial. JAMA Oncol. 2020;6(5):650–9.
16. Ost P, Reynders D, Decaestecker K, Fonteyne V, Lumen N, De Bruycker A, et al. Surveillance or metastasis-directed therapy for oligometastatic prostate cancer recurrence: a prospective, randomized, multicenter phase II trial. J Clin Oncol Off J Am Soc Clin Oncol. 2018;36(5):446–53.
17. Yamada Y, Rogers L, Demanes DJ, Morton G, Prestidge BR, Pouliot J, et al. American brachytherapy society consensus guidelines for high-dose-rate prostate brachytherapy. Brachytherapy. 2012;11(1):20–32.
18. Tran C, Ouk S, Clegg NJ, Chen Y, Watson PA, Arora V, et al. Development of a second-generation antiandrogen for treatment of advanced prostate cancer. Science. 2009;324(5928):787–90.
19. Teo MY, Morris MJ. Prostate-specific membrane antigen-directed therapy for metastatic castration-resistant prostate cancer. Cancer J Sudbury Mass. 2016;22(5):347–52.
20. de Bono J, Mateo J, Fizazi K, Saad F, Shore N, Sandhu S, et al. Olaparib for metastatic castration-resistant prostate cancer. N Engl J Med. 2020;382(22):2091–102.
21. Sfakianos JP, Kim PH, Hakimi AA, Herr HW. The effect of restaging transurethral resection on recurrence and progression rates in patients with nonmuscle invasive bladder cancer treated with intravesical bacillus Calmette-Guérin. J Urol. 2014;191(2):341–5.
22. Herr HW, Sogani PC. Does early cystectomy improve the survival of patients with high risk superficial bladder tumors? J Urol. 2001;166(4):1296–9.
23. Morales A, Herr H, Steinberg G, Given R, Cohen Z, Amrhein J, et al. Efficacy and safety of MCNA in patients with nonmuscle invasive bladder cancer at high risk for recurrence and progression after failed treatment with bacillus Calmette-Guérin. J Urol. 2015;193(4):1135–43.
24. Dalbagni G, Russo P, Bochner B, Ben-Porat L, Sheinfeld J, Sogani P, et al. Phase II trial of intravesical gemcitabine in bacille Calmette-Guérin-refractory transitional cell carcinoma of the bladder. J Clin Oncol Off J Am Soc Clin Oncol. 2006;24(18):2729–34.
25. Bochner BH, Sjoberg DD, Laudone VP. Memorial Sloan Kettering Cancer Center Bladder Cancer Surgical Trials Group. A randomized trial of robot-assisted laparoscopic radical cystectomy. N Engl J Med. 2014;371(4):389–90.
26. Choudhury A, Porta N, Hall E, Song YP, Owen R, MacKay R, et al. Hypofractionated radiotherapy in locally advanced bladder cancer: an individual patient data meta-analysis of the BC2001 and BCON trials. Lancet Oncol. 2021;22(2):246–55.
27. Hafeez S, Webster A, Hansen VN, McNair HA, Warren-Oseni K, Patel E, et al. Protocol for tumour-focused dose-escalated adaptive radiotherapy for the radical treatment of bladder cancer in a multicentre phase II randomised controlled trial (RAIDER): radiotherapy planning and delivery guidance. BMJ Open. 2020;10(12):e041005.
28. Sternberg CN, Yagoda A, Scher HI, Watson RC, Ahmed T, Weiselberg LR, et al. Preliminary results of M-VAC (methotrexate, vinblastine, doxorubicin and cisplatin) for transitional cell carcinoma of the urothelium. J Urol. 1985;133(3):403–7.
29. Song YP, Mistry H, Irlam J, Valentine H, Yang L, Lane B, et al. Long-term outcomes of radical radiation therapy with hypoxia modification with biomarker discovery for stratification: 10-year update of the BCON (bladder carbogen nicotinamide) phase 3 randomized trial (ISRCTN45938399). Int J Radiat Oncol Biol Phys. 2021;110(5):1407–15.

30. Chakravarti A, Winter K, Wu CL, Kaufman D, Hammond E, Parliament M, et al. Expression of the epidermal growth factor receptor and Her-2 are predictors of favorable outcome and reduced complete response rates, respectively, in patients with muscle-invading bladder cancers treated by concurrent radiation and cisplatin-based chemotherapy: a report from the Radiation Therapy Oncology Group. Int J Radiat Oncol Biol Phys. 2005;62(2):309–17.
31. Inoue M, Koga F, Yoshida S, Tamura T, Fujii Y, Ito E, et al. Significance of ERBB2 overexpression in therapeutic resistance and cancer-specific survival in muscle-invasive bladder cancer patients treated with chemoradiation-based selective bladder-sparing approach. Int J Radiat Oncol Biol Phys. 2014;90(2):303–11.
32. Herr HW. Partial nephrectomy for renal cell carcinoma with a normal opposite kidney. Cancer. 1994;73(1):160–2.
33. Motzer RJ, Escudier B, Oudard S, Hutson TE, Porta C, Bracarda S, et al. Efficacy of everolimus in advanced renal cell carcinoma: a double-blind, randomised, placebo-controlled phase III trial. Lancet Lond Engl. 2008;372(9637):449–56.
34. Motzer RJ, Tannir NM, McDermott DF, Arén Frontera O, Melichar B, Choueiri TK, et al. Nivolumab plus Ipilimumab versus sunitinib in advanced renal-cell carcinoma. N Engl J Med. 2018;378(14):1277–90.
35. Siva S, Jackson P, Kron T, Bressel M, Lau E, Hofman M, et al. Impact of stereotactic radiotherapy on kidney function in primary renal cell carcinoma: establishing a dose-response relationship. Radiother Oncol J Eur Soc Ther Radiol Oncol. 2016;118(3):540–6.
36. Siva S, Bressel M, Wood ST, Shaw MG, Loi S, Sandhu SK, et al. Stereotactic radiotherapy and short-course pembrolizumab for oligometastatic renal cell carcinoma-the RAPPORT trial. Eur Urol. 2022;81(4):364–72.
37. Sogani PC, Perrotti M, Herr HW, Fair WR, Thaler HT, Bosl G. Clinical stage I testis cancer: long-term outcome of patients on surveillance. J Urol. 1998;159(3):855–8.
38. Pasalic D, Prajapati S, Ludmir EB, Tang C, Choi S, Kudchadker R, et al. Outcomes and toxicities of proton and photon radiation therapy for testicular seminoma. Int J Part Ther. 2020;7(2):11–20.
39. Apolo AB, Girardi DM, Niglio SA, Nadal R, Kydd AR, Simon N, et al. Final results from a phase I trial and expansion cohorts of Cabozantinib and Nivolumab alone or with Ipilimumab for advanced/metastatic genitourinary tumors. J Clin Oncol Off J Am Soc Clin Oncol. 2024;42(25):3033–46.
40. Canter DJ, Nicholson S, Watkin N, Hall E, Pettaway C, Committee IPACTE. The international penile advanced cancer trial (InPACT): rationale and current status. Eur Urol Focus. 2019;5(5):706–9.
41. He M, Zhang D, Cao Y, Chi C, Zeng Z, Yang X, et al. Chimeric antigen receptor-modified T cells therapy in prostate cancer: a comprehensive review on the current state and prospects. Heliyon. 2023;9(8):e19147.
42. Perera MPJ, Thomas PB, Risbridger GP, Taylor R, Azad A, Hofman MS, et al. Chimeric antigen receptor T-cell therapy in metastatic castrate-resistant prostate cancer. Cancer. 2022;14(3):503.
43. Dorff TB, Blanchard MS, Adkins LN, Luebbert L, Leggett N, Shishido SN, et al. PSCA-CAR T cell therapy in metastatic castration-resistant prostate cancer: a phase 1 trial. Nat Med. 2024;30(6):1636–44.
44. Zhang Z, Li D, Yun H, Liu W, Chai K, Tong J, et al. CAR-T cells in the treatment of urologic neoplasms: present and future. Front Oncol. 2022;12:915171.
45. Pantuck M, Palaskas N, Drakaki A. Next generation T-cell therapy for genitourinary malignancies, part B: overcoming obstacles and future strategies for success. Cancer Treat Res Commun. 2018;17:1–7.
46. Zhang G, Wang Y, Lu S, Ding F, Wang X, Zhu C, et al. Molecular understanding and clinical outcomes of CAR T cell therapy in the treatment of urological tumors. Cell Death Dis. 2024;15(5):359.

Epidemiology, Genetics/Molecular and Screening of Urogenital Cancers

2

Kannan Periasamy and Namrata Das

2.1 Kidney Cancer

2.1.1 Epidemiology of Cancers of the Kidney

Cancers of the kidney and renal pelvis have consistently remained one of the ten most common cancers globally. In terms of incidence, it made up 4.2% of all new cancer cases in 2023, ranking seventh overall. Over the last few decades, there has been a consistent rise in the occurrence of renal cell cancer (RCC), which is partly due to incidental findings on imaging studies performed for other reasons. However, it lies outside the top ten sites in terms of cancer mortality and was responsible for 2.5% of cancer deaths in 2023. There has been a steady improvement in survival over years across all stages, with an overall 5-year survival of 77% [1, 2].

In terms of sex distribution, kidney cancers are more common in males (23.5/100,000 persons) than females (11.7/100,000 persons). It also increases with age, with the median age of diagnosis being 65 years. Incidence rates of RCC vary by geographic region. More cases have been reported in developed countries, particularly North America and Western Europe. Environmental and lifestyle factors, such as smoking and diet, have been hypothesized to be the cause behind this [2, 3].

RCC comprises 85% of all kidney cancers, with clear cell carcinoma being the commonest histological subtype. The other less common histologies are papillary, chromophobe, collecting duct, medullary, etc. The prognosis of chromophobe RCC is favourable as compared to clear cell, whereas studies have reported variable outcomes for the papillary subtype [4].

K. Periasamy (✉)
Radiation Oncology, JIPMER, Puducherry, India

N. Das
Radiation Oncology, AIIMS, New Delhi, India

R. Madan, S. Goyal (eds.), *Essentials of Radiotherapy in Uro-Genital Malignancies*, https://doi.org/10.1007/978-981-95-5945-9_2

2.1.2 Risk Factors

Multiple lifestyle risk factors have been linked with RCC [3, 5]. Modifiable risk factors include obesity, smoking and hypertension. A family history of kidney cancer can also increase an individual's risk. The commonest hereditary type of RCC is associated with von Hippel-Lindau (VHL) disease, where RCC is associated with other vascular tumours [6].

2.1.3 Genetics and Molecular Aspects of Kidney Cancer

Nearly 80% of kidney cancers are clear cell carcinomas, followed by papillary, chromophobe, collecting duct, etc. The histological heterogeneity is reflected in the molecular pathways of pathogenesis as well. Mutations in the VHL gene, a tumour suppressor gene, are commonest for clear cell carcinomas. In addition, alterations in epigenetic regulation through mutations in PRBM1, BAP1 (histone deubiquitinase) and SETD2 (histone methyltransferase) have been found in 41%, 15% and 12% of cases, respectively. Alterations in the PI3/AKT pathway are also associated with RCC and reflect the benefit of using mTOR inhibitors in targeting it.

2.1.4 Hereditary RCC Syndromes

Around 2–4% of RCC cases are hereditary and are often associated with specific genetic syndromes [6, 7].

1. *Von Hippel-Lindau (VHL) Disease:* Individuals with VHL disease have a high risk of developing multiple clear cell RCC tumours, cysts and other tumours like phaeochromocytoma, hemangioblastoma, etc. RCC develops in 25–45% of patients and is almost always bilateral and multifocal.
2. *Hereditary Papillary Renal Carcinoma:* This syndrome is linked to mutations in genes like MET and fumarate hydratase (FH), leading to Type 1 papillary RCC. The presentation again is bilateral and multifocal.
3. *Birt-Hogg-Dubé (BHD) Syndrome:* Birt-Hogg-Dubé (BHD) Syndrome is linked to mutations in the FLCN gene and can lead to the development of different types of kidney tumours.

2.1.5 Screening for Kidney Cancer

Screening for kidney cancers is recommended only in a group of high-risk individuals who have hereditary renal cancer syndromes like VHL disease. The modality of imaging is ultrasound or CT. Genetic counselling forms an integral part for these patients.

2.2 Bladder Cancer

2.2.1 Epidemiology of Bladder Cancer

Bladder cancer is the tenth most frequently occurring cancer across the globe. In terms of gender, it claims the fourth position for men and the 11th position for women in terms of cancer incidence [8]. There is a wide geographical variation in bladder cancer prevalence. Similar to kidney cancers, higher numbers occur in developed nations like the United States, Canada and Western Europe. It is also a disease of the old; almost always patients are above 60 years which also has treatment implications [9].

2.2.2 Risk Factors

Multiple studies have elucidated specific risk factors for bladder cancer, with exposure of certain carcinogens to the bladder epithelium being a putative mechanism for some. Firstly, smoking has been proven to confer a three-fold increased risk of bladder cancer in both men and women [10]. Secondly, occupational exposure to certain carcinogens has been linked to the development of bladder cancer, and certain industries have been historically marked for the same. Painters, drill press operators, etc., who are exposed to aromatic hydrocarbons from industrial chemicals have an increased risk [11]. Apart from these, male sex, age above 55 years and a family history of bladder cancer all elevate the risk.

2.2.3 Genetics of Bladder Cancer

Molecular Subtypes

Bladder cancer is associated with molecular heterogeneity which is reflective in its natural course of disease and outcomes. It has a high mutational burden akin to melanomas and lung cancers which makes immunotherapy an attractive therapeutic strategy. Nearly 25% of all bladder cancers are muscle invasive bladder cancers (MIBC), and it is this group which is the focus of research. The TCGA analysis of 412 cases by multiple analytic platforms found 34 significantly mutated genes and 158 genes that were epigenetically silenced. APOBEC mutation was associated with improved survival (5-year survival 75%), and the PPARG gene was identified as a key gene in pathogenesis [12, 13].

Attempts were made to consolidate data across multiple studies, and a consensus molecular classification of MIBC was published in 2019. Around 1750 transcriptomic profiles across 18 datasets were grouped into 6 molecular classes based on gene expression patterns: luminal papillary (24%), luminal nonspecified (8%), luminal unstable (15%), stroma-rich (15%), basal/squamous (35%), and neuroendocrine-like (3%). Seven key genes are altered in varying proportion across these six groups: FGFR3, CDKN2A, PPARG, ERBB2, E2F3, TP53, and RB1.

2.2.4 Screening for Bladder Cancer

No benefit from mass screening of bladder cancer is established. If it is considered in individuals with high risk due to occupational exposures or a family history of bladder cancer, screening strategies in the form of urine cytology, cystoscopy and CT urography may be considered on an individual basis.

2.3 Prostate Cancer

2.3.1 Epidemiology of Prostate Cancer

Prostate cancer is a disease with a disproportionately low mortality when compared to incidence rates. It ranks second in terms of cancer incidence and fifth when it comes to mortality for men worldwide. Incidence is three times higher in developed countries as compared to developing nations (37.5 versus 11.3 per 100,000 people, respectively) [8].

In terms of cancer incidence age standardized ratios (ASRs), prostate cancer comes after lung cancer in countries with high human development index (37.5 versus 39 per 100,000). In lower HDI nations, prostate cancer ranks first, followed by lung cancer (11.3 versus 10.3 per 100,000 persons).

Prostate cancer is a disease of older men with frequency increasing with age with a median age of diagnosis of 67 years. There are notable racial and ethnic variations in incidence. As per US data, the overall incidence was 113 per 100,000 persons (2016–2022). However, the incidence was highest in the African American population, with an incidence of 183 per 100,000 persons [15].

Risk Factors and Protective Factors

1. *Age:* Aging is the single most significant risk factor for prostate cancer. The risk of developing prostate cancer increases significantly with age, particularly in older men. As men advance in age, their risk of developing prostate cancer rises exponentially. Most cases are diagnosed in men over the age of 50, and the median age at diagnosis is approximately 66 years old.
2. *Family History:* A family history of prostate cancer can significantly increase an individual's risk, especially if the affected relatives are first-degree relatives (e.g., father or brother).
3. *Race and Ethnicity:* As mentioned earlier, African American men are at an elevated risk of developing prostate cancer. The reasons for these disparities are complex and may involve genetic, environmental, and healthcare access factors [21].
4. *Genetics:* Mutations in specific genes, such as BRCA1, BRCA2, and specific DNA repair genes, have been linked to an increased risk of prostate cancer. These genetic factors are more relevant in hereditary forms of the disease.

5. *Diet and Lifestyle*: Dietary factors, such as consuming a diet high in red meat and low in fruits and vegetables, have been associated with an increased risk of prostate cancer. Obesity and a sedentary lifestyle have also been linked to a higher risk.
6. *Geographic and Environmental Factors:* Exposure to certain environmental factors and pollutants may play a role in prostate cancer risk, though the evidence is not yet conclusive.

2.3.2 Genetics of Prostate Cancer

Prostate cancer does not always run an indolent course. The clinical course is varied across individuals, and in some, there can be rapid, non-treatment responsive disease. The molecular underpinnings of such heterogeneity have been understood in the past two decades due to breakthroughs in next-generation sequencing. This has helped decipher the genome and transcriptome of prostate cancer and analyse large volumes of data rapidly. Multiple cancer pathways, including that of androgen receptor signalling, WNT, cell cycle progression, PI3K, DNA repair etc., have been found to harbour a wide array of genomic lesions ranging from mutations, translocations, epigenomic changes, somatic copy number alterations (SCNA), etc. [16]

2.3.3 Molecular Subtypes

Initial studies in the form of whole genome sequencing [17] and whole exome sequencing [18] had identified recurrent translocations in the ETS family, SPOP mutations, etc. The Cancer Genome Atlas (TCGA) consolidated data from 333 primary prostate cancers and found that nearly three quarters of patients can be categorized in one of seven molecular classes defined by fusions: (1) ERG, (2) ETV1/4, (3) FLI1; mutations: (4) SPOP, (5) FOXA1, (6) FOXA1 or (7) IDH1 mutations [16].

The commonest molecular aberration in prostate cancer in up to 50% of cases is a genetic rearrangement in the ETS family transcription factor. It loses its androgen-mediated regulation, resulting in unchecked AR-driven pathway stimulation [19]. SPOP is a protein that serves in the degradation of AR and downstream pathway regulators. Point mutations cause an upregulation in androgen signalling [20]. FOXA1 similarly is a transcription factor involved in AR signalling. Disruptions in the androgen signalling pathway by different driver molecular aberrations play a key role in prostate cancer pathogenesis.

2.3.4 Metastatic CRPC Pathogenesis

Metastatic CRPC portends a poor prognosis. Aggressive tumours accumulate more genetic aberrations with time. ETS translocations, SPOP mutations and NKX3–1 loss are initial events which are followed by PTEN and p53 loss in CRPC. Overall, genes commonly found to be affected are AR (62%), ETS family (56%), p53 (53%) and PTEN (40%) in metastatic CRPC [16, 21, 22].

2.3.5 Clinical Implications

2.3.5.1 Risk Stratification in Early Stage Disease

The development of tissue-based prognostic assays or gene expression classifiers (GECs) has aided prostate cancer risk stratification and therefore decision-making. Tests like Decipher, Oncotype Dx Prostate, Ki67, Prolaris and PTEN are available commercially which have been validated in clinical studies. These can be helpful in deciding intervention versus active surveillance in very low- and low-risk disease. A prospective trial showed an increase in adoption of active surveillance using GECs [23]. These tests are also helpful in predicting prognosis and guiding management following radical prostatectomy. In a clinical utility study, the decipher assay changed treatment recommendations in 39% of post-prostatectomy patients. Patients who were identified as high risk by the assay and offered adjuvant radiotherapy had a 2-year PSA recurrence of 3% versus 25% amongst those who did not receive treatment [24].

2.3.5.2 Avenues for Targeted Treatment

Amongst the many pathways, aberrations in the DNA damage repair (DDR), particularly in the BRCA2 gene, have been established through multiple studies. Around 23% patients harbour mutations in DDR with 8% being germline mutations [16]. Overall, patients with germline BRCA2 mutations have been shown to have a poorer prognosis. The prognostic implication of other DDR genes and the difference in prognosis with somatic versus germline mutations is under research [25]. In the PROfound trial, a FoundationOne CDx NGS-based assay was used to identify patients with aberrations in 1 of 15 genes that directly or indirectly play a role in the homologous recombination pathway. These patients of CRPC had progressed after either abiraterone or enzalutamide and were given the PARP inhibitor olaparib [26]. A benefit of progression-free survival was seen with olaparib which then provided approval of FoundationOne CDx and BRCAanalysis diagnostic companions in all metastatic CRPC patients. Guidelines are now recommending germline testing in all metastatic and advanced disease patients since it opens up avenues of targeted treatment [27].

2.3.5.3 Genetic Testing

Prostate cancer has a heritable component, with personal and family history of cancer increasing its risk. Men from families suffering from Hereditary Breast and Ovarian Cancer (HBOC) and even Lynch syndrome have been found to be at an increased risk for prostate cancer [28, 29]. This led to research in identifying cancer predisposition genes for prostate cancer. Germline mutation in the HOXB13 gene was one of the first to be specific for prostate cancer [30]. Building on that, in a study of more than a hundred patients of prostate cancer and an additional cancer, a multi-gene panel was used to identify the common pathogenic germline variants. Around 10% of patients were found to have pathogenic mutations in cancer-predisposing genes—BRCA2, ATM, MLH1, BRIP1, PALB2 and FGFR3 [31].

Guidelines presently recommend germline testing in patients with a positive family history (breast, ovary, endometrial, pancreatic, colorectal), Ashkenazi Jewish ancestry, personal history of breast cancer and all patients with advanced prostate cancer regardless of family history. Pretext and post-test counselling remains an integral part of genetic counselling.

2.3.6 Screening for Prostate Cancer

Prostate cancer is a site where large randomized trials on the benefits and economics of screening have been studied. Blood serum levels of PSA, a protein secreted by the prostate gland are the commonest method of screening. Depending upon the level of PSA, age and dynamics, the next step is confirmation by a multi-parametric MRI. Screening by performing digital rectal cancer exams can also be done, but it is not a stand-alone option. The debate on whether routine screening is required for all is still not there, and recommendations vary from country to research bodies.

2.3.7 Prostate Cancer Screening Trials

In the general population, screening has not been shown to provide a survival benefit. PSA screening led to an overall increased rate of diagnosis of prostate cancer (relative risk (RR):1.3) which was more for early disease (RR:1.79) as compared to advanced disease (RR: 0.8) in a Cochrane review. In this review of five randomized trials totalling 341,342 patients, prostate mortality was not improved with screening [32]. There was a slight difference in the reporting of the outcomes of the US Prostate, Lung, Colorectal and Ovarian (PLCO) screening trial versus the European Randomized Study of Screening for Prostate Cancer (ERSPC). Whereas the former did not report a benefit in cancer-specific mortality, the European trial reported a 20% benefit with 4 yearly screenings in the 55–69 age group [33, 34]. The ERSPC trial did note an increased rate of overdiagnosis from screening. The detriments of screening include false positive results leading to additional unwarranted investigations and overtreatment leading to treatment complications like incontinence, erectile dysfunction, etc. Most guidelines stress the importance of counselling prior to performing a screening test, a clear explanation of possible harms and benefits and encouraging informed decision-making.

Recommendations on screening Most countries and research bodies do not recommend prostate cancer screening for all. However, informed decision-making and screening of high-risk populations are encouraged. For instance:

1. U.S. Preventive Services Task Force (USPSTF) Recommendations: Routine PSA screening was not advised by USPSTF as per their recommendations in 2012. However, this was revised in 2018, with screening being made an informed, personalized decision for men between 55 and 69 years of age [35].
2. EAU-EANM-ESTRO-ESUR-SIOG guidelines: Screening is offered to well-informed men over 50 years overall, over 45 years who are at high risk (African descent, family history) and over 40 years with BRCA2 mutation [36].

2.3.8 Hormonal Dependence in Prostate Cancer

Hormonal dependence in prostate cancer, also known as androgen dependence, is a critical aspect of the disease's biology and therapeutic approach. Androgen signalling plays centre stage in prostate cancer in spite of molecular heterogeneity in pathogenesis. Testosterone suppression will result in response rates in almost all patients making medical and surgical castration key treatment strategies, particularly for advanced stages of presentation. Nonetheless, with time, castration-resistant prostate cancer (CRPC) invariably returns with new genetic alterations restoring the androgen signalling pathway [37]. Understanding these alternate pathways has helped develop newer agents that target this androgen signalling axis at different points. These new drugs, the androgen receptor signal inhibitors (ARSIs), have improved survival in advanced stages.

2.3.9 Mechanisms of Hormonal Dependence in Prostate Cancer

The hypothalamic-pituitary-gonadal axis controls testosterone production. Pulsatile release of gonadotropin-releasing hormone (GnRH) by the hypothalamus stimulates the pituitary to release luteinizing hormone and follicular-stimulating hormone. This ultimately leads to testosterone production from the testes which is also converted to dihydrotestosterone (DHT). Both testosterone and DHT ultimately act on the androgen receptors present on prostate cancer cells. These are ligand-dependent nuclear transcription factors which dimerize on binding of DHT and enter the nucleus to bind to DNA targets.

Overall, the prostate gland is androgen sensitive. There are multiple ways in which alteration of this signalling pathway can lead to an increase in downstream androgen signalling and proliferation cancer cells.

2.3.9.1 Androgen Receptor Activation

In prostate cancer, the AR pathway becomes dysregulated, leading to increased sensitivity to androgen signalling. Androgen receptor activation by testosterone or DHT in prostate cancer cells promotes cell proliferation and survival, contributing to tumour growth. Inherent amplification of the androgen receptor gene and its increased protein expression are mechanisms of pathogenesis in CRPC despite castrate levels of testosterone [38].

2.3.9.2 Androgen Biosynthesis

Prostate cancer cells can synthesize their own androgens locally, even in the absence of circulating testosterone produced by the testes. This phenomenon is known as intracrine androgen production. Key enzymes involved in intracrine androgen synthesis include cytochrome P450 17A1 (CYP17A1) and 5-alpha-reductase, which convert precursor steroids into active androgens [39].

2.3.9.3 Androgen Receptor Mutations and Amplification

Mutations in the androgen receptor gene can lead to a hyperactive receptor that is more responsive to androgens. These mutations can render prostate cancer cells more hormone-dependent. Gene amplification, where multiple copies of the AR gene are present in cancer cells, can also increase AR protein levels and androgen sensitivity. In CRPC, 40–70% patients have genomic alterations in the AR pathway with amplification of Xq11–12 which is the locus of the AR gene [16].

2.3.9.4 Androgen Receptor Splice Variants

Prostate cancer cells can produce androgen receptor splice variants (e.g., AR-V7) that lack the ligand-binding domain [40].

2.3.9.5 Alternate Pathways of Androgen Biosynthesis

Apart from the de novo synthesis of DHT from cholesterol, there are other alternate pathways of DHT production from extragonadal steroids that the tumour cells exploit to maintain high intratumoral androgen levels. One amongst them is the conversion of adrenal dehydroepiandrosterone (DHEA) to DHT via multiple enzymes. The production of DHEA in the adrenal gland requires the enzyme CYP17A1 (17-hydroxylase). This is suppressed by the drug abiraterone, thereby suppressing the extragonadal DHT production, a key mechanism in CRPC [41].

2.3.9.6 Increased Glucocorticoid Receptor Signalling

This has also been shown to be responsible for treatment resistance in CRPC. Both glucocorticoid receptor (GR) and AR share sequence homology, which allows GR to recognize ligands that bind to AR and cause downstream signalling. It has been observed that in patients with Enzalutamide (a new-generation reversible ARSi) resistance, there is upregulation of GR. The BET family proteins have been implicated for this, and further research might help develop newer therapeutic strategies [42].

2.3.10 Hormonal Therapies for Prostate Cancer

Blockage of androgen signalling is a key step in the management of prostate cancer. Androgen Deprivation Therapy (ADT) encompasses a wide gamut of strategies, starting from surgical castration to remove the source of testosterone to the usage of medical means like LHRH agonists and antagonists.

However, resistance eventually develops. Understanding the genetics and molecular mechanisms has helped develop new drugs in the last couple of decades. These include newer androgen receptor antagonists (e.g. enzalutamide), CYP17A1 inhibitors (e.g. abiraterone), PARP inhibitors for BRCA-positive tumours etc.

2.4 Testicular Cancer

2.4.1 Epidemiology of Testicular Cancer

Testicular cancer is the commonest solid tumour in men between 20 and 34 years. Overall it is a rare tumour with an incidence of 6 per 100,000 men [43]. Worldwide there is wide variation in the incidence, with high numbers seen in the Northern European population (8–9 per 100,000) versus the Asian, African populations (<1 per 100,000) [44]. Around 95% are germ cell tumours (GCTs) which portend excellent prognosis and 5-year survival rates of more than 95% [45].

2.4.2 Genetics of Testicular Cancer

Testicular germ cell tumours (TGCT) are broadly classified as seminomas and non-seminomas. Post-pubertal TGCT, which is the commonest type, arises from precursor lesions known as intratubular germ cell neoplasia (IGCN). Whole genome sequencing has shown low mutational burden for TGCT. On analysis of genomic data of 42 patients, chromosome 12p gain and mutations in KIT and CDC27 were the common [46, 47].

2.4.3 Risk Factors

Undescended testis (cryptorchidism) is linked to increased TGCT; whether it is causal or shares common etiological risk factors is unclear. The relative risk of TGCT in men with undescended testis is 4.8 as per a meta-analysis. However, a personal history of the same is present in only 10% of men with TGCT. A personal or family history of testicular cancer also has proven to increase risk [48].

2.5 Penile Cancer

2.5.1 Epidemiology of Penile Cancer

Penile cancers comprise primarily of squamous cell carcinomas. These are globally rare cancers (0.8 per 100,000 men), with the bulk of patients in India, Africa and South America. Low socioeconomic status and levels of hygiene have been associated with increased incidence in these parts. Incidence increases with age above

60 years; early-stage of diagnosis with absence of lymph node metastasis confers a good prognosis. The five-year survival drops to zero in patients with pelvic nodal metastasis [49].

2.5.2 Risk Factors

Phimosis is the strongest risk factor for developing penile cancers. Studies have shown a relative risk as high as 64 of developing penile cancer in men with this condition. Neonatal circumcision has been found to reduce the risk of developing penile cancer, probably being linked to lowering the risk of developing HPV infection. HPV infection has been established to be the causative agent in up to 50% of cases. This, along with poor hygiene, multiple female sexual partners etc. are all interlinked with the development of penile cancer [49, 50].

2.5.3 Genetics of Penile Cancer

Penile squamous cell carcinomas (SCC) follow the same molecular pathways of pathogenesis as SCC from other sites. HPV mediated downstream signalling, additional p50, NOTCH1 mutations are the major pathways. Additionally, the understanding that high PD-1 expression is present in many patients have opened up avenues of research with checkpoint inhibitors [51].

References

1. Siegel RL, Miller KD, Wagle NS, et al. Cancer statistics, 2023. CA Cancer J Clin. 2023;73:17–48.
2. SEER cancer stat facts: kidney and renal pelvis cancer. Bethesda, MD: National Cancer Institute. https://seer.cancer.gov/statfacts/html/kidrp.html.
3. Capitanio U, Bensalah K, Bex A, et al. Epidemiology of renal cell carcinoma. Eur Urol. 2019;75:74–84.
4. Moch H, Gasser T, Amin MB, et al. Prognostic utility of the recently recommended histologic classification and revised TNM staging system of renal cell carcinoma: a Swiss experience with 588 tumors. Cancer. 2000;89:604–14.
5. Chow WH, McLaughlin JK, Mandel JS, et al. Obesity and risk of renal cell cancer. Cancer Epidemiol Biomarkers Prev. 1996;5:17–21.
6. Schmidt LS, Linehan WM. Genetic predisposition to kidney cancer. Semin Oncol. 2016;43:566–74.
7. Cancer Genome Atlas Research Network. Comprehensive molecular characterization of clear cell renal cell carcinoma. Nature. 2013;499:43–9.
8. Sung H, Ferlay J, Siegel RL, et al. Global cancer statistics 2020: GLOBOCAN estimates of incidence and mortality worldwide for 36 cancers in 185 countries. CA Cancer J Clin. 2021;71:209–49.
9. Antoni S, Ferlay J, Soerjomataram I,et al. Bladder cancer incidence and mortality: a global overview and recent trends. Eur Urol. 2017;71:96–108.

10. Freedman ND, Silverman DT, Hollenbeck AR, et al. Association between smoking and risk of bladder cancer among men and women. JAMA. 2011;306:737–45.
11. Silverman DT, Levin LI, Hoover RN, et al. Occupational risks of bladder cancer in the United States: I. White men. J Natl Cancer Inst. 1989;81:1472–80.
12. Robertson AG, Kim J, Al-Ahmadie H, et al. Comprehensive molecular characterization of muscle-invasive bladder cancer. Cell. 2017;171:540–556.e25.
13. Muto S, Horie S, Takahashi S, et al.. Genetic and epigenetic alterations in normal bladder epithelium in patients with metachronous bladder cancer. Cancer Res. 2000;60: 4021–5.
14. Kamoun A, de Reyniès A, Allory Y, et al. A consensus molecular classification of muscle-invasive bladder cancer. Eur Urol. 2020;77:420–33.
15. Cancer of the prostate - cancer stat facts. SEER. https://seer.cancer.gov/statfacts/html/prost.html.
16. Robinson D, Van Allen EM, Wu YM, et al. Integrative clinical genomics of advanced prostate cancer. Cell. 2015;162:454.
17. Berger MF, Lawrence MS, Demichelis F, et al. The genomic complexity of primary human prostate cancer. Nature. 2011;470:214–20.
18. Barbieri CE, Baca SC, Lawrence MS, et al. Exome sequencing identifies recurrent SPOP, FOXA1 and MED12 mutations in prostate cancer. Nat Genet. 2012;44:685–9.
19. Tomlins SA, Rhodes DR, Perner S, et al. Recurrent fusion of TMPRSS2 and ETS transcription factor genes in prostate cancer. Science. 2005;310:644–8.
20. Geng C, He B, Xu L, et al. Prostate cancer-associated mutations in speckle-type POZ protein (SPOP) regulate steroid receptor coactivator 3 protein turnover. Proc Natl Acad Sci USA. 2013;110:6997–7002.
21. Baca SC, Prandi D, Lawrence M, et al. Punctuated evolution of prostate cancer genomes. Cell. 2013;153:666–77.
22. Hong MKH, Macintyre G, Wedge DC, et al. Tracking the origins and drivers of subclonal metastatic expansion in prostate cancer. Nat Commun. 2015;6:6605.
23. Hu JC, Tosoian JJ, Qi J, et al. Clinical utility of gene expression classifiers in men with newly diagnosed prostate cancer. JCO Precis Oncol. 2018;2
24. Marascio J, Spratt DE, Zhang J, et al. Prospective study to define the clinical utility and benefit of Decipher testing in men following prostatectomy. Prostate Cancer Prostatic Dis. 2020;23:295–302.
25. Nombela P, Lozano R, Aytes A,et al. BRCA2 and other DDR genes in prostate cancer. Cancer. 2019;11
26. de Bono J, Mateo J, Fizazi K, et al. Olaparib for metastatic castration-resistant prostate cancer. N Engl J Med. 2020;382:2091–102.
27. Schaeffer E, Srinivas S, Antonarakis ES, et al. NCCN guidelines insights: prostate cancer, version 1.2021. J Natl Compr Cancer Netw. 2021;19:134–43.
28. Castro E, Goh C, Leongamornlert D, et al. Effect of BRCA mutations on metastatic relapse and cause-specific survival after radical treatment for localised prostate cancer. Eur Urol. 2015;68:186–93.
29. Raymond VM, Mukherjee B, Wang F, et al. Elevated risk of prostate cancer among men with Lynch syndrome. J Clin Oncol. 2013;31:1713–8.
30. Ewing CM, Ray AM, Lange EM, et al. Germline mutations in HOXB13 and prostate-cancer risk. N Engl J Med. 2012;366:141–9.
31. Pilié PG, Johnson AM, Hanson KL, et al. Germline genetic variants in men with prostate cancer and one or more additional cancers. Cancer. 2017;123:3925–32.
32. Ilic D, Neuberger MM, Djulbegovic M, et al. Screening for prostate cancer. Cochrane Database Syst Rev. 2013;2013:CD004720.
33. Andriole GL, Crawford ED, Grubb RL 3rd, et al. Mortality results from a randomized prostate-cancer screening trial. N Engl J Med. 2009;360:1310–9.
34. Schröder FH, Hugosson J, Roobol MJ, et al. Screening and prostate-cancer mortality in a randomized European study. N Engl J Med. 2009;360:1320–8.

35. US Preventive Services Task Force, Grossman DC, Curry SJ, et al. Screening for prostate cancer: US preventive services task force recommendation statement. JAMA. 2018;319:1901–13.
36. Mottet N, van den Bergh RCN, Briers E, et al. EAU-EANM-ESTRO-ESUR-SIOG guidelines on prostate cancer-2020 update. Part 1: screening, diagnosis, and local treatment with curative intent. Eur Urol. 2021;79:243–62.
37. Sharifi N, Gulley JL, Dahut WL. Androgen deprivation therapy for prostate cancer. JAMA. 2005;294:238–44.
38. Waltering KK, Helenius MA, Sahu B, et al. Increased expression of androgen receptor sensitizes prostate cancer cells to low levels of androgens. Cancer Res. 2009;69:8141–9.
39. Labrie F. Intracrinology in action: importance of extragonadal sex steroid biosynthesis and inactivation in peripheral tissues in both women and men. J Steroid Biochem Mol Biol. 2015;145:131–2.
40. Antonarakis ES, Lu C, Wang H, et al. AR-V7 and resistance to enzalutamide and abiraterone in prostate cancer. N Engl J Med. 2014;371:1028–38.
41. Mostaghel EA. Abiraterone in the treatment of metastatic castration-resistant prostate cancer. Cancer Manag Res. 2014;6:39–51.
42. Shah N, Wang P, Wongvipat J, et al. Regulation of the glucocorticoid receptor via a BET-dependent enhancer drives antiandrogen resistance in prostate cancer. Elife. 2017;6
43. Znaor A, Lortet-Tieulent J, et al. International variations and trends in testicular cancer incidence and mortality. Eur Urol. 2014;65:1095–106.
44. Chia VM, Quraishi SM, Devesa S, et al. International trends in the incidence of testicular cancer, 1973-2002. Cancer Epidemiol Biomarkers Prev. 2010;19:1151–9.
45. SEER cancer statistics factsheets: testicular cancer. National Cancer Institute. Bethesda, MD; 2020. https://seer.cancer.gov/statfacts/html/testis.html.
46. Litchfield K, Summersgill B, Yost S, et al. Whole-exome sequencing reveals the mutational spectrum of testicular germ cell tumours. Nat Commun. 2015;6:5973.
47. Sheikine Y, Genega E, Melamed J, et al. Molecular genetics of testicular germ cell tumors. Am J Cancer Res. 2012;2:153–67.
48. McGlynn KA, Cook MB. Etiologic factors in testicular germ-cell tumors. Future Oncol. 2009;5:1389–402.
49. Giona S. The epidemiology of penile cancer. Exon Publications; 2022.
50. de Martel C, Plummer M, Vignat J, et al. Worldwide burden of cancer attributable to HPV by site, country and HPV type. Int J Cancer. 2017;141:664–70.
51. Chahoud J, Pickering CR, Pettaway CA. Genetics and penile cancer: recent developments and implications. Curr Opin Urol. 2019;29:364–70.

Management of Very Low- and Low-Risk Prostate Cancer

3

Renu Madan, Girdhar Bora, Shikha Goyal,
and Narendra Kumar

3.1 Introduction

Prostate cancer is a global health challenge. In 2015, there were an estimated 1,600,000 new cases and 3,66,000 deaths worldwide [1]. With the widespread adoption of prostate-specific antigen (PSA) testing, many prostate cancers are now diagnosed at an early and localized stage. Among these, low-risk prostate cancer represents a subset of patients characterized by indolent behaviour, low likelihood of progression, and favourable prognosis. The clinical dilemma in managing this group lies in balancing the risks of overtreatment against the potential for disease progression [2]. The outcome in these patients remains excellent, with a 15-year prostate cancer-specific survival rate of >95% regardless of the treatment [2].

3.2 Spectrum of the Disease and Clinical Presentations

The spectrum of the prostate cancer varies from screen-detected asymptomatic or low-risk cancer to symptomatic, aggressive and high-risk cancer. Many patients diagnosed in the early stage are asymptomatic and diagnosed on widespread use of serum PSA testing. A few patients may also present with lower urinary tract symptoms such as frequency, urgency, nocturia and hesitancy; however, these symptoms are more common in benign prostatic conditions.

R. Madan (✉) · S. Goyal · N. Kumar
Department of Radiotherapy and Oncology, Postgraduate Institute of Medical Education and Research (PGIMER), Chandigarh, India

G. Bora
Department of Urology, Postgraduate Institute of Medical Education and Research, Chandigarh, India

R. Madan, S. Goyal (eds.), *Essentials of Radiotherapy in Uro-Genital Malignancies*, https://doi.org/10.1007/978-981-95-5945-9_3

3.3 Diagnosis and Work Up

Initial evaluation for carcinoma of the prostate includes Digital Rectal Examination (DRE), PSA testing, imaging, Gleason's score/grade group and the number and extent of cores involved in the pre-treatment biopsy.

3.3.1 PSA Testing

PSA is the most commonly used test for the screening and early diagnosis of prostate cancer. There is no single threshold to define an abnormal PSA test, and generally, repeat testing is advised at a few weeks' interval to confirm the rise.

3.3.2 Digital Rectal Examination (DRE)

The majority of the prostate cancers occur in peripheral zone of prostate, which makes DRE an important tool for evaluation of the abnormal nodules and asymmetry in the prostate.

3.4 Imaging

3.4.1 Ultrasound

It is usually the first investigation and provides anatomical information. Trans-rectal ultrasound (TRUS) is used to guide the prostate biopsy.

3.4.2 Computed Tomography (CT) Scan

CT scan of the abdomen and pelvis provides a high information regarding gross extracapsular spread, lymph node metastasis and visceral metastasis; however, it has limitations in evaluating the prostate gland and may overlook small extracapsular extensions.

3.4.3 Magnetic Resonance Imaging (MRI)

T2-weighted MRI of the pelvis is the best to differentiate prostate from the periprostatic tissue. Multiparametric MRI (mpMRI) of the prostate is defined as at least one additional sequence (diffusion-weighted or dynamic contrast-enhanced) in addition to the T2-weighted MRI. It helps in the evaluation of disease extension and intra-prostatic lesions. One meta-analysis reported that mpMRI has a sensitivity of 44–87% to detect prostate cancer with a negative predictive value of 63–98% [3].

However, for pelvic lymph nodes, mpMRI is as effective as a CT scan. Based on the likelihood of cancer, prostate imaging reporting and data system (PI-RADS) categorise prostatic lesions on a five-point scale as below [4]:

1. PIRADS-1: The risk of clinically significant cancer is highly unlikely.
2. PIRADS-2: The risk of clinically significant cancer is unlikely.
3. PIRADS-3: The risk of clinically significant cancer is equivocal.
4. PIRADS-4: The risk of clinically significant cancer is likely to be present.
5. PIRADS-5: The risk of clinically significant cancer is highly likely to be present.

3.4.4 Bone Imaging

Bone imaging using a bone scan with or without soft tissue imaging can be used for the initial evaluation of the patients having a high risk of bone metastasis. Bone imaging is not required in low-risk prostate cancer patients.

3.4.5 Whole Body Imaging

Whole-body imaging using PET/CT scan is generally not required in low-risk prostate cancer patients. FDG PET has a limited utility in prostate cancer. Wherever required, prostate-specific membrane antigen (PSMA) positron emission tomography (PET) scans with different radioisotopes such as ^{68}Ga and ^{18}F are performed due to higher sensitivity compared to FDG or choline PET CT.

3.4.6 PSA Density

PSA density can be used to differentiate if the PSA rise is due to a benign or a malignant condition. PSA density is defined as a ratio of serum PSA and prostate volume measured by TRUS or prostate MRI. Since PSA is expressed by both benign and malignant prostate cells, an elevated PSA in a small prostate is more worrisome compared to that in a larger prostate. A higher PSA density of >0.15 ng/ml/cc is more suggestive of prostate cancer.

3.4.7 Ratio of Free to Total PSA

Prostate cancer is associated with lower percentage of free (f) PSA compared to total (t) PSA. A value of f/t PSA <10–15% is highly suggestive of prostate cancer, whereas f/t PSA value of >25% is more likely due to benign condition [5]. Ratio of f/t PSA can also be used to decide if a repeat biopsy is indicated in an older patient with previous negative biopsy.

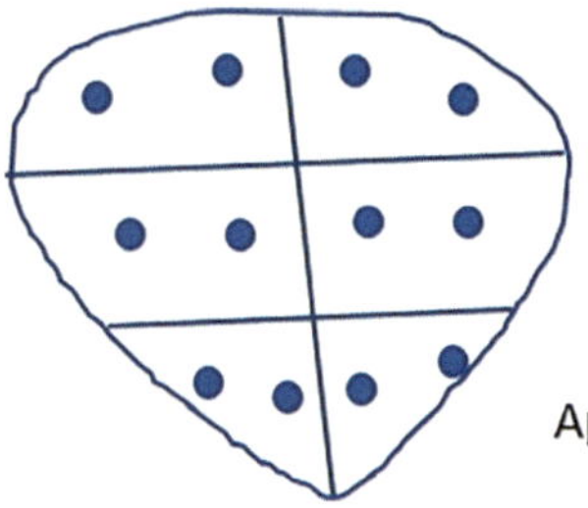

Fig. 3.1 12 Core biopsy, representing sampling of medial and lateral aspects of each apex, mid zone and base. (Adapted from Asian Journal of Andrology 25(1):p 43–49, Jan–Feb 2023. https://doi.org/10.4103/aja2021128)

3.4.8 Biopsy

The results of PSA testing and imaging are used to decide if a biopsy is required or not. However, biopsy in a suspected low-risk cancer patients can be omitted if the life expectancy is less than 10 years, since these patients may not require any treatment.

The initial approach of finger-guided biopsy was described in 1930s, which involves the biopsy of palpable nodule via transrectal route. In 1980s, with the availability of needle guides for ultrasound, systematic sampling of entire prostate became feasible which is considered as a standard of care in current era. While the transrectal biopsy remains the most common approach, transperineal biopsy is an alternative approach to reduce the risk of infection.

Traditional 12-core biopsy includes sampling of medial and lateral aspects of each apex, mid zone and base (Fig. 3.1) on both the right and left sides [6]. TRUS-guided 6-core biopsy includes taking one sample from each apex, mid-gland and base on either side. Studies have shown that a 12-core biopsy increases the cancer detection by 31% compared to the 6-core biopsy [7]. 18-core biopsy may be effective in detecting pre-malignant pathology; however, it does not significantly improve the cancer detection rate compared to the 12-core biopsy.

Pre-biopsy MRI should be performed in a clinically suspected prostate cancer patient. In the event of any abnormal lesion on MRI, a targeted biopsy should be performed along with the systematic biopsies. There is an increasing evidence that MRI-guided targeted biopsy increases the cancer detection rate compared to traditional 12-core systematic biopsy and can prevent unnecessary biopsy in some individuals [8, 9]. However, due to the issues related to the availability, cost and quality of the MRI, the data to recommend the routine use of MRI prior to biopsy is insufficient [10]. When performing MRI-targeted biopsy, it is often required to take 4–6 cores of biopsy around the target to identify the most aggressive form of the cancer [11].

Fine needle aspiration (FNA) has limited role in prostate cancer diagnosis except in confirming the metastatic disease in a patient with a known history of prostate cancer.

3.5 Pathology of Prostate Cancer

Adenocarcinoma of the prostate is the most common histology, accounting for >95% of the prostate cancers. Other histologies include neuroendocrine carcinoma, urothelial carcinoma, squamous cell carcinoma, lymphoma and sarcoma. Acinar adenocarcinoma is more common compared to the ductal adenocarcinoma [12]. Histopathologically, adenocarcinoma is composed of small infiltrating glands with prominent nucleoli. Immunohistochemistry (IHC) may complement if there is a diagnostic dilemma.

On IHC, adenocarcinoma is positive for alpha-methylacyl-CoA racemase (AMACR) and negative for p63 and high molecular weight cytokeratin (34bE12) antibodies [13–15]. IHC for PSA and NKX3.1 has a limited role in the diagnosis since both are expressed by benign and malignant cells. However, these markers help in determining if the lesions in the other organs (suspected metastatic lesions) are of prostatic origin or not; hence; PSA and NKX3.1 positive cells derived from lymph nodes, bone and other organs are more likely to represent the metastatic disease from prostate cancer.

3.5.1 Gleason Score and Grade Grouping

The Gleason score (GS) and grade group correlate with the clinical behaviour and outcome.

Prostate cancer is graded from grade 1 to 5 based on the cell architecture, growth pattern and degree of differentiation, with grade-1 being the well differentiated and grade-5 being the poorly differentiated cancer. The Gleason score ranges from 6 to 10 and is calculated by adding the numerical values of the two most prevalent (primary and secondary) differentiation pattern. For example, if a biopsy consists of predominantly grade-4 and secondarily grade-3 pattern, the composite GS will be $4 + 3 = 7$; however, if the biopsy consists of predominantly grade-3 and secondarily grade-4 pattern, the composite GS will be $3 + 4 = 7$. The former group with GS 4 + 3 will have a poorer outcome compared to GS 3 + 4 [16]. In some cases, tumour may also contain a small component (<5%) of a higher-grade tumour, in addition to the two predominant pattern, known as tertiary tumour grade. Traditionally, tertiary Gleason grade has an insignificant contribution in GS. However, in 2005, ISUP recommended that if a GS on biopsy is 3 + 4 or 4 + 3 and the tertiary pattern is 5, the cancer should be classified as GS 8 or 9 since the outcome in these patients is poorer compared to those without tertiary care pattern of 5 [17].

International Society of Urological Pathology (ISUP) has adopted a 5-tier grading system based on the GS, as mentioned below [18].

- Grade group 1 = GS 3 + 3.
- Grade group 2 = GS 3 + 4.
- Grade group 3 = GS 4 + 3.
- Grade group 4 = GS 4 + 4 or 3 + 5 or 5 + 3.
- Grade group 5 = GS 4 + 5 or 5 + 4 or 5 + 5.

Studies have reported increasing prostate cancer specific mortality with increasing overall grade group [19].

3.5.2 Staging of Prostate Cancer

Tables 3.1 and 3.2 are showing TNM staging and stage grouping of prostate cancer, respectively.

3.5.3 What are the Criteria for Very Low-/Low-Risk Prostate Cancer?

Patients with localized prostate cancer can be stratified into low, intermediate and high risk based on serum PSA, GS and T-stage [20].

Very low risk group should have all of the following factors:

1. cT1c
2. Gleason grade group-1
3. PSA level <10 ng/ml
4. <3 positive biopsy cores and <50% cancer in each core
5. PSA density- <0.15 ng/ml/gm

Low-risk prostate cancer should have all of the following factors

1. cT1c-T2a
2. PSA level <10 ng/ml
3. Gleason grade group- 1

Table 3.1 TNM staging of prostate cancer

Clinical (cT)	
T category	
TX	Primary tumour cannot be assessed
T0	No evidence of primary tumour
T1	Clinically inapparent tumour that is not palpable
T1a	Tumour incidental histologic finding in 5% or less of tissue resected
T1b	Tumour incidental histologic finding in more than 5% of tissue resected
T1c	Tumour identified by needle biopsy found in one or both sides, but not palpable
T2	Tumour is palpable and confined within prostate
T2a	Tumour involves one-half of one side or less
T2b	Tumour involves more than one-half of one side but not both sides
T2c	Tumour involves both sides
T3	Extraprostatic tumour that is not fixed or does not invade adjacent structures
T3a	Extraprostatic extension (unilateral or bilateral)
T3b	Tumour invades seminal vesicle(s)
T4	Tumour is fixed or invades adjacent structures other than seminal vesicles, such as external sphincter, rectum, bladder, levator muscles and/or pelvic wall
Pathologic (pT)	
T category	
T2	Organ confined
T3	Extraprostatic extension
T3a	Extraprostatic extension (unilateral or bilateral) or microscopic invasion of bladder neck
T3b	Tumour invades seminal vesicle(s)
T4	Tumour is fixed or invades adjacent structures other than seminal vesicles, such as external sphincter, rectum, bladder, levator muscles and/or pelvic wall
N category	
NX	Regional lymph nodes were not assessed
N0	No positive regional lymph nodes
N1	Metastases in regional lymph node(s)
M category	*M criteria*
M0	No distant metastasis
M1	Distant metastasis
M1a	Nonregional lymph node(s)
M1b	Bone(s)
M1c	Other site(s) with or without bone disease

Table 3.2 AJCC stage grouping of prostate cancer

WHEN T IS…	AND N IS…	AND M IS…	AND PSA IS…	AND GRADE GROUP IS…	THEN THE STAGE GROUP IS…
cT1a-c, cT2a	N0	M0	<10 ng/mL	1	I
pT2	N0	M0	<10 ng/mL	1	I
cT1a-c, cT2a	N0	M0	≥10, <20 ng/mL	1	IIA
pT2	N0	M0	≥10, <20 ng/mL	1	IIA
cT2b-c	N0	M0	<20 ng/mL	1	IIA
T1-2	N0	M0	<20 ng/mL	2	IIB
T1-2	N0	M0	<20 ng/mL	3	IIC
T1-2	N0	M0	<20 ng/mL	4	IIC
T1-2	N0	M0	≥20 ng/mL	1–4	IIIA
T3-4	N0	M0	Any	1–4	IIIB
Any T	N0	M0	Any	5	IIIC
Any T	N1	M0	Any	Any	IVA
Any T	Any	M1	Any	Any	IVB

With permission, License number and date—6034750546459 dated 23-05-25, Licensed Content Publisher—John Wiley and Sons, License content title- Prostate cancer—major changes in the American Joint Committee on Cancer eighth edition cancer staging manual
Abbreviation: *PSA* indicates prostate-specific antigen
Note that, when either PSA or grade group is not available, grouping should be determined by T category and/or either PSA or grade group, as available

3.6 Management

Management of prostate cancer depends on two factors (i) life expectancy and (ii) stage/risk category. Active surveillance is recommended for majority of the very low risk prostate cancer patients. For patients with low-risk prostate cancer and a life expectancy of ≥10 years, treatment options include radical prostatectomy, radiotherapy or active surveillance. Observation is an option for low-risk and very low-risk patients having a life expectancy of <10 years. Hormonal therapy is not recommended in the low-risk group of patients.

3.6.1 Active Surveillance

Active surveillance (AS) is widely accepted as the preferred management strategy for patients with very low-risk prostate cancer and a life expectancy greater than 10 years. AS includes regular monitoring with PSA testing, digital rectal examination (DRE) and periodic biopsies. The goal of active surveillance is to avoid treatment complications in men with indolent cancer. AS can be distinguished from observation or watchful waiting by postponement of the curative treatment till the disease progression. The term observation means that the patient is not a candidate for definitive therapy and palliative treatment is offered when the patient becomes symptomatic.

3.6.1.1 Recommendations for Active Surveillance [20]

1. PSA testing—every 6 monthly or when clinically indicated.
2. DRE—annually or when clinically indicated.
3. Repeat prostate biopsy—annually or when clinically indicated.
4. Repeat mpMRI—annually or when clinically indicated.
5. Metastatic staging evaluation should not be performed.
6. Surveillance protocol may be modified based on the risk reclassification and life expectancy.
7. Transition to observation when life expectancy is <10 years.

The advantages of AS include avoidance of definitive treatment in 50–68% patients for at least 10 years, thus maintaining quality of life and avoiding side effects of the treatment.

The disadvantage of AS is that approximately 32–50% patients on active surveillance undergo definitive treatment by 10 years; however, outcome is not compromised by the delayed treatment [21, 22].

3.6.2 Definitive Therapy

Though active surveillance is preferred for the majority of the low-risk patients, definitive treatment in the form of radical prostatectomy or radiotherapy (RT) can be offered to those with a high risk of progression such as high PSA density, high number of positive cores (i.e. >3) and high genomic risk. Definitive therapy is also considered in patients who are psychologically not comfortable living with a cancer or in those who are reluctant for regular follow-up [23, 24]. Another indication of definitive therapy is the disease progression on active surveillance, i.e. conversion to high grade group, increased tumour volume and increased PSA density.

Both radiation and surgery have shown equivalent disease control rates. Patients with bothersome urinary symptoms are more likely to be benefited from surgery compared to RT.

3.6.3 Radiotherapy

Both external beam radiotherapy (EBRT) and brachytherapy can be used as single modality for low risk prostate cancer patients [25]. Conformal RT techniques including intensity modulated radiotherapy (IMRT) and image-guided radiotherapy (IGRT) have replaced older two-dimensional techniques. IMRT is considered standard of care since it has a favorable toxicity profile compared to 3DCRT.

3.6.4 Brachytherapy

Brachytherapy alone is an option for low-risk prostate cancer patients. However, those with previous history of transurethral resection of prostate (TURP) and with a large prostate are more likely to develop brachytherapy-related complications and are generally considered a contraindication of brachytherapy [26]. Detailed brachytherapy is discussed elsewhere in the book.

3.7 Radiotherapy Planning and EBRT Contouring Guidelines

CT-based contouring guidelines lead to a large inter-observer variation [27]. Incorporation of MRI to CT reduces inter-observer variation in target volume delineation [28]. MRI helps in

(i) Better identification of caudal aspect of prostatic apex, external urethral sphincter and prostatic urethra.
(ii) Improved delineation of lateral border of prostate particularly at the level of apex.
(iii) Better delineation of posterior border and base of the prostate.
(iv) Better delineation of seminal vesicle (SV).
(v) Identification of extracapsular extension (ECE).
(vi) Prevents unnecessary exposure of vascular structure and anterior fibromuscular stroma (AFMS).

To minimize the inter-observer variation, EORTC-ACROP group formulated contouring guidelines based on MRI and CT scan [29].

For RT planning, multi-parametric or functional MRI is not required since only anatomical information is needed for the contouring; hence, a T2-weighted MRI in the transverse plane is sufficient. However, if a boost to the intra-prostatic lesion is planned, multi-parametric MRI should be performed [30]. Ideally, both CT and MRI should be done in similar positions and with similar bladder-rectal protocols. CT-MRI fusion can be done based on the bony structures, i.e. pubic bones. Alternatively, prostate fiducials can be placed at least 7 days prior to the planning CT. Due to the inevitable difference in bladder and rectal filling between CT and MRI, fusion based on the implanted fiducials is considered superior compared to bony matching [31]. Once both the images are fused, the prostate contours of MRI can be extrapolated on CT. Early results with PET-based target delineation are promising but not recommended at present [32].

3.7.1 Planning CT

Planning CT should be taken prior to RT at a slice thickness of ≤ 5 mm, in supine position. Bladder should be comfortably full. The patients should be asked to drink approx. 350 ml of water during the hour prior to planning CT [33]. Bowel preparation is suggested and rectum should ideally be empty of faeces and flatus. Routine use of enema is recommended. For positioning and immobilization, footpads/footstocks should be used. Anterior and lateral tattoos should be placed at the level of symphysis pubis for set up. Planning CT should be taken from the sacro-iliac joints to 1 cm below the ischial tuberosities. An MRI prostate can be done before RT planning for better prostate definition.

3.7.2 Target Volume Definition

Gross target volume (GTV) consists of only prostate. Clinical target volume (CTV) consists of prostate with or without proximal 2 cm of seminal vesicles depending on the institutional protocols [33]. Lymph nodes need not to be included in the target volume in low-risk prostate cancer patients. Three planning target volumes (PTVs) are generated according to the CHHiP protocol:

PTV 1 consists of prostate and proximal 2 cm of SV + 1 cm margin all around.
PTV 2 consists of prostate + 1 cm margin all around, except 5 mm posteriorly towards rectum.
PTV 3 consists of prostate + 0.5 cm margin all around, except 0 mm posteriorly towards rectum.

Organ at risks (OARs) including bladder, rectum, femoral heads, penile bulb, urethra and bowel should be outlined. Standard plan evaluation criteria should be used. Image-guided radiotherapy (IGRT), preferably with daily CBCT, is recommended for the treatment delivery. Studies have shown that the use of IGRT significantly reduces grade 2 or more genitourinary and gastro-intestinal toxicities compared to non-IGRT techniques [34, 35].

3.7.3 Radiobiology and Radiotherapy Dose

In general, increased fractionation provides a therapeutic advantage between tumour control and late side effects. The α/β ratio of late responding tissues is considered low (usually 3) and that for early responding tissues and most of the tumours is considered high (usually 8–10). Previous studies have shown a low α/β ratio of prostate cancer, ranging from 1.4 to 1.93, compared to surrounding normal tissue complications such as proctitis [36–42].

Cancers with a low α/β ratio such as prostate cancer have at least equal or better tumour response to hypo-fractionated RT compared to the conventional fractionation, i.e. 1.8–2 Gy/fraction though a few studies have demonstrated small increase in acute toxicities with hypo-fractionated RT in prostate cancer patients. Extreme hypo-fractionated RT using stereotactic body radiotherapy (SBRT) has also been explored. Hypofractionated RT is also advantageous in cost, resource utilisation and patient convenience [34, 43–45].

In the mid-90s, conventional fractionation schedule of 60–70 Gy/6–7 weeks was the most commonly used schedule for prostate cancer patients [46]. Gradually, the practice changed to hypo-fractionated RT with dose fractionation ranging from 50 Gy/20 fractions/4 weeks [47], 50 Gy/16 fractions/21 days [48] and 36 Gy/6 fractions/5 weeks [49].

In one of the first randomized trials comparing 66 Gy/33 fractions/45 days and 55.2 Gy/20 fractions/28 days, 5 years biochemical/clinical failure rates were higher in hypo-fractionated arm; though there was no difference in overall survival (OS) and late toxicities [50]. Another study comparing 64 Gy/32 fractions and 55 Gy/20 fractions in early stage prostate cancer showed similar rates of PSA control at 4 years, in both the treatment arms, though there was some increase in the rectal toxicity in the hypofractionated arm [51]. All these studies are compatible with an α/β ratio of 1.5–3 Gy. More recent randomized controlled trials have shown that the efficacy of hypofractionated RT is not inferior to that of conventional fractionation RT [43, 52–54]. A 2019 Cochrane review of 10 trials with 8278 patients reported that moderate hypofractionation up to fraction size of 3.4 Gy results in similar oncological outcome with little or no increase in acute or late toxicity [55]. One study compared 75.6 Gy/42 fractions with 72 Gy/30 fractions and found the superior local control with hypofractionation [44]. According to Dearnaley and colleagues, hypofractionated RT (60 Gy/20 fractions) is non-inferior to conventional RT (74 Gy/37 fractions) with comparable 5-years biochemical control rates of 88.3% and 90.6% in 74 Gy versus 60 Gy arm respectively [33]. At present, the ideal dose fractionation schedule for prostate cancer is not known. However, based on the largest available evidence, a dose of 70 Gy/28 fractions or 60 Gy/20 fractions is generally recommended and used by majority of the radiation oncologists [56]. Figure 3.2 is showing dose colour wash of a patient with low-risk prostate cancer treated in accordance with CHHiP protocol. Figure 3.3 is showing radiotherapy treatment verification of a prostate cancer patient with cone beam CT (CBCT).

Prostate cancer also exhibits a radiation dose-response relationship. In a meta-analysis, 10 Gy increment in biologically effective dose (BED) from 140 to 200 Gy, at α/β of 1.5, was associated with 5-unit improvement in percent freedom from biochemical failure (FFBF) [57]. However, there were no additional benefits of BED >200 Gy.

3.7.4 Role of Boost to Intra-Prostatic Disease

Majority of the patients fail locally in the original intra-prostatic lesion. Dose escalation to this area, which has a high risk of local failure, using MRI or PET CT has failed to show any conclusive results. Groenendaal and colleagues developed a model to incorporate the MRI data into treatment planning for focal boost to the intra-prostatic lesion [58]. The FLAME trial demonstrated that MRI-based focal tumour boost up to 95 Gy by simultaneous integrated boost (SIB) significantly

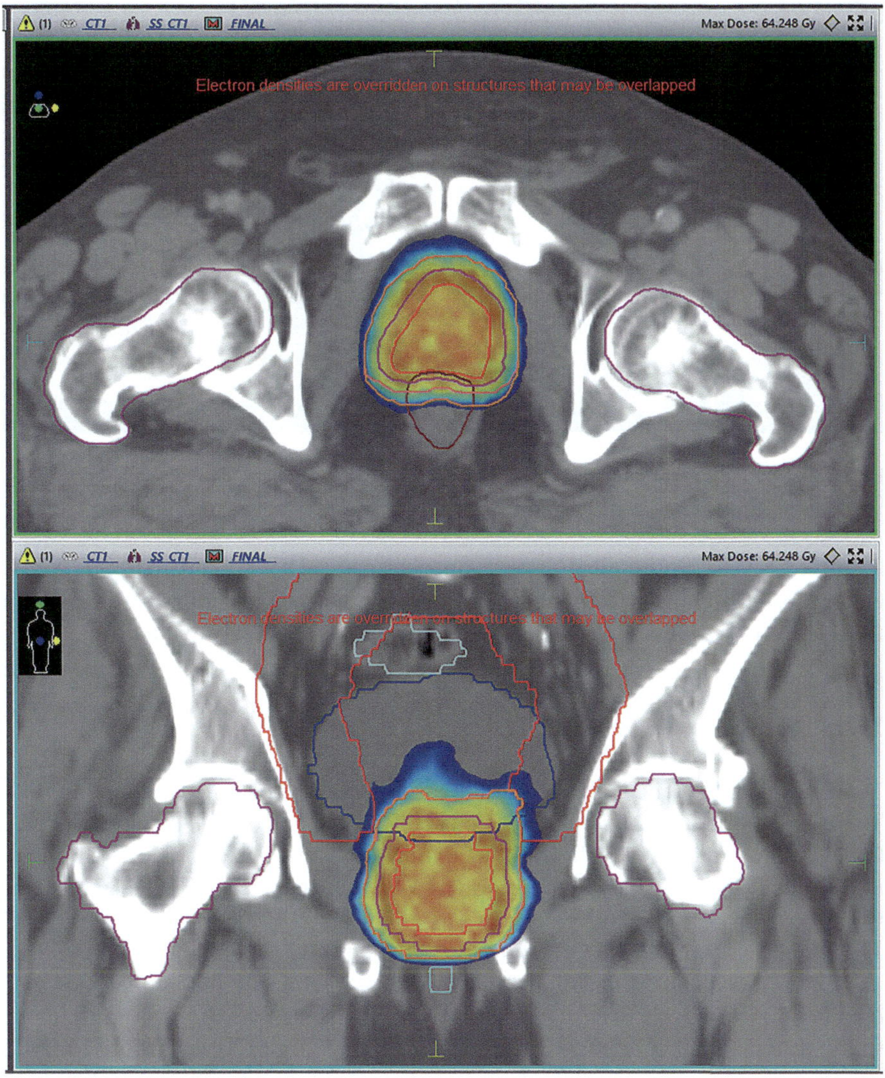

Fig. 3.2 Dose colour wash of a patient with low-risk prostate cancer treated in accordance with CHHiP protocol

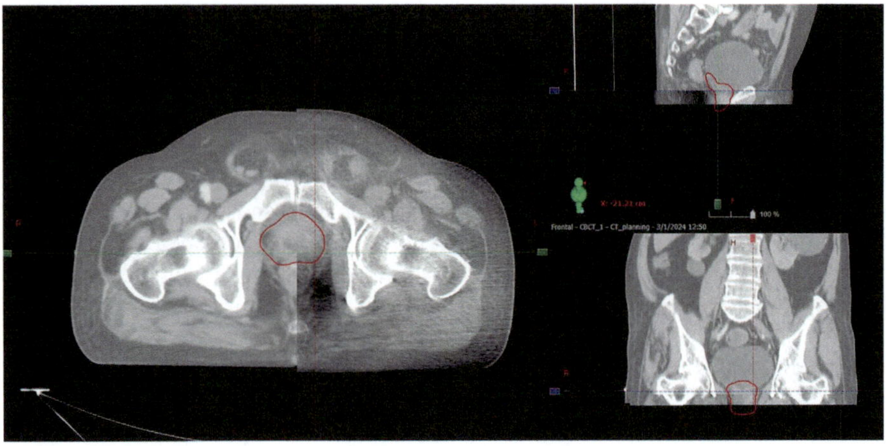

Fig. 3.3 Radiotherapy treatment verification of a prostate cancer patient with cone beam CT (CBCT)

improved 5-year biochemical disease-free survival (bDFS) compared to 77 Gy to entire prostate in intermediate- and high-risk prostate cancer. However, the data for focal boost to intra-prostatic lesion in low-risk disease is not available [59].

3.7.5 EBRT Toxicities

Toxicities of EBRT include gastrointestinal, urinary and erectile dysfunction [60]. There is a conflicting data if hypofractionated RT increases overall treatment-related toxicity. Few studies have shown non-significant increase in toxicities with hypofractionated RT [52]. One study reported 5-year incidence of RTOG grade 2 or worse bowel and bladder adverse events as 13·7% and 9·1% in the 74 Gy group and 11·9% and 11·7% in the 60 Gy group respectively [33].

A 2019 Cochrane review of 10 trials with 8278 patients reported that moderate hypofractionation adds to a little or no increase in acute or late toxicity [55]. In one study, patients with compromised urinary function before RT were more likely to have worse urinary function after hypofractionated RT. [43] In Dutch HYPRO trial, hypofractionated RT was associated with increased risk of acute grade ≥2 gastrointestinal and genitourinary toxicity [61]. RTOG 0415 trial showed that hypofractionated RT was associated with increased physician-reported grade 2–3 gastrointestinal and genitourinary toxicities at a median follow-up of 5.9 years [62]. The drawback of most of trials is a limited follow up, rarely exceeding more than 5 years.

3.7.6 Stereotactic Body Radiation Therapy (Ultrahypofractionated RT)

Stereotactic body radiation therapy (SBRT) is an extreme form of hypofractionation, where entire radiotherapy dose is delivered in fewer fractions, i.e. 5–7. It is a viable option for carefully selected low-risk prostate cancer patients [56]. PACE-A trial compared surgery to SBRT, whereas PACE B trial compared conventionally fractionated RT (2–3 Gy per fraction) to SBRT in low- and intermediate-risk prostate cancer [63, 64]. In the SBRT arm, a dose of 36.25 Gy in 5 fractions was prescribed to PTV, and the treatment was delivered daily or on alternate days. Five-year biochemical or clinical relapse-free survival was 95.8% and 94.6% in SBRT versus conventional or moderately hypofractionated arm, respectively. The incidence of grade 2 or worse genitourinary and gastrointestinal toxicities was 7.3% and 0.8% in SBRT arm compared to 4.5% and 0.3% in conventional or moderately hypofractionated arm. In contrast to HYPO RT PC trial, the authors in PACE studies did not report any significant increase in RTOG grade 2 or worse genitourinary or gastrointestinal toxicities in SBRT arm. A systematic review of over 6000 patients from 38 studies confirmed that SBRT yields favourable tumour control and quality of life without significantly increasing toxicities [65]. Despite the favourable results, median follow-up is generally limited to less than 5 years in most of the studies. Currently, two ongoing randomized trials are comparing conventional RT with SBRT in prostate cancer (NCT03367702 and NCT01794403).

3.7.7 Particle Therapy

There are no randomized trials comparing proton and photon for prostate cancer. One systematic review reported that outcomes were similar in proton and photon, and proton therapy does not yield any additional advantages [66].

The guidelines from American Urological Association (AUA), American Society for Radiation Oncology (ASTRO) and American Society of Clinical Oncology (ASCO) suggest that proton therapy does not offer any additional advantage over photon beam therapy. However, physical characteristics of 'Bragg peak' helps in reducing gastro-intestinal and genitourinary toxicities [67, 68].

Carbon ion, an alternative type of particle therapy, has been evaluated for the treatment of prostate cancer in Japan [69]. In their analysis of 2157 patients, 5-year biochemical relapse-free survival was 92%, 89% and 92% for low-, intermediate- and high-risk prostate cancer patients. None of the patients developed grade 3 toxicities, with grade 2 toxicities occurring in a small proportion of patients.

3.7.8 Radical Prostatectomy

In the Prostate Cancer Research International Active Surveillance (PRIAS) study, approximately 60% of men eventually received active treatment over a 10-year period, with many undergoing radical prostatectomy due to disease progression or pathological upgrading [70].

3.8 Pathological Upgrading and Disease Progression

Biopsy-based risk stratification may underestimate cancer aggressiveness. Studies show that restaging biopsies result in upgrading or upstaging in approximately 25% of patients eligible for AS [71]. For example, Berglund et al. (2008) found a significant rate of pathological upgrading upon immediate repeat biopsy [72]. This diagnostic uncertainty drives interest in surgical management to provide definitive pathological staging.

3.9 Evidence from Population-Based and Clinical Studies

Population-based studies from Sweden suggest that 50% of men with low-risk prostate cancer are either upgraded or upstaged at radical prostatectomy [73]. While similar data from the United States are limited and generally drawn from academic centres with small cohorts, they highlight the limitations of current risk stratification models [74].

Several randomized clinical trials have sought to clarify the benefits of radical prostatectomy in localized disease:

SPCG-4 (Scandinavian Prostate Cancer Group Study Number 4): Found a survival benefit for radical prostatectomy over watchful waiting [75].

PIVOT (Prostate Cancer Intervention Versus Observation Trial): Did not demonstrate a significant survival advantage of radical prostatectomy over observation in low-risk patients [76].

PROTECT (Prostate Testing for Cancer and Treatment Trial): Showed similar mortality outcomes between active monitoring, radical prostatectomy, and radiotherapy over a 15-year period, though radical prostatectomy reduced the risk of disease progression [2].

These differing outcomes underscore the absence of consensus on the optimal management for very low-risk prostate cancer and highlight the importance of individualized treatment planning.

3.10 Surgical Considerations in Very Low-Risk Prostate Cancer

The main concern about performing radical prostatectomy in low-risk cases is overtreatment and functional complications. Trials like PIVOT, SPCG-4, and PROTECT show differing outcomes regarding survival and progression. Therefore, shared decision-making is essential [2, 76]. To minimize harm, the *pentafecta outcome*—no complications, continence, potency, negative margins and biochemical recurrence-free survival—should be pursued. Intrafascial NVB preservation is most suitable in very low-risk disease, as neurovascular bundles are uninvolved. Advanced techniques such as high anterior release, anterior hood preservation and Retzius-sparing RARP can be used safely without oncologic compromise.

3.11 Surgical Approaches to Radical Prostatectomy

3.11.1 Open Radical Prostatectomy

Open radical prostatectomy, particularly the retropubic approach, has been a standard for decades. The procedure involves a midline abdominal incision, dissection of the Retzius space, and removal of the prostate and seminal vesicles. Walsh and Donker's introduction of the anatomic nerve-sparing technique in 1982 revolutionized outcomes, enabling better preservation of erectile function [77].

3.11.2 Laparoscopic Radical Prostatectomy

Laparoscopic RP is a minimally invasive alternative, offering reduced blood loss and quicker recovery. However, due to the steep learning curve and the technical challenges of intracorporeal suturing, its use has declined with the advent of robotic assistance [78].

3.11.3 Robot-Assisted Radical Prostatectomy (RARP)

RARP has become the most common technique, accounting for over 90% of procedures [79]. It offers enhanced visualization, precision, and ergonomics, contributing to lower complication rates and better functional outcomes. The introduction of the da Vinci Surgical System in the early 2000s transformed the surgical landscape. Recently various other robotic surgical system has been introduced, which further enhanced the use of this technology.

3.11.4 Preoperative Preparation

Prior to surgery, patients are counselled on key lifestyle changes: a heart-healthy diet, regular exercise, smoking cessation, and weight loss if needed. Specifically for RARP, Kegel exercises (three times daily) and walking 1–2 miles per day are emphasized [80].

3.11.5 Patient Positioning

Under general anaesthesia, the patient is placed in lithotomy position with hips flexed to avoid nerve injury. Pneumoperitoneum is created, standard robotic ports are placed and the patient is moved to steep Trendelenburg to shift abdominal contents away from the pelvis, and robot is then docked [81].

3.12 Surgical Steps Are Discussed Below [82]

3.12.1 Approach

Two common approaches are used:

- *Posterior-first*: Dissection between the bladder and rectum is performed first.
- *Anterior-first*: Procedure begins by dropping the bladder.

3.12.2 Bladder Mobilization

The peritoneum is incised, bladder is dropped, pubic bone is identified and anterior prostatic fat (APF) is removed for visualization of prostate.

3.12.3 Endopelvic Fascia

Fascia is incised laterally to protect the neurovascular bundles (NVBs).

3.12.4 Bladder Neck Dissection

The anterior bladder neck is dissected with minimal cautery. The full posterior bladder wall is preserved to aid in Rocco stitch placement.

3.12.5 Seminal Vesicles & Rectum

Seminal vesicles are mobilized gently, Denonvilliers' fascia lifted and rectum retracted while dissecting the prostate-rectum plane.

3.12.6 Prostatic Pedicles & NVBs

Minimal traction, no cautery and precise dissection reduce NVB injury.

3.12.7 Dorsal Venous Complex (DVC) & Urethra

Sharp DVC transection and oversewing with 3-0 barbed sutures have improved early continence and potency. Urethral length is preserved through careful apical dissection.

3.12.8 Anastomosis (Rocco & Van Velthoven)

A Rocco stitch stabilizes the posterior bladder neck. A single-knot Van Velthoven anastomosis is performed using two running sutures.

3.13 Postoperative Care

Early ambulation is prioritized, with catheter removal after 6–10 days. Continence is monitored via daily pad logs.

3.14 Comparative Effectiveness

A Bayesian network meta-analysis found radical prostatectomy and brachytherapy offered the best oncologic outcomes among treatments for low-risk prostate cancer. However, radical prostatectomy and brachytherapy had higher cancer-specific mortality than EBRT and AS. All-cause mortality was similar across modalities [83].

3.15 Patient Selection and Shared Decision-Making

Younger patients with anxiety about progression or unfavourable pathology may choose radical prostatectomy, while older men or those with comorbidities may opt for AS. Shared decision-making should emphasize limitations of current models, prognosis, and possible functional impairments from surgery [84].

Other approaches including cryotherapy, photodynamic therapy and high intensity focussed ultrasound (HIFU) have been explored in localised prostate cancer, however; these are not recommended over surgery or radiation therapy. Androgen deprivation therapy (ADT) alone is not recommended for the initial treatment of localised prostate cancer unless for palliation of symptoms in patients with limited life expectancy.

3.16 Conclusion

Low-risk prostate cancer patients have excellent outcomes irrespective of the treatment modality. The choice of therapy depends on the ratio of possible benefit and risk of potential overtreatment and side effects. It is important to discuss pros and cons of each modality with the patients in a multidisciplinary tumor board.

References

1. Global Burden of Disease Cancer Collaboration, Fitzmaurice C, Allen C, Barber RM, Barregard L, Bhutta ZA, et al. Global, regional, and National Cancer Incidence, mortality, years of life lost, years lived with disability, and disability-adjusted life-years for 32 cancer groups, 1990 to 2015: a systematic analysis for the global burden of disease study. JAMA Oncol. 2017;3(4):524–48.
2. Hamdy FC, Donovan JL, Lane JA, Metcalfe C, Davis M, Turner EL, et al. Fifteen-year outcomes after monitoring, surgery, or radiotherapy for prostate cancer. N Engl J Med [Internet]. 2023 Apr 27 [cited 2025 Apr 16];388(17). Available from: https://pubmed.ncbi.nlm.nih.gov/36912538/.
3. Fütterer JJ, Heijmink SWTPJ, Scheenen TWJ, Veltman J, Huisman HJ, Vos P, et al. Prostate cancer localization with dynamic contrast-enhanced MR imaging and proton MR spectroscopic imaging. Radiology. 2006;241(2):449–58.
4. Turkbey B, Rosenkrantz AB, Haider MA, Padhani AR, Villeirs G, Macura KJ, et al. Prostate imaging reporting and data system version 2.1: 2019 update of prostate imaging reporting and data system version 2. Eur Urol. 2019;76(3):340–51.
5. Catalona WJ, Partin AW, Slawin KM, Brawer MK, Flanigan RC, Patel A, et al. Use of the percentage of free prostate-specific antigen to enhance differentiation of prostate cancer from benign prostatic disease: a prospective multicenter clinical trial. JAMA. 1998;279(19):1542–7.
6. Ukimura O, Coleman JA, de la Taille A, Emberton M, Epstein JI, Freedland SJ, et al. Contemporary role of systematic prostate biopsies: indications, techniques, and implications for patient care. Eur Urol. 2013;63(2):214–30.
7. Eichler K, Hempel S, Wilby J, Myers L, Bachmann LM, Kleijnen J. Diagnostic value of systematic biopsy methods in the investigation of prostate cancer: a systematic review. J Urol. 2006;175(5):1605–12.
8. Drost FJH, Osses DF, Nieboer D, Steyerberg EW, Bangma CH, Roobol MJ, et al. Prostate MRI, with or without MRI-targeted biopsy, and systematic biopsy for detecting prostate cancer. Cochrane Database Syst Rev. 2019;4(4):CD012663.
9. Kasivisvanathan V, Rannikko AS, Borghi M, Panebianco V, Mynderse LA, Vaarala MH, et al. MRI-targeted or standard biopsy for prostate-cancer diagnosis. N Engl J Med. 2018;378(19):1767–77.
10. Fulgham PF, Rukstalis DB, Turkbey IB, Rubenstein JN, Taneja S, Carroll PR, et al. AUA policy statement on the use of multiparametric magnetic resonance imaging in the diagnosis, staging and Management of Prostate Cancer. J Urol. 2017;198(4):832–8.
11. Brisbane WG, Priester AM, Ballon J, Kwan L, Delfin MK, Felker ER, et al. Targeted prostate biopsy: umbra, penumbra, and value of perilesional sampling. Eur Urol. 2022;82(3):303–10.
12. Chow K, Bedő J, Ryan A, Agarwal D, Bolton D, Chan Y, et al. Ductal variant prostate carcinoma is associated with a significantly shorter metastasis-free survival. Eur J Cancer. 2021;148:440–50.
13. Yang XJ, Lecksell K, Gaudin P, Epstein JI. Rare expression of high-molecular-weight cytokeratin in adenocarcinoma of the prostate gland: a study of 100 cases of metastatic and locally advanced prostate cancer. Am J Surg Pathol. 1999;23(2):147–52.

14. Rubin MA, Zhou M, Dhanasekaran SM, Varambally S, Barrette TR, Sanda MG, et al. Alpha-Methylacyl coenzyme a racemase as a tissue biomarker for prostate cancer. JAMA. 2002;287(13):1662–70.
15. Shah RB, Zhou M, LeBlanc M, Snyder M, Rubin MA. Comparison of the basal cell-specific markers, 34betaE12 and p63, in the diagnosis of prostate cancer. Am J Surg Pathol. 2002;26(9):1161–8.
16. Kang DE, Fitzsimons NJ, Presti JC, Kane CJ, Terris MK, Aronson WJ, et al. Risk stratification of men with Gleason score 7 to 10 tumors by primary and secondary Gleason score: results from the SEARCH database. Urology. 2007;70(2):277–82.
17. Epstein JI, Allsbrook WC, Amin MB, Egevad LL. ISUP grading committee. The 2005 International Society of Urological Pathology (ISUP) consensus conference on Gleason grading of prostatic carcinoma. Am J Surg Pathol. 2005;29(9):1228–42.
18. Epstein JI, Egevad L, Amin MB, Delahunt B, Srigley JR, Humphrey PA, et al. The 2014 International Society of Urological Pathology (ISUP) consensus conference on Gleason grading of prostatic carcinoma: definition of grading patterns and proposal for a new grading system. Am J Surg Pathol. 2016;40(2):244–52.
19. Berney DM, Beltran L, Fisher G, North BV, Greenberg D, Møller H, et al. Validation of a contemporary prostate cancer grading system using prostate cancer death as outcome. Br J Cancer. 2016;114(10):1078–83.
20. NCCN [Internet]. [cited 2025 Feb 7]. Guidelines detail. Available from: https://www.nccn.org/guidelines/guidelines-detail?category=1&id=1459.
21. Tosoian JJ, Mamawala M, Epstein JI, Landis P, Wolf S, Trock BJ, et al. Intermediate and longer-term outcomes from a prospective active-surveillance program for favorable-risk prostate cancer. J Clin Oncol Off J Am Soc Clin Oncol. 2015;33(30):3379–85.
22. Cooley LF, Emeka AA, Meyers TJ, Cooper PR, Lin DW, Finelli A, et al. Factors associated with time to conversion from active surveillance to treatment for prostate cancer in a multi-institutional cohort. J Urol. 2021;206(5):1147–56.
23. Bekelman JE, Rumble RB, Chen RC, Pisansky TM, Finelli A, Feifer A, et al. Clinically localized prostate cancer: ASCO clinical practice guideline endorsement of an American urological association/American Society for Radiation Oncology/Society of Urologic Oncology Guideline. J Clin Oncol Off J Am Soc Clin Oncol. 2018;36(32):3251–8.
24. Cooperberg MR, Zheng Y, Faino AV, Newcomb LF, Zhu K, Cowan JE, et al. Tailoring intensity of active surveillance for low-risk prostate cancer based on individualized prediction of risk stability. JAMA Oncol. 2020;6(10):e203187.
25. Sanda MG, Cadeddu JA, Kirkby E, Chen RC, Crispino T, Fontanarosa J, et al. Clinically localized prostate cancer: AUA/ASTRO/SUO guideline. Part II: recommended approaches and details of specific care options. J Urol. 2018;199(4):990–7.
26. Davis BJ, Horwitz EM, Lee WR, Crook JM, Stock RG, Merrick GS, et al. American brachytherapy society consensus guidelines for transrectal ultrasound-guided permanent prostate brachytherapy. Brachytherapy. 2012;11(1):6–19.
27. Boehmer D, Maingon P, Poortmans P, Baron MH, Miralbell R, Remouchamps V, et al. Guidelines for primary radiotherapy of patients with prostate cancer. Radiother Oncol. 2006;79(3):259–69.
28. Rasch C, Barillot I, Remeijer P, Touw A, van Herk M, Lebesque JV. Definition of the prostate in CT and MRI: a multi-observer study. Int J Radiat Oncol Biol Phys. 1999;43(1):57–66.
29. Salembier C, Villeirs G, De Bari B, Hoskin P, Pieters BR, Van Vulpen M, et al. ESTRO ACROP consensus guideline on CT- and MRI-based target volume delineation for primary radiation therapy of localized prostate cancer. Radiother Oncol. 2018;127(1):49–61.
30. Barentsz JO, Weinreb JC, Verma S, Thoeny HC, Tempany CM, Shtern F, et al. Synopsis of the PI-RADS v2 guidelines for multiparametric prostate magnetic resonance imaging and recommendations for use. Eur Urol. 2016;69(1):41–9.
31. Parker CC, Damyanovich A, Haycocks T, Haider M, Bayley A, Catton CN. Magnetic resonance imaging in the radiation treatment planning of localized prostate cancer using intra-

prostatic fiducial markers for computed tomography co-registration. Radiother Oncol. 2003;66(2):217–24.
32. Zamboglou C, Sachpazidis I, Koubar K, Drendel V, Wiehle R, Kirste S, et al. Evaluation of intensity modulated radiation therapy dose painting for localized prostate cancer using 68Ga-HBED-CC PSMA-PET/CT: a planning study based on histopathology reference. Radiother Oncol. 2017;123(3):472–7.
33. Dearnaley D, Syndikus I, Mossop H, Khoo V, Birtle A, Bloomfield D, et al. Conventional versus hypofractionated high-dose intensity-modulated radiotherapy for prostate cancer: 5-year outcomes of the randomised, non-inferiority, phase 3 CHHiP trial. Lancet Oncol. 2016;17(8):1047–60.
34. Aluwini S, Pos F, Schimmel E, van Lin E, Krol S, van der Toorn PP, et al. Hypofractionated versus conventionally fractionated radiotherapy for patients with prostate cancer (HYPRO): acute toxicity results from a randomised non-inferiority phase 3 trial. Lancet Oncol. 2015;16(3):274–83.
35. Wortel RC, Incrocci L, Pos FJ, Lebesque JV, Witte MG, van der Heide UA, et al. Acute toxicity after image-guided intensity modulated radiation therapy compared to 3D conformal radiation therapy in prostate cancer patients. Int J Radiat Oncol Biol Phys. 2015;91(4):737–44.
36. Dasu A, Toma-Dasu I. Prostate alpha/beta revisited -- an analysis of clinical results from 14 168 patients. Acta Oncol. 2012;51(8):963–74.
37. Vogelius IR, Bentzen SM. Meta-analysis of the alpha/beta ratio for prostate cancer in the presence of an overall time factor: bad news, good news, or no news? Int J Radiat Oncol Biol Phys. 2013;85(1):89–94.
38. Miralbell R, Roberts SA, Zubizarreta E, Hendry JH. Dose-fractionation sensitivity of prostate cancer deduced from radiotherapy outcomes of 5,969 patients in seven international institutional datasets: $\alpha/\beta = 1.4$ (0.9–2.2) Gy. Int J Radiat Oncol Biol Phys. 2012;82(1):e17–24.
39. Proust-Lima C, Taylor JMG, Sécher S, Sandler H, Kestin L, Pickles T, et al. Confirmation of a low α/β ratio for prostate cancer treated by external beam radiation therapy alone using a post-treatment repeated-measures model for PSA dynamics. Int J Radiat Oncol Biol Phys. 2011;79(1):195–201.
40. Brenner DJ, Martinez AA, Edmundson GK, Mitchell C, Thames HD, Armour EP. Direct evidence that prostate tumors show high sensitivity to fractionation (low alpha/beta ratio), similar to late-responding normal tissue. Int J Radiat Oncol Biol Phys. 2002;52(1):6–13.
41. D'Souza WD, Thames HD. Is the alpha/beta ratio for prostate cancer low? Int J Radiat Oncol Biol Phys. 2001;51(1):1–3.
42. Fowler J, Chappell R, Ritter M. Is alpha/beta for prostate tumors really low? Int J Radiat Oncol Biol Phys. 2001;50(4):1021–31.
43. Pollack A, Walker G, Horwitz EM, Price R, Feigenberg S, Konski AA, et al. Randomized trial of hypofractionated external-beam radiotherapy for prostate cancer. J Clin Oncol Off J Am Soc Clin Oncol. 2013;31(31):3860–8.
44. Hoffman KE, Voong KR, Pugh TJ, Skinner H, Levy LB, Takiar V, et al. Risk of late toxicity in men receiving dose-escalated hypofractionated intensity modulated prostate radiation therapy: results from a randomized trial. Int J Radiat Oncol Biol Phys. 2014;88(5):1074–84.
45. Norkus D, Karklelyte A, Engels B, Versmessen H, Griskevicius R, De Ridder M, et al. A randomized hypofractionation dose escalation trial for high risk prostate cancer patients: interim analysis of acute toxicity and quality of life in 124 patients. Radiat Oncol Lond Engl. 2013;8:206.
46. Zagars GK, von Eschenbach AC, Johnson DE, Oswald MJ. The role of radiation therapy in stages A2 and B adenocarcinoma of the prostate. Int J Radiat Oncol Biol Phys. 1988;14(4):701–9.
47. Duncan W, Warde P, Catton CN, Munro AJ, Lakier R, Gadalla T, et al. Carcinoma of the prostate: results of radical radiotherapy (1970–1985). Int J Radiat Oncol Biol Phys. 1993;26(2):203–10.
48. Read G, Pointon RC. Retrospective study of radiotherapy in early carcinoma of the prostate. Br J Urol. 1989;63(2):191–5.
49. Collins CD, Lloyd-Davies RW, Swan AV. Radical external beam radiotherapy for localised carcinoma of the prostate using a hypofractionation technique. Clin Oncol. 1991;3(3):127–32.

50. Lukka H, Hayter C, Julian JA, Warde P, Morris WJ, Gospodarowicz M, et al. Randomized trial comparing two fractionation schedules for patients with localized prostate cancer. J Clin Oncol. 2005;23(25):6132–8.
51. Yeoh EEK, Fraser RJ, McGowan RE, Botten RJ, Di Matteo AC, Roos DE, et al. Evidence for efficacy without increased toxicity of hypofractionated radiotherapy for prostate carcinoma: early results of a phase III randomized trial. Int J Radiat Oncol Biol Phys. 2003;55(4):943–55.
52. Lee WR, Dignam JJ, Amin MB, Bruner DW, Low D, Swanson GP, et al. Randomized phase III noninferiority study comparing two radiotherapy fractionation schedules in patients with Low-risk prostate cancer. J Clin Oncol Off J Am Soc Clin Oncol. 2016;34(20):2325–32.
53. Catton CN, Lukka H, Gu CS, Martin JM, Supiot S, Chung PWM, et al. Randomized trial of a Hypofractionated radiation regimen for the treatment of localized prostate cancer. J Clin Oncol. 2017;35(17):1884–90.
54. Avkshtol V, Ruth KJ, Ross EA, Hallman MA, Greenberg RE, Price RA, et al. Ten-year update of a randomized, prospective trial of conventional fractionated versus moderate Hypofractionated radiation therapy for localized prostate cancer. J Clin Oncol. 2020;38(15):1676–84.
55. Hickey BE, James ML, Daly T, Soh FY, Jeffery M. Hypofractionation for clinically localized prostate cancer. Cochrane Database Syst Rev. 2019;9(9):CD011462.
56. Morgan SC, Hoffman K, Loblaw DA, Buyyounouski MK, Patton C, Barocas D, et al. Hypofractionated radiation therapy for localized prostate cancer: executive summary of an ASTRO, ASCO and AUA evidence-based guideline. J Urol. 2019;201(3):528–34.
57. Zaorsky NG, Palmer JD, Hurwitz MD, Keith SW, Dicker AP, Den RB. What is the ideal radiotherapy dose to treat prostate cancer? A meta-analysis of biologically equivalent dose escalation. Radiother Oncol. 2015;115(3):295–300.
58. Groenendaal G, Borren A, Moman MR, Monninkhof E, van Diest PJ, Philippens MEP, et al. Pathologic validation of a model based on diffusion-weighted imaging and dynamic contrast-enhanced magnetic resonance imaging for tumor delineation in the prostate peripheral zone. Int J Radiat Oncol Biol Phys. 2012;82(3):e537–44.
59. Kerkmeijer LGW, Groen VH, Pos FJ, Haustermans K, Monninkhof EM, Smeenk RJ, et al. Focal boost to the Intraprostatic tumor in external beam radiotherapy for patients with localized prostate cancer: results from the FLAME randomized phase III trial. J Clin Oncol. 2021;39(7):787–96.
60. Sanda MG, Dunn RL, Michalski J, Sandler HM, Northouse L, Hembroff L, et al. Quality of life and satisfaction with outcome among prostate-cancer survivors. N Engl J Med. 2008;358(12):1250–61.
61. Incrocci L, Wortel RC, Alemayehu WG, Aluwini S, Schimmel E, Krol S, et al. Hypofractionated versus conventionally fractionated radiotherapy for patients with localised prostate cancer (HYPRO): final efficacy results from a randomised, multicentre, open-label, phase 3 trial. Lancet Oncol. 2016;17(8):1061–9.
62. Bruner DW, Pugh SL, Lee WR, Hall WA, Dignam JJ, Low D, et al. Quality of life in patients with Low-risk prostate cancer treated with Hypofractionated vs. conventional radiotherapy: a phase 3 randomized clinical trial. JAMA Oncol. 2019;5(5):664–70.
63. van As N, Yasar B, Griffin C, Patel J, Tree AC, Ostler P, et al. Radical prostatectomy versus stereotactic radiotherapy for clinically localised prostate cancer: results of the PACE-A randomised trial. Eur Urol. 2024;86(6):566–76.
64. Tree AC, Ostler P, van der Voet H, Chu W, Loblaw A, Ford D, et al. Intensity-modulated radiotherapy versus stereotactic body radiotherapy for prostate cancer (PACE-B): 2-year toxicity results from an open-label, randomised, phase 3, non-inferiority trial. Lancet Oncol. 2022;23(10):1308–20.
65. Jackson WC, Silva J, Hartman HE, Dess RT, Kishan AU, Beeler WH, et al. Stereotactic body radiation therapy for localized prostate cancer: a systematic review and meta-analysis of over 6,000 patients treated on prospective studies. Int J Radiat Oncol Biol Phys. 2019;104(4):778–89.
66. Allen AM, Pawlicki T, Dong L, Fourkal E, Buyyounouski M, Cengel K, et al. An evidence based review of proton beam therapy: the report of ASTRO'S emerging technology committee. Radiother Oncol. 2012;103(1):8–11.

67. Yu JB, Soulos PR, Herrin J, Cramer LD, Potosky AL, Roberts KB, et al. Proton versus intensity-modulated radiotherapy for prostate cancer: patterns of care and early toxicity. J Natl Cancer Inst. 2013;105(1):25–32.
68. Sheets NC, Goldin GH, Meyer AM, Wu Y, Chang Y, Stürmer T, et al. Intensity-modulated radiation therapy, proton therapy, or conformal radiation therapy and morbidity and disease control in localized prostate cancer. JAMA. 2012;307(15):1611–20.
69. Nomiya T, Tsuji H, Kawamura H, Ohno T, Toyama S, Shioyama Y, et al. A multi-institutional analysis of prospective studies of carbon ion radiotherapy for prostate cancer: a report from the Japan carbon ion radiation oncology study group (J-CROS). Radiother Oncol. 2016;121(2):288–93.
70. Bokhorst LP, Valdagni R, Rannikko A, Kakehi Y, Pickles T, Bangma CH, et al. A decade of active surveillance in the PRIAS study: an update and evaluation of the criteria used to recommend a switch to active treatment. Eur Urol. 2016;70(6):954–60.
71. Dall'Era MA, Konety BR, Cowan JE, Shinohara K, Stauf F, Cooperberg MR, et al. Active surveillance for the management of prostate cancer in a contemporary cohort. Cancer. 2008;112(12):2664–70.
72. Berglund RK, Masterson TA, Vora KC, Eggener SE, Eastham JA, Guillonneau BD. Pathological upgrading and up staging with immediate repeat biopsy in patients eligible for active surveillance. J Urol. 2008;180(5):1964–7. discussion 1967–1968.
73. Godtman RA, Holmberg E, Khatami A, Stranne J, Hugosson J. Outcome following active surveillance of men with screen-detected prostate cancer. Results from the Göteborg randomised population-based prostate cancer screening trial. Eur Urol. 2013;63(1):101–7.
74. Cooperberg MR, Broering JM, Carroll PR. Risk assessment for prostate cancer metastasis and mortality at the time of diagnosis. J Natl Cancer Inst. 2009;101(12):878–87.
75. Bill-Axelson A, Holmberg L, Garmo H, Taari K, Busch C, Nordling S, et al. Radical prostatectomy or watchful waiting in prostate cancer - 29-year follow-up. N Engl J Med. 2018;379(24):2319–29.
76. Wilt TJ, Brawer MK, Jones KM, Barry MJ, Aronson WJ, Fox S, et al. Radical prostatectomy versus observation for localized prostate cancer. N Engl J Med. 2012;367(3):203–13.
77. Walsh PC, Donker PJ. Impotence following radical prostatectomy: insight into etiology and prevention. J Urol. 1982;128(3):492–7.
78. Rassweiler J, Seemann O, Schulze M, Teber D, Hatzinger M, Frede T. Laparoscopic versus open radical prostatectomy: a comparative study at a single institution. J Urol. 2003;169(5):1689–93.
79. Ficarra V, Novara G, Rosen RC, Artibani W, Carroll PR, Costello A, et al. Systematic review and meta-analysis of studies reporting urinary continence recovery after robot-assisted radical prostatectomy. Eur Urol. 2012;62(3):405–17.
80. Patel VR, Tully AS, Holmes R, Lindsay J. Robotic radical prostatectomy in the community setting--the learning curve and beyond: initial 200 cases. J Urol. 2005;174(1):269–72.
81. Kaul S, Savera A, Badani K, Fumo M, Bhandari A, Menon M. Functional outcomes and oncological efficacy of Vattikuti institute prostatectomy with veil of Aphrodite nerve-sparing: an analysis of 154 consecutive patients. BJU Int. 2006;97(3):467–72.
82. Su LM, Link RE, Bhayani SB, Sullivan W, Pavlovich CP. Nerve-sparing laparoscopic radical prostatectomy: replicating the open surgical technique. Urology. 2004;64(1):123–7.
83. Chen RC, Basak R, Meyer AM, Kuo TM, Carpenter WR, Agans RP, et al. Association between choice of radical prostatectomy, external beam radiotherapy, brachytherapy, or active surveillance and patient-reported quality of life among men with localized prostate cancer. JAMA. 2017;317(11):1141–50.
84. Hoffman RM, Koyama T, Fan KH, Albertsen PC, Barry MJ, Goodman M, et al. Mortality after radical prostatectomy or external beam radiotherapy for localized prostate cancer. J Natl Cancer Inst. 2013;105(10):711–8.

Intermediate-Risk Prostate Cancer: A Guide for Radiation Oncologists

4

K. N. Yousra Izzuddeen and Adila Amariyil

4.1 Introduction

Prostate cancer is the second most common cancer and the fifth most common cause of cancer-related deaths in men globally [1]. In India, prostate cancer is the third most common cancer in men, after lung and oral cavity cancers [2]. Five-year relative survival for all stages of prostate cancer combined is 97% [3]. Risk stratification is necessary for the optimal treatment of prostate cancer. The NCCN schema for risk stratification based on groups defined by D'Amico et al. is widely employed in clinical practice; however, it is important to note that while it is prognostic, it is not predictive of specific treatment benefits. Intermediate-risk prostate cancer contains a large and heterogeneous population defined by stage, PSA levels and Gleason score. Depending on clinical and pathological characteristics, it is further classified into favourable and unfavourable intermediate groups.

4.2 Classification and Classification and Staging

The AJCC TNM staging for prostate cancer is widely used in clinical practice [4].

Histopathological grading is conducted in tissues obtained from needle biopsy or prostatectomy. The Gleason scoring system was devised by Dr. Donald Gleason using glandular architecture and microscopic appearance. The specimen is assigned two grades based on the most common and second most common glandular patterns. These values are added to calculate the Gleason score. A new

K. N. Yousra Izzuddeen (✉)
Department of Radiation Oncology, Burjeel Medical City, Abu Dhabi, United Arab Emirates

A. Amariyil
Department of Radiation Oncology, AIIMS-NCI Jhajjar, Jhajjar, Haryana, India

R. Madan, S. Goyal (eds.), *Essentials of Radiotherapy in Uro-Genital Malignancies*, https://doi.org/10.1007/978-981-95-5945-9_4

system developed during the 2014 International Society of Urological Pathology (ISUP) Consensus Conference assigns grade groups based on the Gleason score (GS).

Gleason grade groups are as follows [5],

- Grade Group 1: GS ≤ 6; Individual discrete well-formed glands.
- Grade Group 2: GS 3 + 4 = 7; Mainly well-formed glands and a lesser component of poorly formed/fused/cribriform glands.
- Grade Group 3: GS 4 + 3 = 7; mainly poorly formed/fused/cribriform glands with a lesser component of well-formed glands.
- Grade Group 4: GS 8 (4 + 4/3 + 5/5 + 3); only poorly formed/fused/cribriform glands OR mainly well-formed glands with a lesser component lacking glands OR predominantly lacking glands with a lesser component of well-formed glands.
- Grade Group 5: GS 9/10 (4 + 5/5 + 4/5 + 5); mainly poorly formed/fused/cribriform glands with a lessor component lacking gland formation OR mainly lacking gland formation with or without formed/fused/cribriform glands.

Definition Intermediate-risk prostate cancer is defined by the presence of one or more intermediate-risk factors (IRF) in the absence of any high or very high-risk features. The three intermediate risk factors (IRFs) are

1. Stage IIa–IIb,
2. Pathological grade group 2 or 3,
3. PSA value between 10 and 20 ng/mL.

Favourable intermediate-risk subgroup It has only one IRF with grade group 1 or 2 and less than 50% of biopsy cores positive.

Unfavourable intermediate risk group It is characterized by the presence of two or more IRFs or histological grade group 3 or more than 50% positive cores. Patients in the unfavourable intermediate-risk group have worse PSA recurrence-free survival and higher rates of distant metastasis and prostate cancer-specific mortality than the favourable intermediate-risk group [6].

4.3 Diagnostic Tools and Evaluation

4.3.1 Biopsy

Transrectal ultrasound (TRUS)-guided biopsy is the standard practice in diagnosing prostate cancer. MRI/TRUS-targeted biopsy technique increases the detection of clinically significant high-risk prostate cancer. The NCCN recommends an extended pattern minimum 12-core biopsy with six medial cores and six cores from the lateral peripheral zone and lesion-directed biopsy.

4.3.2 Imaging Techniques

Both bone and soft tissue imaging techniques should be used in the initial staging and monitoring of prostate cancer patients due to the predilection of prostate cancer to metastasize to lymph nodes and bone.

- *Multiparametric MRI (mp MRI)* is preferred for soft tissue imaging of the chest and abdomen. It typically includes three sequences: T2-weighted imaging, diffusion-weighted imaging (DWI) and dynamic contrast-enhanced imaging (DCE). The use of mp MRI is supported by evidence due to its ability to detect more poorly differentiated tumours, better assessment of extracapsular extension and aid in targeted biopsy protocols.
- Conventional technetium-99 m-labelled methylene diphosphonate (MDP) bone scan can be used for bone imaging. It provides an indirect measure of tumour activity based on osteoblastic activity by binding to the hydroxyapatite mineral of bone.
- Chest CT and CT or MRI of the abdomen and pelvis can be used for soft tissue imaging of the chest, abdomen and pelvis.
- *Next-generation imaging* using prostate-specific membrane antigen (PSMA) binding radiopharmaceuticals can be used for combined bone and soft tissue imaging. Ga-68 PSMA-11 or F-18 piflufolastat PSMA PET/CT or PET/MRI is encouraged for use in frontline imaging due to increased specificity and sensitivity for low-burden metastasis.

4.4 Treatment Options

4.4.1 Active Surveillance and Observation

Active surveillance is defined as active monitoring of the course of a disease to avoid or delay treatment and its potential side effects. It is useful in patients with seemingly indolent disease and a longer life expectancy. Close monitoring and prompt initiation of treatment at progression is necessary in this group of patients to ensure the chance of cure. Observation on the other hand involves monitoring the course of the disease with history and physical examination and no surveillance biopsies. If the patient on observation develops symptoms, assessment of disease burden followed by initiation of treatment or palliation is to be considered. The goal of observation is to delay non-curative treatment and maintain quality of life in a patient with limited life expectancy where prostate cancer is not likely to be the cause of mortality or significant morbidity.

In intermediate-risk prostate cancer, the role of active surveillance or observation is limited and is to be considered only for carefully selected groups of patients. Active surveillance may be considered for favourable intermediate-risk prostate cancer with a life expectancy of >10 years, particularly in those with a low percentage of Gleason pattern 4, low tumour volume, low PSA density and low genomic risk. NCCN recommendations for active surveillance are summarized below,

- PSA no more often than every 6 months (unless clinically indicated).
- Digital rectal examination (DRE) no more often than every 12 months (unless clinically indicated).
- Repeat biopsy no more often than every 12 months (unless clinically indicated).
- To consider mpMRI no more often than every 12 months (if suspicious lesion on mpMRI, MRI-ultrasound fusion biopsy improves detection of higher grade).
- Patients are to be transitioned into observation once life expectancy is <10 years.

In patients of intermediate-risk prostate cancer with a life expectancy of 5–10 years, observation is preferred. Observation involves PSA and physical examination not more often than every 6 months but will not include surveillance biopsies or radiographic imaging. Studies that evaluated the role of active surveillance/observation in intermediate-risk prostate cancer are summarized below (Table 4.1).

4.4.2 Radical Prostatectomy

Radical prostatectomy is a recommended treatment option for intermediate-risk prostate cancer with expected patient survival of more than 10 years. The recommendation for radical prostatectomy is based on two randomized controlled

Table 4.1 Trials evaluating active surveillance/observation in Intermediate-risk prostate cancer

Trial/ authors	Patients	Treatment	Outcomes	Median follow-up	Remarks
ProtecT (2016, NEJM) [7]	1643 localized prostate cancer patients	Radical prostatectomy vs active monitoring vs RT	No difference in prostate cancer-specific mortality	10 years	Surgery and RT associated with lower rates of disease progression
Klotz et al. (2014, JCO)	993 patients of favourable/ IR	Single arm—Active surveillance	10-year and 15-year cause-specific survival—98.1% and 94.3%	6.4 years	Active surveillance is feasible and safe for favourable risk patients
SPCG-4 (2018, NEJM) [8]	695 localized prostate cancer patients	Radical prostatectomy vs watchful waiting	The relative risk of death is 0.55 with RP	23.6 years	2.9 years of extra life gained through RP
PIVOT (2017, NEJM) [9]	731patients (249 in intermediate risk)	Radical prostatectomy vs observation	All-cause mortality is not significantly different	12.7 years	14.5% (significant) difference in the intermediate-risk group with surgery

trials, the SPCG-4 trial and the PIVOT trial. The long-term follow-up of the SPCG-4 trial reported a cumulative incidence of death from prostate cancer of 19.6% in the radical prostatectomy group and 31.3% in the watchful waiting group in localized prostate cancer [8]. The subgroup analysis of the PIVOT trial favoured radical prostatectomy in intermediate-risk patients compared to observation [9]. Laparoscopic and robot-assisted radical prostatectomy are comparable to open surgery in experienced hands. Nerve-sparing techniques are associated with improved urinary and sexual function. The use of mp MRI to detect extracapsular extension can aid in nerve-sparing surgery. The decision for pelvic LN dissection (PLND) is made with the help of nomograms to predict LN involvement. The NCCN recommends PLND if the probability of nodal metastasis is more than 2%.

There are no published prospective trials comparing radical prostatectomy versus EBRT to date. Indications for adjuvant RT after radical prostatectomy include pT3a disease, positive margins and seminal vesicle involvement.

4.4.3 Radiotherapy

Radiotherapy is recommended for intermediate-risk prostate cancer with a life expectancy of 10 years or higher. The use of radiotherapy in prostate cancer includes external beam radiotherapy (EBRT) and brachytherapy. EBRT techniques include IMRT and SBRT.

4.4.3.1 External Beam Radiotherapy (EBRT)

EBRT for primary prostate cancer has several advantages over radical prostatectomy. The use of EBRT avoids complications associated with surgery, such as the risk of undergoing anaesthesia, bleeding and transfusion reactions. EBRT is associated with a low risk of urinary incontinence and stricture and a good chance of short-term preservation of erectile function.

The recommended dose of radiation is 76–78 Gy in conventional fractionation or an equivalent dose of 60 Gy in 20 fractions with moderate hypofractionation. Ultra hypofractionation with the technique of SBRT is also feasible. Recommended dose fractionation schedules SBRT includes the following—9.5 Gy × 4 fractions, 7.25 Gy–8 Gy × 5 fractions or 6.1 Gy × 7 fractions. Dose escalation is associated with a reduction in biochemical failure and the development of metastases in intermediate-risk prostate cancer patients. Studies that investigated the role of dose escalation in intermediate-risk prostate cancer are summarized below (Table 4.2).

Hypofractionation is favoured in prostate cancer due to the radiobiological advantage of low α/β (the suggested value of α/β in prostate cancer is as low as 1.5 Gy, which is lower than late-reacting tissues). Moderate hypofractionation is the standard of care in prostate cancer. SBRT is well tolerated and effective but lacks long-term survival data. Multiple randomized trials have addressed the role of hypofractionation in prostate cancer which is summarized below (Table 4.3).

Androgen deprivation therapy (ADT) for a short term of 4–6 months should be given with EBRT in patients with intermediate-risk prostate cancer as neoadjuvant/

Table 4.2 Trials Investigating the role of dose escalation in intermediate-risk prostate cancer

Trial/authors	Patients	Arms	ADT	Outcomes	Remarks
RTOG 0126 [10]	1532 (intermediate risk)	70.2 Gy/39# vs 79.2 Gy/44#	None	Improvements in biochemical failure and distant metastases with dose escalation. Did not improve OS	High doses caused more late toxic effects but lower rates of salvage therapy
MRC RT01 [11]	843 (311 intermediate risk)	64 Gy/32# vs 74 Gy/37#	3–6 months	Lower biochemical failure rates in the dose-escalated arm	No benefit in OS at 10 years
Heemsbergen et al. [12]	664 (179 intermediate risk)	68 Gy vs 78 Gy	Allowed (mainly in high-risk)	Lower biochemical and local failure with dose escalation	No difference in OS, a significant benefit in PSA > 10
GETUG 06 [13]	306 (localized prostate cancer)	70 Gy vs 80 Gy	None	Lower biochemical relapse rates in the 80 Gy arm	Slightly higher toxicity (LENT SOMA) in 80 Gy

concomitant/adjuvant therapy. Options for androgen deprivation in intermediate-risk prostate cancer are.

- LHRH (luteinizing hormone-releasing hormone) agonist alone: causes initial stimulation of the production of LH by pituitary, followed by suppression of LH and testosterone to castration levels in 30 days. Options are goserelin, leuprolide and triptorelin.
- LHRH agonist plus first-generation anti-androgen: counteract the effect of adrenal androgen at the target cells by competitive inhibition at the receptor. Together, LHRH agonists and anti-androgens cause powerful androgen blockade. Recommended first-generation anti-androgens are nilutamide, flutamide and bicalutamide.
- LHRH antagonist: blocks the action of LHRH on the pituitary with no initial surge in LH or testosterone levels, e.g. degarelix or relugolix.

Randomized controlled trials addressing the role of ADT in intermediate-risk prostate cancer are summarized in Table 4.4.

4.4.3.2 Brachytherapy

Brachytherapy in prostate cancer involves the interstitial placement of radioactive sources into the prostate tissue. The main advantage of brachytherapy is that the treatment is completed in 1 day and the patient can return to normal

Table 4.3 Trials investigating the role of moderate and ultra hypofractionation in intermediate-risk prostate cancer

Trial/authors	Patients	Arms	ADT	Outcomes	Remarks
Hoffman et al. (JCO, 2018) [14]	206 (147 intermediate risk)	75.6 Gy/42# vs 72 GY/30#	ADT ≤ 4 months in 50 patients	Fewer treatment failures with hypofractionation. No difference in OS	A non-significant increase in late GI toxicity in the hypofractionated arm
HYPRO (2016, *The Lancet Oncology*) [15]	804 (211 intermediate risk)	78 Gy/39# vs 64.6 Gy/19# (3 fractions per week)	537 patients received ADT	Similar biochemical recurrence-free survival	The superiority of the hypofractionated regimen could not be proved
CHHiP (2016, *The Lancet Oncology*) [16]	3216 (73% intermediate risk)	74 Gy/37# vs 60 Gy/20# vs 57 Gy/19#	3–6 months of ADT in most patients	Biochemical recurrence-free survival similar in 74 Gy and 60 Gy arms. 57 Gy is inferior to 74 Gy.	Non-inferiority 60 Gy/20# was proved
PROFIT (2017, JCO) [17]	1206 (intermediate risk)	78 Gy/39# vs 60 Gy/20#	None	Biochemical recurrence-free survival similar between arms	Non-inferiority 60 Gy/20# was proved
HYPO-RT-PC (2019, *The Lancet Oncology*) [18]	1200 (1054 intermediate risk)	42.7 Gy/7# (3 days per week) vs 78 Gy/39#	None	5-year failure-free survival of 84% in both groups	Ultra hypofractionation is non-inferior to conventional fractionation.
PACE-B (2022, *the lancet oncology*) [19]	874	78 Gy/39# (amended to 62 Gy/20#) vs 46.25 Gy/5#	None	Acute toxicities are not increased with SBRT	Data on biochemical recurrence-free survival is yet to mature

Table 4.4 ADT in intermediate-risk prostate cancer

Trial/authors	Patients	Arms	Dose of RT	Outcomes	Remarks
TROG 96.01 (2011, *the lancet oncology*) [20]	818 (130 intermediate risk)	RT alone vs RT + 3-month ADT Vs RT + 6-month ADT	66 Gy/33# in all arms	The addition of 6 months of ADT improved biochemical and local progression, event-free survival, prostate cancer-specific and all-cause mortality	3-month ADT arm had improved biochemical and local progression
D'Amico et al. (2008, JAMA) [21]	206 (PSA >10 ng/mL or GS 7–10; or extracapsular extension; and/or seminal vesicle invasion)	RT alone vs RT + 6-month ADT	—	An increase in all-cause mortality in patients randomized to RT alone	6-month ADT improved survival in patients with unfavourable factors and minimal comorbidities
RTOG 9408 (2011, NEJM & 2022, IJROBP). Secondary analysis in JAMA network open, 2020	1979 (1068 intermediate risk)	RT alone vs RT + 4-month ADT	66.6 Gy/37# in both arms	Short-term ADT resulted in increased OS and decreased disease-specific mortality at 10 years [22]	OS converges at 15 years, estimated additional 6 months of life [23]. A secondary analysis showed benefit only in unfavourable intermediate risk [24]
EORTC 22991 (2016 & 2022, JCO)	819 (613 intermediate risk)	RT alone vs RT + 6-month ADT	70 Gy or 74 Gy or 78 Gy	Improved biochemical and clinical DFS irrespective of dose [25]	On long-term follow-up, EFS and DFS improved with no difference in OS and DMFS [26]
RTOG 9910 (2015, JCO) [27]	1489 (intermediate risk)	RT + 4 months ADT vs RT + 6 months ADT	70.2 Gy/39# 46.8 Gy/26# to pelvic LNs	Extending AS duration did not improve outcomes in intermediate-risk prostate cancer	

activities afterwards. The risk of incontinence is minimal in patients without a previous transurethral resection of the prostate (TURP) and short-term preservation of erectile function is good with brachytherapy. The major disadvantage of brachytherapy is the need for general anaesthesia and associated risks. Higher rates of incontinence in post-TURP patients and progressive worsening of erectile function are also drawbacks of brachytherapy.

Currently, two methods are used for interstitial brachytherapy of the prostate: low dose rate (LDR) and high dose rate (HDR). LDR brachytherapy involves the placement of permanent seed implants in the prostate (dose rate 0.4–2 Gy/h). The radionuclides used for LDR brachytherapy and dose recommendations are summarized below (Table 4.5).

HDR brachytherapy involves the temporary insertion of a radiation source and delivery of radiation at a higher dose rate of >12 Gy/h. It requires remote afterloading of high-activity sources. Iridium 192 is the commonly used HDR source. NCCN recommends an HDR boost of 15 Gy in a single fraction or 10.75 per fraction for two fractions along with EBRT in unfavourable intermediate risk. Monotherapy can be considered in the favourable intermediate-risk group. Studies evaluating the role of brachytherapy in intermediate-risk prostate cancer are summarized below:

- A prospective phase II trial by *Frank et al.* [29] reported efficacy and toxicity outcomes of brachytherapy in patients with intermediate-risk prostate cancer. 300 patients of ≤ stage T2b prostate cancer with GS 6 and PSA 10–15 or GS 7 and PSA <10 were treated with LDR brachytherapy alone. After a median follow-up of 5.1 years, 5-year rates of overall and biochemical progression-free survival were 94.9% and 92.7% respectively.
- The *ASCENDE-RT trial* [30] (Androgen Suppression Combined with Elective Nodal and Dose Escalated Radiation Therapy) included patients with high- and intermediate-risk disease (122 patients out of 398 harboured intermediate risk). Patients were randomized to receive either 78 Gy EBRT or 46 Gy EBRT with an LDR brachytherapy boost of 115 Gy along with ADT. After a median follow-up of 6.5 years, the primary outcome of biochemical progression-free survival favoured the dose-escalated arm.
- *Brachytherapy alone as a treatment: The latest randomized controlled trial, NRG Oncology RTOG 0232* [31], with a median follow-up of 12 years, randomizes patients with intermediate-risk cancer to receive combination treatment of EBRT (45 Gy in 25 fractions over 5 weeks) to prostate and seminal vesicles followed by brachytherapy boost (110 Gy if I-125, 100 Gy

Table 4.5 LDR brachytherapy radionuclide characteristics [28] (NCCN Guidelines version 4.2023)

Radionuclide	Half-life	Average energy	Monotherapy seed strength	Dose (monotherapy)	Dose (boost)
Iodine-125	59.4 days	28.4 keV	0.3–0.6 mCi	145 Gy	110–115 Gy
Palladium-103	17 days	20.7 keV	1.1–2.2 mCi	125 Gy	90–100 Gy
Cesium-131	9.7 days	30.4 keV	2.5–3.9 mCi	115 Gy	85 Gy

if Pd-103) versus brachytherapy alone (145 Gy if I-125, 125 Gy if Pd-103). They showed there was no difference in freedom from progression between both the arms, but Grade 2 and 3 GU/GI toxicities were significantly higher in the combination arm. This points towards offering brachytherapy alone as a curative treatment option for patients with intermediate-risk prostate cancer.

4.5 Radiotherapy Planning

EBRT using conformal techniques like IMRT is recommended in carcinoma of the prostate for optimal target coverage and sparing of OARs. The process of conformal radiotherapy involves simulation, target and OAR delineation and treatment planning and delivery.

- *Simulation*: Planning CT scans are taken in a supine position with both arms resting above the head after immobilizing the patient with a six-clamp pelvic thermoplastic mask or vacuum bag/cushion. The bladder can be comfortably full or follow a bladder protocol before simulation and each treatment, and the rectum should be empty of both faeces and flatus. Contrast-enhanced CTs are useful for the delineation of pelvic nodal volume. A slice thickness of <5 mm is recommended. Scans from lower sacroiliac joints to 1 cm below ischial tuberosities are usually sufficient.
- *Target and OAR delineation*: The CTV includes prostate ± seminal vesicle with differential margins. Nodal irradiation may be considered in unfavourable risk patients with a high chance of pelvic nodal involvement, although the evidence for this is still evolving. The use of T2 weighted MRI can aid in better delineation of the prostate and seminal vesicle. Urinary bladder, rectum, bowel, urethral bulb and bilateral femoral heads are to be contoured as organs at risk.
- *Treatment planning and delivery*: Forward or inverse planning IMRT is preferred for optimal target coverage and OAR sparing. Simulated integrated boost (SIB) technique can aid in dose escalation. Accuracy of treatment delivery should be verified by daily prostate localization using the technique of image-guided radiotherapy (IGRT) using cone beam CT/ ultrasound/ implanted fiducials and electromagnetic tracking. Perirectal spacers implanted between the prostate and rectum are known to reduce rectal dose and toxicities.

4.6 Latest Evidence/Future Perspectives

Genetic testing in patients with intermediate-risk cancer Germline mutations of BRCA, ATM and CHEK-2 have been shown to be associated with higher risk for patients on active surveillance. Tissue-based molecular assays like Oncotype DX, Decipher, and Polaris, are now available that can help in better prognostication and risk stratification and would help to tailor decision-making in this sub-group of patients [32]. Further research and implementation of routine genetic testing would refine treatment options and outcomes.

Particle Beam therapy Ultra-hypofractionated proton beam radiotherapy alone, at a dose of 36.25 GyE in 5 fractions over 10 days, may also be cautiously considered a treatment option [33]. Being a relatively newer concept, longer follow-up data is being eagerly awaited. There has been ongoing interest and research in using carbon ion therapy using doses between 54 and 75 GyE in 20 fractions in prostate cancer, showing promising results and avenues for future research.

4.7 Conclusions

- Management of intermediate-risk prostate cancer is largely a shared decision-making process between the oncologist and the patient and should be individualized after active discussion in detail regarding various treatment options.
- Active surveillance is emerging as a management option in favourable intermediate-risk prostate cancer.
- Major treatment options include radical radiotherapy and radical prostatectomy.
- Moderate hypofractionated RT is the standard of care in carcinoma of the prostate.
- Ultra hypofractionation with the technique of SBRT is an emerging promising treatment option.
- ADT for a short duration of 4–6 months should be added to radical radiotherapy.
- Brachytherapy alone may be a treatment option for those patients with favourable intermediate risk disease who opt for radiotherapy as the treatment modality.
- Further research and implementation of genetic testing may further fine-tune management options.

References

Guidelines: The NCCN Guidelines version 4.2023 prostate cancer.

1. Sung H, Ferlay J, Siegel RL, Laversanne M, Soerjomataram I, Jemal A, et al. Global cancer statistics 2020: GLOBOCAN estimates of incidence and mortality worldwide for 36 cancers in 185 countries. CA Cancer J Clin. 2021;71(3):209–49.
2. Mathur P, Sathishkumar K, Chaturvedi M, Das P, Sudarshan KL, Santhappan S, Nallasamy V, John A, Narasimhan S, Roselind FS, ICMR-NCDIR-NCRP Investigator Group. Cancer statistics, 2020: report from National Cancer Registry Programme, India. JCO Glob Oncol. 2020;6:1063–75.
3. Siegel RL, Miller KD, Wagle NS, Jemal A. Cancer statistics, 2023. CA Cancer J Clin. 2023;73(1):17–48.
4. Buyyounouski MK, Choyke PL, McKenney JK, Sartor O, Sandler HM, Amin MB, Kattan MW, Lin DW. Prostate cancer - major changes in the American Joint Committee on Cancer eighth edition cancer staging manual. CA Cancer J Clin. 2017;67(3):245–53.

5. Epstein JI, Egevad L, Amin MB, Delahunt B, Srigley JR, Humphrey PA, Grading Committee. The 2014 International Society of Urological Pathology (ISUP) Consensus Conference on Gleason Grading of Prostatic Carcinoma: Definition of Grading Patterns and Proposal for a New Grading System. Am J Surg Pathol. 2016;40(2):244.
6. Zumsteg ZS, Spratt DE, Pei I, Zhang Z, Yamada Y, Kollmeier M, et al. A new risk classification system for therapeutic decision making with intermediate-risk prostate cancer patients undergoing dose-escalated external-beam radiation therapy. Eur Urol. 2013;64(6):895–902.
7. Hamdy FC, Donovan JL, Lane JA, Mason M, Metcalfe C, Holding P, et al. 10-year outcomes after monitoring, surgery, or radiotherapy for localized prostate cancer. N Engl J Med. 2016;375(15):1415–24.
8. Bill-Axelson A, Holmberg L, Garmo H, Taari K, Busch C, Nordling S, Häggman M, Andersson SO, Andrén O, Steineck G, Adami HO, Johansson JE. Radical prostatectomy or watchful waiting in prostate cancer - 29-year follow-up. N Engl J Med. 2018;379(24):2319–29.
9. Wilt TJ, Jones KM, Barry MJ, Andriole GL, Culkin D, Wheeler T, et al. Follow-up of prostatectomy versus observation for early prostate cancer. N Engl J Med. 2017;377(2):132–42.
10. Michalski JM, Moughan J, Purdy J, Bosch W, Bruner DW, Bahary JP, et al. Effect of standard vs dose-escalated radiation therapy for patients with intermediate-risk prostate cancer: the NRG oncology RTOG 0126 randomized clinical trial. JAMA Oncol. 2018;4(6):e180039.
11. Dearnaley DP, Jovic G, Syndikus I, Khoo V, Cowan RA, Graham JD, et al. Escalated-dose versus control-dose conformal radiotherapy for prostate cancer: long-term results from the MRC RT01 randomised controlled trial. Lancet Oncol. 2014;15(4):464–73.
12. Heemsbergen WD, Al-Mamgani A, Slot A, Dielwart MFH, Lebesque JV. Long-term results of the Dutch randomized prostate cancer trial: impact of dose-escalation on local, biochemical, clinical failure, and survival. Radiother Oncol. 2014;110(1):104–9.
13. Beckendorf V, Guerif S, Le Prisé E, Cosset JM, Bougnoux A, Chauvet B, et al. 70 Gy versus 80 Gy in localized prostate cancer: 5-year results of GETUG 06 randomized trial. Int J Radiat Oncol. 2011;80(4):1056–63.
14. Hoffman KE, Voong KR, Levy LB, Allen PK, Choi S, Schlembach PJ, Lee AK, McGuire SE, Nguyen Q, Pugh TJ, Frank SJ, Kudchadker RJ, Du W, Kuban DA. Randomized trial of hypofractionated, dose-escalated, intensity-modulated radiation therapy (IMRT) versus conventionally fractionated IMRT for localized prostate cancer. J Clin Oncol. 2018;36(29):2943–9. https://doi.org/10.1200/JCO.2018.77.9868. Epub 2018 Aug 14
15. Incrocci L, Wortel RC, Alemayehu WG, Aluwini S, Schimmel E, Krol S, et al. Hypofractionated versus conventionally fractionated radiotherapy for patients with localised prostate cancer (HYPRO): final efficacy results from a randomised, multicentre, open-label, phase 3 trial. Lancet Oncol. 2016 Aug;17(8):1061–9.
16. Dearnaley D, Syndikus I, Mossop H, Khoo V, Birtle A, Bloomfield D, et al. Conventional versus hypofractionated high-dose intensity-modulated radiotherapy for prostate cancer: 5-year outcomes of the randomised, non-inferiority, phase 3 CHHiP trial. Lancet Oncol. 2016;17(8):1047–60.
17. Catton CN, Lukka H, Gu CS, Martin JM, Supiot S, Chung PWM, et al. Randomized trial of a hypofractionated radiation regimen for the treatment of localized prostate cancer. J Clin Oncol Off J Am Soc Clin Oncol. 2017;35(17):1884–90.
18. Widmark A, Gunnlaugsson A, Beckman L, Thellenberg-Karlsson C, Hoyer M, Lagerlund M, et al. Ultra-hypofractionated versus conventionally fractionated radiotherapy for prostate cancer: 5-year outcomes of the HYPO-RT-PC randomised, non-inferiority, phase 3 trial. Lancet. 2019;394(10196):385–95.
19. Tree AC, Ostler P, van der Voet H, Chu W, Loblaw A, Ford D, et al. Intensity-modulated radiotherapy versus stereotactic body radiotherapy for prostate cancer (PACE-B): 2-year toxicity results from an open-label, randomised, phase 3, non-inferiority trial. Lancet Oncol. 2022;23(10):1308–20.
20. Denham JW, Steigler A, Lamb DS, Joseph D, Turner S, Matthews J, et al. Short-term neoadjuvant androgen deprivation and radiotherapy for locally advanced prostate cancer: 10-year data from the TROG 96.01 randomised trial. Lancet Oncol. 2011;12(5):451–9.

21. D'Amico AV, Chen MH, Renshaw AA, Loffredo M, Kantoff PW. Androgen suppression and radiation vs radiation alone for prostate cancer: a randomized trial. JAMA. 2008;299(3):289–95.
22. Jones CU, Hunt D, McGowan DG, Amin MB, Chetner MP, Bruner DW, et al. Radiotherapy and short-term androgen deprivation for localized prostate cancer. N Engl J Med. 2011;365(2):107–18.
23. Jones CU, Pugh SL, Sandler HM, Chetner MP, Amin MB, Bruner DW, et al. Adding short-term androgen deprivation therapy to radiation therapy in men with localized prostate cancer: long-term update of the NRG/RTOG 9408 randomized clinical trial. Int J Radiat Oncol Biol Phys. 2022;112(2):294–303.
24. Zumsteg ZS, Spratt DE, Daskivich TJ, Tighiouart M, Luu M, Rodgers JP, et al. Effect of androgen deprivation on long-term outcomes of intermediate-risk prostate cancer stratified as favorable or unfavorable: a secondary analysis of the RTOG 9408 randomized clinical trial. JAMA Netw Open. 2020;3(9):e2015083.
25. Bolla M, Neven A, Maingon P, Carrie C, Boladeras A, Andreopoulos D, et al. Short androgen suppression and radiation dose escalation in prostate cancer: 12-year results of EORTC trial 22991 in patients with localized intermediate-risk disease. J Clin Oncol Off J Am Soc Clin Oncol. 2021;39(27):3022–33.
26. Bolla M, Neven A, Maingon P, Carrie C, Boladeras A, Andreopoulos D, et al. Short androgen suppression and radiation dose escalation in prostate cancer: 12-year results of EORTC trial 22991 in patients with localized intermediate-risk disease. J Clin Oncol [Internet]. 2021 [cited 2023 Oct 3]. Available from: https://ascopubs.org/doi/pdf/10.1200/JCO.21.00855?role=tab.
27. Pisansky TM, Hunt D, Gomella LG, Amin MB, Balogh AG, Chinn DM, et al. Duration of androgen suppression before radiotherapy for localized prostate cancer: radiation therapy oncology group randomized clinical trial 9910. J Clin Oncol Off J Am Soc Clin Oncol. 2015;33(4):332–9.
28. Davis BJ, Horwitz EM, Lee WR, Crook JM, Stock RG, Merrick GS, Butler WM, Grimm PD, Stone NN, Potters L, Zietman AL, Zelefsky MJ, American Brachytherapy Society. American brachytherapy society consensus guidelines for transrectal ultrasound-guided permanent prostate brachytherapy. Brachytherapy. 2012;11(1):6–19. https://doi.org/10.1016/j.brachy.2011.07.005.
29. Frank SJ, Pugh TJ, Blanchard P, Mahmood U, Graber WJ, Kudchadker RJ, et al. Prospective phase 2 trial of permanent seed implantation prostate brachytherapy for intermediate-risk localized prostate cancer: efficacy, toxicity, and quality of life outcomes. Int J Radiat Oncol Biol Phys. 2018;100(2):374–82.
30. Morris WJ, Tyldesley S, Rodda S, Halperin R, Pai H, McKenzie M, et al. Androgen suppression combined with elective nodal and dose escalated radiation therapy (the ASCENDE-RT trial): an analysis of survival endpoints for a randomized trial comparing a low-dose-rate brachytherapy boost to a dose-escalated external beam boost for high- and intermediate-risk prostate cancer. Int J Radiat Oncol Biol Phys. 2017;98(2):275–85.
31. Michalski JM, Winter KA, Prestidge BR, Sanda MG, Amin M, Bice WS, et al. Effect of brachytherapy with external beam radiation therapy versus brachytherapy alone for intermediate-risk prostate cancer: NRG oncology RTOG 0232 randomized clinical trial. J Clin Oncol Off J Am Soc Clin Oncol. 2023;41(24):4035–44.
32. Basourakos SP, Tzeng M, Lewicki PJ, Patel K, Hussein Al Awamlh A, B, Venkat S, et al. Tissue-based biomarkers for the risk stratification of men with clinically localized prostate cancer. Front Oncol. 2021;11:676716.
33. Kubeš J, Haas A, Vondráček V, Andrlík M, Navrátil M, Sláviková S, et al. Ultrahypofractionated proton radiation therapy in the treatment of low and intermediate-risk prostate cancer-5-year outcomes. Int J Radiat Oncol Biol Phys. 2021;110(4):1090–7.

Management of High-Risk Prostate Cancer

5

Shikha Goyal and Renu Madan

5.1 Introduction

High-risk prostate cancer implies an aggressive subset of localized prostate cancer that is defined by the presence of one or more adverse characteristics such as advanced clinical T stage, high Gleason's score, or high prostate-specific antigen (PSA) levels. It requires prompt and aggressive treatment and may involve multimodality management for optimal disease control. It poses a significant challenge, with a high risk of recurrence, metastases, and cancer-specific mortality despite advances in diagnostic and treatment strategies.

5.2 Definition and Risk Stratification

The initial widely used risk stratification proposed by D'Amico used three risk groups based on the disease characteristics defined earlier [1]: (a) Low risk: AJCC (1992) stage T1c or T2a, PSA ≤10 ng/mL, and biopsy Gleason's score ≤6 (5-year risk of biochemical failure <25%), (b) Intermediate risk: stage T2b, or PSA >10 but ≤20 ng/mL, or Gleason score 7 (5-year risk of biochemical failure 25–50%), and (c) High risk: stage T2c or above, PSA >20 ng/mL, or Gleason's score >7 (5-year risk of biochemical failure 25–50%).

In 2010, the National Comprehensive Cancer Network (NCCN) risk classification system moved T2c to intermediate-risk category while categorizing erstwhile high-risk patients as high risk of recurrence (T3a) or very high risk of recurrence (T3b or T4) [2].

The latest NCCN classification retains the two high-risk groups but defines them as follows:

S. Goyal (✉) · R. Madan
Department of Radiotherapy and Oncology, Post Graduate Institute of Medical Education and Research (PGIMER), Chandigarh, India

R. Madan, S. Goyal (eds.), *Essentials of Radiotherapy in Uro-Genital Malignancies*, https://doi.org/10.1007/978-981-95-5945-9_5

High risk: one or more high risk features (cT3-T4, Grade group 4 or 5 (Gleason's score 8–10), PSA >20 ng/mL), and
Very high risk: at least two of these features (cT3-4, Grade group 4 or 5, PSA >40 ng/mL).

Bone and soft tissue imaging - either a combination of bone scan and contrast enhanced computed tomography (CECT) of chest and abdomen, a prostate specific membrane antigen positron emission tomography-CECT (PSMA PET-CECT) or PET-magnetic resonance imaging (PET-MRI) is recommended as part of staging evaluation of these patients [3].

These risk categories do not account for the actual volume or burden of disease; patients with involvement of a single core vs. multiple cores would be classified in the same category.

A risk score was developed at UCSF—CAPRA (Cancer of the Prostate Risk Assessment), also including patient age and number of positive biopsy cores in addition to the other three parameters to overcome some of these shortcomings. The score ranges from 0 to 10 a score of 6 or above is deemed high risk; a score of 3–5 is intermediate risk, and that from 0 to 2 is low risk. The score is predictive of post-operative pathologic outcomes and PSA relapse rates but can also be applied to other treatment modalities to determine distant metastases and mortality risk [4, 5]. A CAPRA score of 6 and above predicts a cancer-specific survival probability of 93.4% at 5 years and 79.1% at 10 years. Probability of remaining metastasis-free at 5 years is 90.4% and 83.4% at 10 years.

Another tool that estimates the risk of biochemical or clinical progression post-prostatectomy is a nomogram developed by Stephenson at MSKCC; it incorporates surgical margins, nodal involvement, and year of surgery as well as use of adjuvant radiotherapy, in addition to the routine characteristics for risk stratification [6].

De novo high-risk disease is hormone sensitive by definition and does not mandate estimation of serum testosterone levels.

A reliable risk stratification approach helps determine the optimal treatment modality as well as surveillance strategy for an individual patient.

5.3 Clinical Presentation and Diagnosis

Most prostate cancer detected at localized stage is asymptomatic. Patients may be evaluated after an abnormal PSA test during a routine health check or surveillance in those at higher risk of developing prostate cancer due to family history. Alternatively, patients may undergo physical examination or ultrasounds of the prostate for evaluation of lower urinary tract symptoms attributable to benign prostatic hyperplasia and may be detected to have suspicious nodules on digital rectal examination or abnormal ultrasound findings directing further investigations such as biopsy and MRI. A very small proportion may present with acute urinary retention, constipation, declining renal function due to obstructive uropathy, haematuria, or pelvic pain.

Biopsy is essential for diagnosis and Gleason's scoring, while a multiparametric MRI aids local staging. In high-risk patients, evaluation for regional or distant disease is necessary, and PSMA PET-CECT is now the standard modality for staging. MRI and PET can also help detect more clinically significant cancers by guiding biopsies if performed in patients with high PSA values prior to biopsy. A combination of PET and MRI is deemed more sensitive than either modality alone for detecting extraprostatic extension and seminal vesicle involvement [7]. One-third of high-risk patients may return node-positive on PET, and nearly half of these nodal metastases may be non-regional; nearly one-sixth of patients may harbour bone metastases, thus changing the risk category, stage, and proposed management [8].

5.4 Treatment Options

The various treatment options for high/very high risk prostate cancer may include

Local therapies:

1. External beam radiation therapy (EBRT)
2. Brachytherapy (low dose rate or high dose rate)
3. Radical prostatectomy (open vs. minimally invasive)

Systemic therapies:

1. Androgen deprivation therapy (ADT) including newer agents
2. Chemotherapy

Most of the practiced approaches use a combination of two or more of the above strategies. There is no single preferred approach and may depend on the clinical situation, available expertise, patient preferences based on expected side effect profile, in addition to the available clinical data.

5.4.1 Ratiotherapy (RT) + ADT Combinations

5.4.1.1 RT Alone vs. RT + Long-Term ADT (LTADT)

RTOG 85-31 randomized high-risk (T3), post-prostatectomy (15%, seminal vesicle involved or margin positive), or node-positive (26.9%) patients to RT alone (60–70 Gy @ 1.8–2 Gy/Fr) or RT with lifelong goserelin started during last week of RT. Lifelong goserelin arm had higher overall survival (OS) (49% vs. 39%), cancer-specific survival (CSS) (84% vs. 78%), and lesser distant metastases (DM) (24% vs. 38%). OS gain was maximum in Gleason's 7–10 (39% vs. 25%) [9].

The randomized EORTC study compared 70 Gy EBRT to EBRT plus goserelin for 3 years starting on first day of RT in patients with locally advanced disease (3.5% node positive). Combination arm showed higher 10-year OS (58.1% vs.

39.8%), CSS (89.7% vs. 69.6%), and disease-free survival (DFS) (47.7% vs. 22.7%) but had similar cardiovascular mortality [10].

5.4.1.2 LTADT Alone vs. LTADT + RT

The Scandinavian phase 3 trial, SPCG-7, compared endocrine treatment alone {3 months of combined androgen blockade (CAB) with leuprolide and flutamide followed by continuous flutamide} and same endocrine therapy combined with RT {three dimensional conformal radiotherapy (3DCRT), at least 70 Gy, starting after CAB} in high-risk patients with PSA <70 ng/dl. RT combination arm had significantly lower 10-year PSA recurrence (25.9% vs. 74.7%; $p < 0.0001$), prostate cancer-specific mortality (PCSM) (11.9% vs. 23.9%, RR 0.44) and overall mortality (29.6% vs. 39.4%, RR 0.68), but with slightly higher urinary, rectal, and sexual symptoms [11].

Another intergroup trial compared lifelong ADT with lifelong ADT plus RT (65–69 Gy) in high-risk patients and concluded that the combination arm had better OS and CSS but slightly higher bowel toxicity [12].

5.4.1.3 RT+ Short-Term ADT (STADT) vs. RT + LTADT

RTOG 92-02, a phase 3 study included patients with PSA <150 ng/ml and no extra-pelvic nodes (4.2% were pelvic node-positive) and randomized them into short-term ADT (STADT: 4 months of goserelin and flutamide before and during RT 65–70 Gy) or long-term ADT (STADT + RT 65-70 Gy + 2 years of additional goserelin). Long-term ADT arm had significantly better 10-year CSS (88.7% vs. 83.9%), lower DM (14.8% vs. 22.8%), and lower biochemical recurrence (BCR) (51.9% vs. 68.1%) but similar OS (53.9% vs. 51.6%) overall but better OS in Gleason's 8–10 cohort (45.1% vs. 31.9%) [13].

Another EORTC study compared ADT of 6 months with EBRT (70 Gy) to similar treatment with additional 2.5 years of ADT and found that the shorter ADT duration was inferior in terms of 5-year overall mortality (19% vs. 15.2%, HR 1.45, p=0.65 for noninferiority) and CSS (95.3% vs. 96.8%) without any significant difference in cardiovascular mortality [14].

Even when using contemporary escalated RT dose of 76 Gy, longer ADT (2 years vs. 4 months) allowed better biochemical control and higher metastases-free survival (MFS) and OS in high-risk patients [15].

Attempts to reduce the duration of ADT succeeded following the superiority trial comparing 36 vs. 18 months of ADT (including 4 months of pre-RT CAB) along with EBRT 70 Gy. Longer duration ADT was not superior with 5-year OS of 91% vs. 83% ($p = 0.07$), and quality of life (QOL) scores favouring shorter ADT duration. Both arms had similar DSS despite higher BCR in the 18-month arm (31% vs. 25%). Shorter ADT duration also demonstrated a higher (58% vs. 48%) and quicker (median time 2.1 vs. 4.0 years from end of ADT) testosterone recovery [16].

In elderly men aged 75 years or older, cardiovascular mortality becomes a competing risk; thus, LTADT does not contribute to better OS and should be used judiciously [17]. Use of radiotherapy, however, does not lead to disproportionately higher toxicities compared to younger men and should be considered, especially in patients with a reasonable life expectancy [18].

Adding zoledronate to LTADT (18 months) does not improve survival [19].

5.4.2 ADT Alone

Concerns about the side effects of RT and the delay in response from RT in prostate cancer prompts several patients and practitioners to choose ADT alone in high-risk prostate cancer, especially in elderly and those with limited life expectancy. Orchiectomy has proven similar to a combined orchiectomy and radiotherapy approach and superior to radiotherapy alone in preventing distant metastases and in overall survival in older studies [20]. However, the aforementioned phase 3 data have shown that RT reduces cancer deaths with minimal impact on long-term morbidity when added to long-term ADT and should be considered when not contraindicated.

5.4.3 Surgery

The role of surgery has evolved in prostate-confined high-risk disease (high PSA or Gleason's score) due to increasing experience with complex surgeries, desire to avoid the systemic side effects of ADT when given in combination with RT, and availability of effective salvage options after post-surgery relapses. Modern surgical techniques with nerve sparing can give urinary continence rates exceeding 90% and preserved potency in over 60%. Nearly 50% of patients required salvage therapy (ADT, RT, or combination) [21]. Minimally invasive approaches are deemed equivalent to open prostatectomy [22]. The procedure entails radical prostatectomy (RP) (removal of prostate and seminal vesicles) and extended lymphadenectomy addressing obturator, internal, and external iliac lymph nodes till common iliac bifurcation, although less extensive lymphadenectomy has also been explored with similar oncologic outcomes but better biochemical control in grade group 3–5 patients with extended lymphadenectomy [23].

5.4.4 Surgery vs. Non-surgical Approaches

There are no prospective studies comparing RP with RT (with ADT) in high-risk prostate cancer. Retrospective data give different inferences based on the database studies. A SEER Medicare database reported the best survival outcomes with EBRT plus brachytherapy (+/− ADT), intermediate with RP, and the worst with EBRT plus ADT [24]. Another report from the National Cancer Database reported poorer outcomes with EBRT plus brachytherapy compared to RP [25]. RT has reportedly worse survival than RP as per a meta-analysis across all risk groups; the difference did not change in high-risk group either (HR 1.88 for overall mortality and 1.83 for PCSM) [26]. A recently published systematic review of phase 2 or 3 studies comparing EBRT with RP reported similar overall survival, cancer-specific survival, and distant metastases rates with both approaches. However, side effect profile was different, with higher urinary incontinence and sexual dysfunction in RP patients and higher bowel symptoms in EBRT patients. However, this review included data mostly for low or intermediate risk patients [27]. A recent report comparing data from two randomized trials (CALGB-90203, NRG/RTOG-0521) suggests a higher risk of DM (23% vs. 16%) at 8 years after RP than after EBRT with LTADT; this difference disappears when EBRT is compared to RP patients who have received neoadjuvant chemohormonal therapy [28]. SPCG-15 is a randomized trial evaluating these two approaches and may solve the dilemma in future.

5.4.5 Novel Systemic Therapy Approaches

Systemic therapy agents such as chemotherapy (docetaxel) and androgen receptor pathway inhibitors (abiraterone, enzalutamide, apalutamide, darolutamide) have shown excellent control in advanced/metastatic disease and possibly may improve DM rates in high-risk prostate cancer as well when added to traditional approaches. Docetaxel as adjuvant therapy (6 cycles, after completion of RT) in high-risk disease was evaluated in RTOG 05-21; docetaxel improved 4-year OS by 4% while significantly adding to 6-year DFS and MFS, albeit at the cost of significantly higher hematologic toxicity (44.3% vs. 1.8% ≥grade 3) [29]. Survival gain was also observed with docetaxel in STAMPEDE trial [30]. Docetaxel was also evaluated in GETUG-12, with better relapse-free survival (RFS), but no benefit in DM or CSS even on long-term follow-up [31]. On the other hand, a French study did not find even biochemical control improvement with docetaxel [32].

Abiraterone for 2 years has also demonstrated failure-free survival (FFS) benefit in patients with high-risk disease in STAMPEDE [33].

Other agents including immunotherapy are also being investigated. However, the choice of adding these treatments should be personalized based on individual patient characteristics.

5.4.6 Advances in Radiotherapy

5.4.6.1 RT Techniques

Prostate RT to high doses is limited by rectal tolerance. Even for conventionally fractionated dose of 64 Gy, 3DCRT leads to significantly lower proctitis and rectal bleeding rates without changing tumor control [34]. Improving conformality with intensity modulation (IMRT) has led to further reduction in both acute and late gastrointestinal toxicity irrespective of treatment volume—prostate only or prostate with pelvic nodes [35]. Use of daily image guidance (IGRT) enables reduction in margins for prostate motion and positional changes due to bladder or rectal filling; this reduces the volume of rectum and bladder exposed to higher doses and enables delivery of higher RT doses to prostate [36]. In the older machines, fiducial markers implanted in prostate helped image matching prior to RT with orthogonal images, while currently, cone-beam CT helps 3D visualization of prostate and surrounding structures to monitor positional shifts and volume change. Several modalities of online image guidance using ultrasound, infrared, electromagnetic transducers, X-rays, or MRI are available; some measure interfractional motion, while others can monitor and correct for intrafraction motion as well. In addition to image guidance, a stringent protocol for rectal and bladder preparation ensures accurate treatment delivery and has resulted in better biochemical and local control rates [37, 38].

5.4.6.2 RT Dose Escalation

Attempts at dose escalation (78 vs. 70 Gy) using 3DCRT but without ADT at MD Anderson showed benefit in 8-year FFS (63% vs. 26%) and freedom from DM (96% vs. 83%) in high-risk patients with PSA >10 ng/ml but at the cost of higher 10-year rectal toxicity (7% vs. 1% grade 3) [39]. The GETUG-06 trial also evaluated dose escalation from 70 to 80 Gy without ADT and showed a reduction in 5-year BCR from 32% to 23.5%; the difference was higher with PSA >15 ng/dl. Dose escalation led to higher grade 2 or more acute and delayed urinary toxicity, while rectal toxicity rates were not different, nor was QOL [40].

However, incorporation of highly conformal RT modalities such as proton therapy has enabled dose escalation to doses of 79.2 Gy vs. 70.2 Gy (50.4 Gy using 3DCRT, subsequent boost with proton therapy) without ADT and led to higher 5-year freedom from BCR (83.3% vs. 67.6%) with minimal acute and late grade 3 morbidity of ≤2%; however, the dose escalation did not yield any OS benefit [41]. The Dutch trial and MRC trials using dose escalation with conformal techniques showed similar improvements in biochemical and local control despite allowing ADT in high-risk patients [42, 43].

Retrospective multi-institutional data demonstrate that both EBRT with IMRT (dose 74–80 Gy) and high-dose-rate brachytherapy boost are good options to improve biochemical and local control with similar toxicities [44].

When comparing RT doses of 68–74 Gy and ADT duration of 6–18 months, local failure rates decline progressively with higher RT doses and ADT duration, but at a higher risk of urethral strictures [45]. Dose escalation to even higher doses up to 95 Gy to intraprostatic lesions has become feasible with modern techniques and shows promise in improving both local and distant control despite use of ADT for 1 year and comparator RT arm with dose of 77 Gy in 35 fractions [46]. Another recent trial that used a comparator arm of 78 Gy along with ADT and evaluated low-dose-rate brachytherapy boost demonstrated reduced BCR for both intermediate- and high-risk categories, again at the cost of higher acute and late grade 3 GU toxicity [47, 48].

A meta-analysis of seven trials demonstrated the benefit of dose escalation in all risk categories and established a dose-response relationship; each Gy of additional RT dose reduces biochemical failures by 1.8%, leading to a 19% improvement with a 10-Gy higher dose (70–80 Gy) [49].

Dose escalation uniformly reduces biochemical failures independent of ADT and possibly DM at the cost of higher toxicity, thereby reducing need of salvage therapy. However, there is no OS gain; therefore, it should be considered with caution in patients who are elderly or have significant comorbid conditions, especially when involving bladder (benign prostatic hyperplasia with significant symptoms, previous TUR channelling, urethral stricture) or rectum (haemorrhoids), and when image guidance is not available.

5.4.6.3 RT Volume

Several trials of conventional and conformal radiotherapy era have used cone-down boost to prostate after an initial dose of 46–60 Gy to pelvis (including pelvic nodes and prostate with seminal vesicles). However, other institutions continued to treat prostate alone with high doses, especially when ADT was being used. Two randomized trials addressed the issue of appropriate target volume. The GETUG-01 study compared prostate-alone RT (66–70 Gy) with prostate plus pelvic nodal RT (66–70 Gy to prostate, 46 Gy to pelvic nodes) [50]. RTOG 94-13 trial compared prostate-only RT (70.2 Gy) with prostate plus pelvic-nodal RT (70.2 Gy to prostate, 50.4 Gy to pelvic nodes) [51]. The latter study also compared neoadjuvant or adjuvant ADT approaches in a 2 × 2 factorial manner. Both studies failed to show any advantage with pelvic RT in terms of biochemical control or event-free survival. Both these trials have been criticized for several reasons including patient selection, technique/volume and dose of RT, and shorter ADT duration. The POP-RT trial corrected several of these shortcomings and used a moderate hypofractionation approach with image guidance, PSMA PET-CT-based staging and a 2-year ADT duration for high-risk patients with contemporary doses and volumes, comparing prostate-only vs. additional pelvic nodal RT (68 Gy in 25 fractions to prostate, 45 Gy in 25 fractions to pelvic nodes). This study was able to demonstrate a superior BCR-free survival and DFS in the pelvic nodal RT arm compared to prostate-only RT arm, but both arms had similar OS, late toxicity, and QOL [52, 53].

5.4.6.4 RT Fractionation

Traditionally, EBRT approach for prostate cancer has used conventional fractionation (CF) (1.8–2 Gy per fraction for total doses of 64–80 Gy), with dose escalation being enabled by several technological improvements. Radiobiologically, prostate cancer responds better to a higher dose per fraction, and thus hypofractionation (HF) approaches became popular. Both moderate and extreme HF approaches have been utilized in high-risk disease as well.

HYPRO trial compared CF (78 Gy in 39 fractions) with moderate HF (64.6 Gy in 19 fractions) for intermediate- to high-risk patients with concurrent ADT given for median 32 months. Seven-year RFS was 67.6% vs. 71.7%, and the difference was statistically non-significant. There was no OS difference [54].

Hypo-RT-PC included both intermediate- and high-risk patients and compared CF (78 Gy in 39 fractions) to ultra-HF (42·7 Gy in 7 fractions, 3 fractions per week) and established non-inferiority of latter regime in terms of FFS (84% at 5 years in both, HR 1.002) with increased 1-year urinary toxicity [55].

In both these trials, RT clinical target volume (CTV) was confined to prostate +/− seminal vesicles but excluded pelvic nodes. Planning target volume (PTV) margins for setup error and internal motion (3–10 mm), especially towards rectum (0–5 mm), were smaller compared to historic approaches.

After POP-RT demonstrated improved locoregional control with addition of pelvic nodal RT and ultra-HF demonstrated acceptable biochemical control and toxicity in a single-arm study of high/very high risk and node-positive patients, the same investigators are evaluating this strategy in a phase 3 study for high-risk and node-positive patients—the standard arm has POP-RT fractionation (68 Gy in 25 fractions), while the investigational arm uses 36.25 Gy in 5 fractions (nodal volume received 25 Gy with additional boost for positive nodes) given on alternate days. The primary endpoint is 4-year biochemical FFS [56, 57].

5.4.6.5 Treatment Protocol at Our Institute

We use a moderately HF approach adapted from CHHIP trial for patients with high−/very high-risk disease. Patients are simulated after a standard bowel and bladder protocol in supine position, with 3 mm CT slice thickness. Nodal CTV is delineated according to NRG Oncology guidelines, with cranial limit till aortic bifurcation, including common iliac group of nodes [58]. Prostate and seminal vesicles (SV) are delineated with the aid of co-registered T2-weighted MRI sequences. There are typically four PTVs: PTV 44 Gy (nodal CTV plus 5 mm margin), PTV 48 Gy (CTV prostate + SV with 1 cm margin), PTV 57.6 Gy {CTV prostate + SV (if involved) with 1 cm margin except 5 mm posteriorly} and PTV 60 Gy {CTV prostate + SV (if involved) with 5 mm margin except 1 mm posteriorly}. Dose prescription is given in 20 fractions, and 95% of each volume is prescribed to receive the prescribed dose. Organs at risk include rectum, bladder, both femur heads, penile bulb, and bowel, and appropriate dose constraints are given as per QUANTEC recommendations. Once approved, treatment is carried out with daily image guidance for five fractions per week (Figs. 5.1 and 5.2).

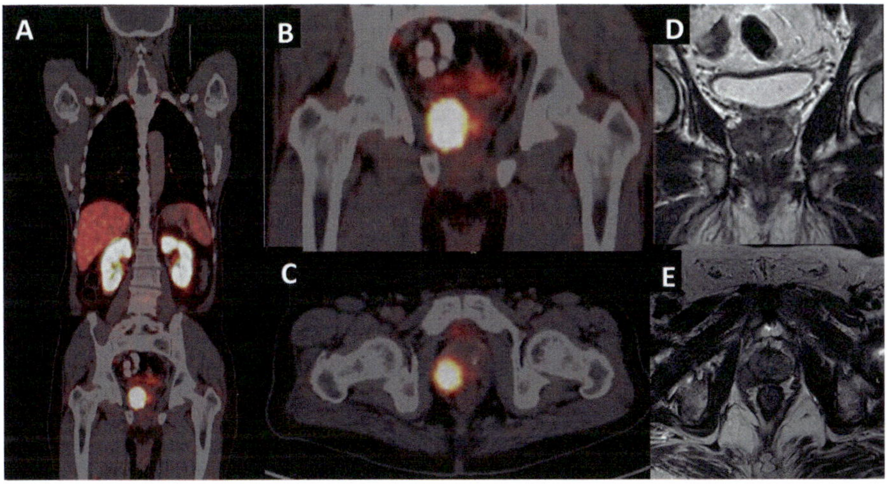

Fig. 5.1 (**a**) PSMA PET-CT whole-body images for a carcinoma prostate patient. (**b**, **c**) PSMA-avid right peripheral zone lesion is seen with extracapsular extension abutting right levator ani muscle and invasion of right seminal vesicle in coronal and axial views, respectively. (**d**, **e**) Corresponding T2w MRI images in coronal and axial orientation demonstrating the same lesion as a T2 hypointense nodule

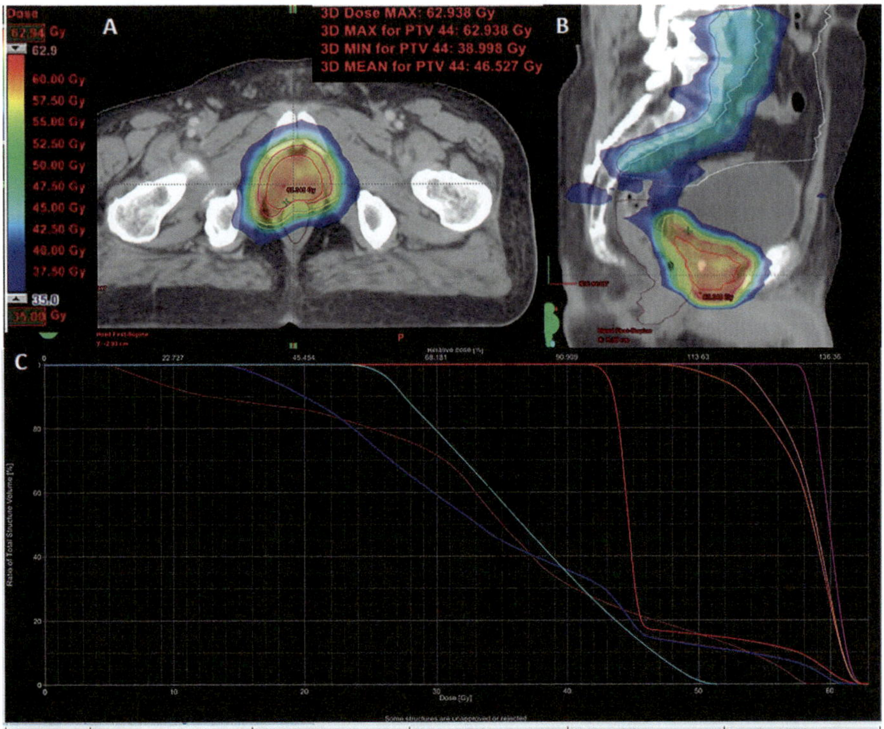

DVH Line	Structure	Volume [cm³]	Min Dose [Gy]	Max Dose [Gy]	Mean Dose [Gy]
	RECTUM	55.0	4.685	59.301	34.726
	PTV 60	90.0	56.669	62.938	59.873
	PTV 57.6	161.3	50.442	62.938	58.469
	PTV 48	176.4	44.162	62.938	57.840
	PTV 44	1156.6	38.998	62.938	46.527
	PENILE BULB	0.8	23.186	51.408	36.792
	BLADDER	272.9	13.433	62.155	34.880

Fig. 5.2 (**a**) Axial and (**b**) sagittal dose colour wash of the same patient as in Fig. 5.1, showing the dose distribution with relative sparing of organs at risk. (**c**) Dose volume histogram for the same plan

5.5 Personalization Through Genomics

A tumour RNA expression profile resulting in a cell cycle progression score is combined with CAPRA score in the Prolaris assay that is superior to clinicopathologic factors and CAPRA score alone in determining prognosis including risk of metastases in intermediate- and high-risk disease [59]. Decipher genomic classifier may also predict DM and survival in post-prostatectomy or biopsy specimens [60]. NRG-GU009 is a phase 3 trial evaluating modification of concurrent therapy with radical RT based on Decipher score—patients with lower scores are offered 12 instead of 24 months of ADT, while those with higher scores receive apalutamide in addition to 24 months of ADT.

5.6 Conclusions

High-risk prostate cancer poses a formidable challenge, but in the present era, diagnosis, staging, and treatment modalities have enabled better BCR-free rates as well as OS gains. Choice among several therapeutic options is based on several parameters and should involve a multidisciplinary consultation involving the patient, but the strongest factor is the expected post-therapy morbidity. Genomics may help personalize therapy in future, allowing for treatment intensification in those at most risk and de-intensification in those at least risk of progression.

References

1. D'Amico AV, Whittington R, Malkowicz SB, et al. Biochemical outcome after radical prostatectomy, external beam radiation therapy, or interstitial radiation therapy for clinically localized prostate cancer. JAMA. 1998;280(11):969–74.
2. Mohler J, Bahnson RR, Boston B, et al. NCCN clinical practice guidelines in oncology: prostate cancer. J Natl Compr Cancer Netw. 2010;8(2):162–200.
3. NCCN clinical practice guidelines in oncology—Prostate cancer version 1.2025—December 4, 2024. https://www.nccn.org/professionals/physician_gls/pdf/prostate.pdf.
4. Cooperberg MR, Pasta DJ, Elkin EP, et al. The University of California, san Francisco cancer of the prostate risk assessment score: a straightforward and reliable preoperative predictor of disease recurrence after radical prostatectomy [published correction appears in J Urol. 2006 Jun;175(6):2369]. J Urol. 2005;173(6):1938–42.
5. Cooperberg MR, Broering JM, Carroll PR. Risk assessment for prostate cancer metastasis and mortality at the time of diagnosis. J Natl Cancer Inst. 2009;101(12):878–87.
6. Stephenson AJ, Scardino PT, Eastham JA, et al. Postoperative nomogram predicting the 10-year probability of prostate cancer recurrence after radical prostatectomy. J Clin Oncol. 2005;23(28):7005–12.
7. Jochumsen MR, Bouchelouche K. PSMA PET/CT for primary staging of prostate cancer - an updated overview. Semin Nucl Med. 2024;54(1):39–45.
8. Klingenberg S, Jochumsen MR, Ulhøi BP, et al. ^{68}Ga-PSMA PET/CT for primary lymph node and distant metastasis NM staging of high-risk prostate cancer. J Nucl Med. 2021;62(2):214–20.
9. Pilepich MV, Winter K, Lawton CA, et al. Androgen suppression adjuvant to definitive radiotherapy in prostate carcinoma--long-term results of phase III RTOG 85–31. Int J Radiat Oncol Biol Phys. 2005;61(5):1285–90.
10. Bolla M, Van Tienhoven G, Warde P, et al. External irradiation with or without long-term androgen suppression for prostate cancer with high metastatic risk: 10-year results of an EORTC randomised study. Lancet Oncol. 2010;11(11):1066–73.
11. Widmark A, Klepp O, Solberg A, et al. Endocrine treatment, with or without radiotherapy, in locally advanced prostate cancer (SPCG-7/SFUO-3): an open randomised phase III trial [published correction appears in Lancet. 2009;373(9670):1174]. Lancet 2009;373(9660):301–08.
12. Mason MD, Parulekar WR, Sydes MR, et al. Final report of the intergroup randomized study of combined androgen-deprivation therapy plus radiotherapy versus androgen-deprivation therapy alone in locally advanced prostate cancer. J Clin Oncol. 2015;33(19):2143–50.
13. Horwitz EM, Bae K, Hanks GE, et al. Ten-year follow-up of radiation therapy oncology group protocol 92-02: a phase III trial of the duration of elective androgen deprivation in locally advanced prostate cancer. J Clin Oncol. 2008;26(15):2497–504.
14. Bolla M, de Reijke TM, Van Tienhoven G, et al. Duration of androgen suppression in the treatment of prostate cancer. N Engl J Med. 2009;360(24):2516–27.

15. Zapatero A, Guerrero A, Maldonado X, et al. High-dose radiotherapy with short-term or long-term androgen deprivation in localised prostate cancer (DART01/05 GICOR): a randomised, controlled, phase 3 trial [published correction appears in Lancet Oncol. 2015 Jun;16(6):e262].
16. Nabid A, Carrier N, Martin AG, et al. Duration of androgen deprivation therapy in high-risk prostate cancer: a randomized phase III trial. Eur Urol. 2018;74(4):432–41.
17. Yamazaki H, Masui K, Suzuki G, et al. Effect of androgen deprivation therapy on other-cause of mortality in elderly patients with clinically localized prostate cancer treated with modern radiotherapy: is there a negative impact? J Clin Med. 2019;8(3):338.
18. Payne HA, Hughes S. Radical radiotherapy for high-risk prostate cancer in older men. Oncologist. 2012;17(Suppl 1):9–15.
19. Denham JW, Joseph D, Lamb DS, et al. Short-term androgen suppression and radiotherapy versus intermediate-term androgen suppression and radiotherapy, with or without zoledronic acid, in men with locally advanced prostate cancer (TROG 03.04 RADAR): 10-year results from a randomised, phase 3, factorial trial. Lancet Oncol. 2019;20(2):267–81.
20. Fellows GJ, Clark PB, Beynon LL, et al. Treatment of advanced localized prostatic cancer by orchiectomy, radiotherapy, or combined treatment. A Medical Research Council Study. Urological Cancer Working Party--Subgroup on Prostatic Cancer. Br J Urol. 1992;70(3):304–9.
21. Loeb S, Smith ND, Roehl KA, Catalona WJ. Intermediate-term potency, continence, and survival outcomes of radical prostatectomy for clinically high-risk or locally advanced prostate cancer. Urology. 2007;69(6):1170–5.
22. Harty NJ, Kozinn SI, Canes D, Sorcini A, Moinzadeh A. Comparison of positive surgical margin rates in high risk prostate cancer: open versus minimally invasive radical prostatectomy. Int Braz J Urol. 2013;39(5):639–46. discussion 647-8.
23. Lestingi JFP, Guglielmetti GB, Trinh QD, et al. Extended versus limited pelvic lymph node dissection during radical prostatectomy for intermediate- and high-risk prostate cancer: early oncological outcomes from a randomized phase 3 trial. Eur Urol. 2021;79(5):595–604.
24. Jayadevappa R, Lee DI, Chhatre S, Guzzo TJ, Malkowicz SB. Comparative effectiveness of treatments for high-risk prostate cancer patients. Urol Oncol. 2019;37(9):574.e11–8.
25. Berg S, Cole AP, Krimphove MJ, et al. Comparative effectiveness of radical prostatectomy versus external beam radiation therapy plus brachytherapy in patients with high-risk localized prostate cancer. Eur Urol. 2019;75(4):552–5.
26. Wallis CJD, Saskin R, Choo R, Herschorn S, Kodama RT, Satkunasivam R, Shah PS, Danjoux C, Nam RK. Surgery versus radiotherapy for clinically-localized prostate cancer: a systematic review and meta-analysis. Eur Urol. 2016;70(1):21–30.
27. Hekman L, Barrett A, Ross D, et al. A systematic review of clinical trials comparing radiation therapy versus radical prostatectomy in prostate cancer. Clin Genitourin Cancer. 2024;22(5):102157.
28. ASCO GU Symposium 2025, available online at https://s3.amazonaws.com/files.oncology-meetings.org/prod/s3fs-public/2025-02/GU25-Prostate-Cancer-Localized.pdf.
29. Rosenthal SA, Hu C, Sartor O, et al. Effect of chemotherapy with docetaxel with androgen suppression and radiotherapy for localized high-risk prostate cancer: the randomized phase III NRG oncology RTOG 0521 trial [published correction appears in J Clin Oncol. 2021;39(17):1949].
30. James ND, Sydes MR, Clarke NW, et al. Addition of docetaxel, zoledronic acid, or both to first-line long-term hormone therapy in prostate cancer (STAMPEDE): survival results from an adaptive, multiarm, multistage, platform randomised controlled trial. Lancet. 2016;387(10024):1163–77.
31. Fizazi K, Faivre L, Lesaunier F, et al. Androgen deprivation therapy plus docetaxel and estramustine versus androgen deprivation therapy alone for high-risk localised prostate cancer (GETUG 12): a phase 3 randomised controlled trial. Lancet Oncol. 2015;16(7):787–94.
32. Oudard S, Latorzeff I, Caty A, et al. Effect of adding docetaxel to androgen-deprivation therapy in patients with high-risk prostate cancer with rising prostate-specific antigen levels after primary local therapy: a randomized clinical trial. JAMA Oncol. 2019;5(5):623–32.

33. James ND, de Bono JS, Spears MR, et al. Abiraterone for prostate cancer not previously treated with hormone therapy. N Engl J Med. 2017;377(4):338–51.
34. Dearnaley DP, Khoo VS, Norman AR, et al. Comparison of radiation side-effects of conformal and conventional radiotherapy in prostate cancer: a randomised trial. Lancet. 1999;353(9149):267–72.
35. Sharma NK, Li T, Chen DY, Pollack A, Horwitz EM, Buyyounouski MK. Intensity-modulated radiotherapy reduces gastrointestinal toxicity in patients treated with androgen deprivation therapy for prostate cancer. Int J Radiat Oncol Biol Phys. 2011;80(2):437–44.
36. Zelefsky MJ, Kollmeier M, Cox B, et al. Improved clinical outcomes with high-dose image guided radiotherapy compared with non-IGRT for the treatment of clinically localized prostate cancer. Int J Radiat Oncol Biol Phys. 2012;84(1):125–9.
37. Guckenberger M, Pohl F, Baier K, Meyer J, Vordermark D, Flentje M. Adverse effect of a distended rectum in intensity-modulated radiotherapy (IMRT) treatment planning of prostate cancer. Radiother Oncol. 2006;79(1):59–64.
38. Maggio A, Gabriele D, Garibaldi E, et al. Impact of a rectal and bladder preparation protocol on prostate cancer outcome in patients treated with external beam radiotherapy. Auswirkungen des Rektum-Blasen-Vorbereitungsprotokolls auf die Ergebnisse einer externen Strahlentherapie bei Patienten mit Prostatakarzinom. Strahlenther Onkol. 2017;193(9):722–32.
39. Kuban DA, Tucker SL, Dong L, et al. Long-term results of the M. D. Anderson randomized dose-escalation trial for prostate cancer. Int J Radiat Oncol Biol Phys. 2008;70(1):67–74.
40. Beckendorf V, Guerif S, Le Prisé E, et al. 70 Gy versus 80 Gy in localized prostate cancer: 5-year results of GETUG 06 randomized trial. Int J Radiat Oncol Biol Phys. 2011;80(4):1056–63.
41. Zietman AL, Bae K, Slater JD, Shipley WU, et al. Randomized trial comparing conventional-dose with high-dose conformal radiation therapy in early-stage adenocarcinoma of the prostate: long-term results from proton radiation oncology group/american college of radiology 95-09. J Clin Oncol. 2010;28(7):1106–11.
42. Heemsbergen WD, Al-Mamgani A, Slot A, Dielwart MF, Lebesque JV. Long-term results of the Dutch randomized prostate cancer trial: impact of dose-escalation on local, biochemical, clinical failure, and survival. Radiother Oncol. 2014;110(1):104–9.
43. Dearnaley DP, Jovic G, Syndikus I, et al. Escalated-dose versus control-dose conformal radiotherapy for prostate cancer: long-term results from the MRC RT01 randomised controlled trial. Lancet Oncol. 2014;15(4):464–73.
44. Yamazaki H, Suzuki G, Masui K, et al. Radiotherapy for clinically localized T3b or T4 very-high-risk prostate cancer-role of dose escalation using high-dose-rate brachytherapy boost or high dose intensity modulated radiotherapy. Cancers (Basel). 2021;13(8):1856.
45. Denham JW, Steigler A, Joseph D, et al. Radiation dose escalation or longer androgen suppression for locally advanced prostate cancer? Data from the TROG 03.04 RADAR trial. Radiother Oncol. 2015;115(3):301–7.
46. Groen VH, Haustermans K, Pos FJ, et al. Patterns of failure following external beam radiotherapy with or without an additional focal boost in the randomized controlled FLAME trial for localized prostate cancer. Eur Urol. 2022;82(3):252–7.
47. Morris WJ, Tyldesley S, Rodda S, et al. Androgen suppression combined with elective nodal and dose escalated radiation therapy (the ASCENDE-RT trial): an analysis of survival endpoints for a randomized trial comparing a low-dose-rate brachytherapy boost to a dose-escalated external beam boost for high- and intermediate-risk prostate cancer. Int J Radiat Oncol Biol Phys. 2017;98(2):275–85.
48. Rodda S, Tyldesley S, Morris WJ, et al. ASCENDE-RT: an analysis of treatment-related morbidity for a randomized trial comparing a low-dose-rate brachytherapy boost with a dose-escalated external beam boost for high- and intermediate-risk prostate cancer. Int J Radiat Oncol Biol Phys. 2017;98(2):286–95.
49. Viani GA, Stefano EJ, Afonso SL. Higher-than-conventional radiation doses in localized prostate cancer treatment: a meta-analysis of randomized, controlled trials. Int J Radiat Oncol Biol Phys. 2009;74(5):1405–18.

50. Roach M, Moughan J, Lawton CAF, et al. Sequence of hormonal therapy and radiotherapy field size in unfavourable, localised prostate cancer (NRG/RTOG 9413): long-term results of a randomised, phase 3 trial. Lancet Oncol. 2018;19(11):1504–15.
51. Pommier P, Chabaud S, Lagrange JL, et al. Is there a role for pelvic irradiation in localized prostate adenocarcinoma? Update of the long-term survival results of the GETUG-01 randomized study. Int J Radiat Oncol Biol Phys. 2016;96(4):759–69.
52. Murthy V, Maitre P, Kannan S, et al. Prostate-only versus whole-pelvic radiation therapy in high-risk and very high-risk prostate cancer (POP-RT): outcomes from phase III randomized controlled trial. J Clin Oncol. 2021;39(11):1234–42.
53. Maitre P, Maheshwari G, Sarkar J, et al. Late urinary toxicity and quality of life with pelvic radiation therapy for high-risk prostate cancer: dose-effect relations in the POP-RT randomized phase 3 trial. Int J Radiat Oncol Biol Phys. 2024;120(2):537–43.
54. de Vries KC, Wortel RC, Oomen-de Hoop E, Heemsbergen WD, Pos FJ, Incrocci L. Hyprofractionated versus conventionally fractionated radiation therapy for patients with intermediate- or high-risk, localized, prostate cancer: 7-year outcomes from the randomized, multicenter, open-label, phase 3 HYPRO trial. Int J Radiat Oncol Biol Phys. 2020;106(1):108–15.
55. Widmark A, Gunnlaugsson A, Beckman L, et al. Ultra-hypofractionated versus conventionally fractionated radiotherapy for prostate cancer: 5-year outcomes of the HYPO-RT-PC randomised, non-inferiority, phase 3 trial. Lancet. 2019;394(10196):385–95.
56. Murthy V, Gupta M, Mulye G, et al. Early results of extreme hypofractionation using stereotactic body radiation therapy for high-risk, very high-risk and node-positive prostate cancer. Clin Oncol (R Coll Radiol). 2018;30(7):442–7.
57. Murthy V, Mallick I, Gavarraju A, et al. Study protocol of a randomised controlled trial of prostate radiotherapy in high-risk and node-positive disease comparing moderate and extreme hypofractionation (PRIME TRIAL). BMJ Open. 2020;10(2):e034623.
58. Hall WA, Paulson E, Davis BJ, et al. NRG oncology updated international consensus atlas on pelvic lymph node volumes for intact and postoperative prostate cancer. Int J Radiat Oncol Biol Phys. 2021;109(1):174–85.
59. Tward JD, Schlomm T, Bardot S, et al. Personalizing localized prostate cancer: validation of a combined clinical cell-cycle risk (CCR) score threshold for prognosticating benefit from multimodality therapy. Clin Genitourin Cancer. 2021;19(4):296–304.e3.
60. Jairath NK, Dal Pra A, Vince R Jr, et al. A systematic review of the evidence for the decipher genomic classifier in prostate cancer. Eur Urol. 2021;79(3):374–83.

Metastatic Prostate Cancer: Hormone Sensitive

6

Sweety Gupta, R. Lekshmi, and Deepak Sundriyal

6.1 Introduction

According to the GLOBOCAN 2022 data, prostate cancer ranks fourth in incidence and eighth in mortality worldwide, and in India, it ranks twelfth in incidence and fourteenth in mortality [1]. As most of the patients present in advanced stages in India, the exact incidence of metastatic disease is uncertain, while only 6% is present as metastatic disease in the West [2, 3]. Across various stages of prostate cancer, some patients exhibit metastases visible on traditional imaging methods such as X-rays or bone scans. In contrast, others may require advanced modalities of imaging, like computed tomography (CT) and magnetic resonance imaging (MRI) scans. Some men with advanced prostate cancer show signs of metastatic disease initially, while others develop it after receiving treatment for localized disease [4]. The majority of males in both groups do not receive long-term androgen deprivation therapy (ADT), and serum testosterone levels are usually above 50 ng/dL [4]. These males are considered to have castration-sensitive (also known as noncastrate) prostate cancer (CSPC).

Although there have been significant advancements in the systemic treatment of advanced prostate cancer, metastatic prostate cancer is still an incurable disease. The overall survival rate at 5 years for patients initially diagnosed with metastatic hormone-sensitive prostate cancer (mHSPC) is 30% [5]. The prognosis is typically better for people with low-volume disease than those with high-volume disease. In comparison to individuals with de novo synchronous metastatic disease, the

S. Gupta (✉) · R. Lekshmi
Department of Radiation Oncology, AIIMS Rishikesh, Rishikesh, Uttarakhand, India
e-mail: sweety.rt@aiimsrishikesh.edu.in

D. Sundriyal
Department of Medical Oncology, AIIMS Rishikesh, Rishikesh, Uttarakhand, India
e-mail: deepak.monc@aiimsrishikesh.edu.in

R. Madan, S. Goyal (eds.), *Essentials of Radiotherapy in Uro-Genital Malignancies*, https://doi.org/10.1007/978-981-95-5945-9_6

prognosis is better for patients with metachronous metastatic disease, which is defined as patients with metastatic relapse following definitive local treatment [6].

Though there is an initial high response rate, many patients ultimately develop metastatic castration-resistant prostate cancer (mCRPC). Some evidence indicates that delaying progression might be possible when testosterone levels in the serum are at or below 20 ng/dL [7]. However, even when using androgen deprivation therapy (ADT) exclusively, progression usually happens within a year [7]. Factors such as the disease's extent, the involvement of visceral organs, the timing of metastatic presentation (either de novo/synchronous or recurrent/metachronous), and patient and tumor characteristics (like germline or somatic genetic alterations, presence of androgen-insensitive clones, and small cell or neuroendocrine differentiation) can influence the risk of progression [8]. The primary objective of mHSPC therapy is to extend the patient's life span through sustained tumor control by targeting the key agents of tumor growth, notably the androgen receptor (AR) pathway, cell reproduction, and possibly other mechanisms of tumor growth that are currently targeted in mCRPC in the future. Therapies focusing on the AR pathway encompass androgen deprivation therapy (ADT) and AR pathway inhibitors (ARPIs). ADT is linked with a decrease in the volume of androgen that can bind to the AR, resulting in a reduction of AR-triggered cell signaling and an increase in cell cycle arrest and apoptosis. ARPIs function either by restricting androgen synthesis (as seen in abiraterone acetate) or by competitively binding to the AR (as exhibited by apalutamide, darolutamide, and enzalutamide), leading to disruption of the cell cycle. Drugs like taxanes, such as docetaxel, contribute to microtubule stability, hinder mitosis, and prevent AR translocation from the cytoplasm to the cell nucleus. Integrating treatments with diverse mechanisms of action often provides the best chance for tumor regression.

6.2 Newly Diagnosed Metastatic Prostate Cancer—Important Definitions

To aid in treatment selection for men diagnosed with metastatic prostate cancer, specific definitions are crucial, as illustrated in Tables 6.1 and 6.2.

Table 6.1 Definitions of newly diagnosed metastatic prostate cancer

De novo metastatic prostate cancer defines men diagnosed with synchronous metastatic disease without prior local treatment of the prostate.
Metachronous metastatic prostate cancer defines men diagnosed with metastatic PC after local treatment of the prostate (radiotherapy or prostatectomy)

Table 6.2 Definitions of high-volume and high-risk disease prostate cancer

Term	Definition	References
High-volume disease	Visceral metastases and/or ≥4 bone lesions with ≥1 beyond the vertebral bodies and pelvis	CHAARTED Trial Sweeney NEJM 2015 [9]
High-risk disease	At least 2/3 criteria: • Gleason score ≥8 • ≥3 Bone metastases • Visceral metastases	LATITUDE Trial Fizazi NEJM 2017 [10]

Low-volume and low-risk diseases are defined as those that do not meet the above-mentioned criteria

6.3 Classification of mHSPC Based on the Timing of Metastasis

Metastatic hormone-sensitive prostate cancer (mHSPC) may present in two ways: either as primary metastasis detected at diagnosis, termed synchronous disease, or as a recurrence following local treatment, known as metachronous disease. The prognosis for individuals with synchronous metastatic prostate cancer is markedly less promising, with a significantly shorter duration until resistance emerges (372 versus 1613 days; $p < 0.001$) and a notably shorter median overall survival (OS) of merely 6.2 years compared to 11.6 years in metachronous metastatic patients [11]. Furthermore, the extent to which the tumor spreads significantly impacts the progression of the disease. As a result, it is incorporated into various risk classifications established in the CHAARTED and LATITUDE studies.

6.4 Role of Imaging in mHSPC

Conventional imaging techniques such as CT and Technetium-99 bone scan are commonly used to assess metastatic hormone-sensitive prostate cancer. There is increasing use of more advanced imaging techniques in the context of metastatic hormone-sensitive prostate cancer (mHSPC). Prostate-specific membrane antigen positron emission tomography (PSMA PET) can be used to visualize PSMA expressed on the surface of prostate cancer cells. Initial studies using integrated PET/CT with PSMA-targeting radiotracers such as Ga-68 PSMA-11 and piflufolastat F-18 have demonstrated improved sensitivity and specificity for pelvic lymph nodes and distant metastases compared to conventional imaging and other PET tracers like FDG. However, sensitivity may vary based on PSA levels [12]. Both radionuclide uptake and accompanying CT imaging results are crucial components of the evaluation. PET allows for the early detection of metastases that would not be possible with conventional imaging methods [13]. While magnetic resonance imaging (MRI) can provide valuable information about the extent of the primary tumor or an intraspinal lesion, it is not the standard modality of imaging for assessing metastatic disease [14].

6.5 Treatment Strategies for Metastatic Hormone-Sensitive Prostate Cancer

6.5.1 Systemic Treatment Strategies

6.5.1.1 Androgen Deprivation Therapy (ADT)

Androgen deprivation therapy (ADT), aimed at reducing serum testosterone levels to castrate levels, serves as a cornerstone of systemic treatment for castration-sensitive metastatic prostate cancer. This can be achieved through surgical orchiectomy (castration) or medical castration utilizing gonadotropin-releasing hormone (GnRH) agonists or antagonists. Both surgical and medical approaches effectively lower serum testosterone levels in patients with advanced CSPC, with the choice between the two depending on various factors such as patient preference, cost, and treatment accessibility.

Surgical Castration (Bilateral Orchidectomy)

Surgical castration leads to an immediate decline in testosterone. Surgical castration may be apt for patients with metastatic cord compression or urine outflow tract obstruction, where a prompt relief of symptoms for better clinical outcome is desired [15]. Bilateral orchidectomy is a cost-efficient modality. After surgery, serum testosterone levels swiftly decrease to castrate levels, often resulting in improvements in bone pain and other symptoms associated with the disease. The lower overall cost, avoidance of ongoing medical castration injections, and possibly lesser clinic visits make orchidectomy an attractive option in rising healthcare expenses [15]. Psychological impacts of orchidectomy may be alleviated through the placement of testicular prostheses or by modifying the procedure to a subcapsular orchiectomy, wherein the tunica albuginea and epididymis are preserved, offering a cosmetic enhancement in the scrotum.

Medical Castration

Medical castration can be achieved using either a GnRH (gonadotropin-releasing hormone) agonist or a GnRH antagonist.

6.6 GnRH Agonists

Mechanism of Action The GnRH agonist operates by binding to the GnRH receptor located in the pituitary gland. This binding triggers the release of follicle-stimulating hormone (FSH) and luteinizing hormone (LH), resulting in an initial surge known as the flare-up effect. Concurrently, this process increases the abundance of GnRH receptors (upregulation). Following this initial phase of heightened stimulation, GnRH agonists induce a downregulation of GnRH receptors in the pituitary, consequently reducing the production of luteinizing hormone (LH), follicle-stimulating hormone (FSH), and testosterone, as illustrated in Fig. 6.1.

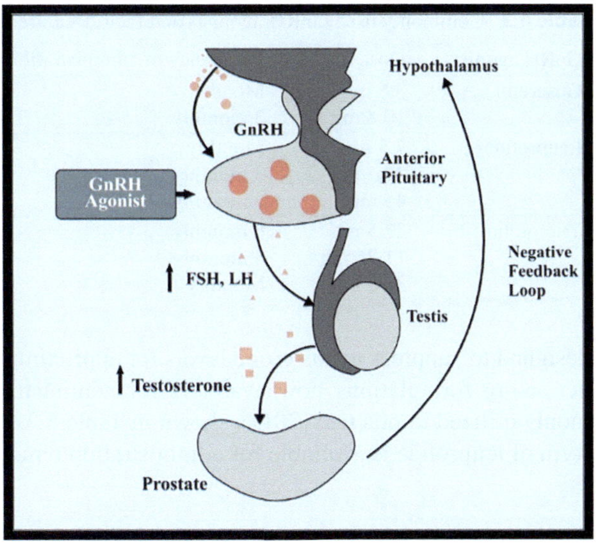

Fig. 6.1 Mechanism of action of GnRH agonist

Synthetic GnRH analogs exhibit increased receptor affinity and enhanced resistance to enzymatic degradation and are nearly 100 times more effective than the natural GnRH molecule [16]. GnRH agonists initially stimulate the release of both LH and FSH from pituitary gonadotropin-producing cells, resulting in heightened production of testosterone from testicular Leydig cells. However, after approximately a week of therapy, GnRH receptors on gonadotropin-producing cells become downregulated, resulting in a decrease in pituitary LH and FSH production [17]. This reduction in serum LH levels prompts a decrease in serum testosterone to castrate levels within 3–4 weeks of initiating treatment. Sustained therapy maintains serum testosterone at castrate levels. While testosterone production usually rebounds after discontinuation of GnRH agonist therapy, it may not always return to baseline levels. It can be influenced by factors such as the duration of treatment and patient age [18].

Flare Phenomenon The transient surge in LH following the initiation of GnRH therapy may trigger a temporary increase in serum testosterone, potentially stimulating prostate cancer growth. While rare, this "flare" can exacerbate bone pain, bladder obstruction, or other cancer-related symptoms. Thus, GnRH monotherapy is contraindicated in patients with urinary tract obstruction or painful bone metastases. The flare phenomenon in metastatic disease can be effectively prevented by administering antiandrogen therapy for a brief period, typically 2 weeks, which inhibits the effects of elevated serum testosterone [19].

Formulations GnRH agonists available for parenteral administration include leuprolide, goserelin, triptorelin, and buserelin, with buserelin also available in both parenteral and nasal formulations. Depot formulations of these agents were initially

Table 6.3 Commonly used GnRH agonists and their dose, frequency, mode of administration

GnRH agonists	Dose	Frequency of administration	Mode of administration
Goserelin	3.6 mg 10.8 mg	Monthly 3 monthly	Subcutaneous
Leuprolide	7.5 mg 22.5 mg 45 mg	Monthly 3 monthly 6 monthly	Intramuscular
Triptorelin	22.5 mg 11.25 mg 3.75 mg	6 monthly 3 monthly Monthly	Intramuscular

designed to suppress testosterone levels for approximately 1 month, with even longer-acting formulations now available for administration every 3 months, commonly utilized in practice [20] as shown in Table 6.3. Additionally, a subcutaneous form of leuprolide is available for administration 6 monthly.

6.7 GnRH Antagonists

Mechanism of Action GnRH antagonists bind to GnRH receptors on gonadotropin-producing cells of the pituitary, suppressing the release of LH or FSH, thus effectively lowering testosterone levels, as shown in Fig. 6.2.
Pure GnRH antagonists were formulated to suppress testosterone while avoiding the flare phenomenon associated with GnRH agonists. They are associated with the elevation of liver enzymes, and monitoring of LFT is thus crucial during treatment [21]. Examples of GnRH antagonists include degarelix and relugolix, as shown in Table 6.4.

Antiandrogens

- *First-generation antiandrogens*—Bicalutamide, Flutamide, Nilutamide.
- *Second-generation antiandrogens*—Enzalutamide, Apalutamide, Darolutamide.

The second-generation drugs also inhibit nuclear translocation. They are used along with GnRH agonists to prevent flare reactions.

Commonly used antiandrogens are illustrated in Table 6.5.

Mechanism of Action Binds to androgen receptors and inhibits testosterone binding to the androgen receptors, as shown in Fig. 6.3.

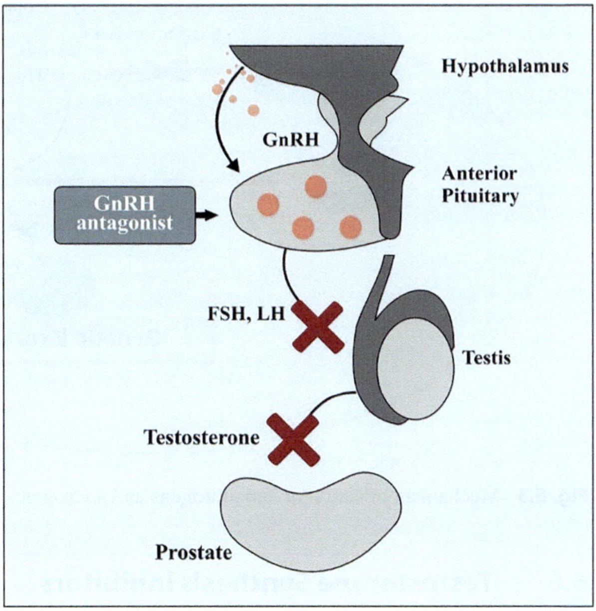

Fig. 6.2 Mechanism of action of GnRH antagonist

Table 6.4 Commonly used GnRH antagonists and their dose, frequency, mode of administration

GnRH antagonists	Dose	Frequency of administration	Mode of administration
Degarelix	240 mg loading dose 80 mg maintenance dose	Monthly	Subcutaneous
Relugolix	300 mg loading dose on the first day 120 mg maintenance dose	Daily	Oral

Table 6.5 Commonly used antiandrogens and their doses

Antiandrogens	Dose
Bicalutamide	50 mg daily with GnRH agonist 150 mg daily as monotherapy
Enzalutamide	160 mg daily
Apalutamide	Correct dose of Apalutamide 240 mg once daily

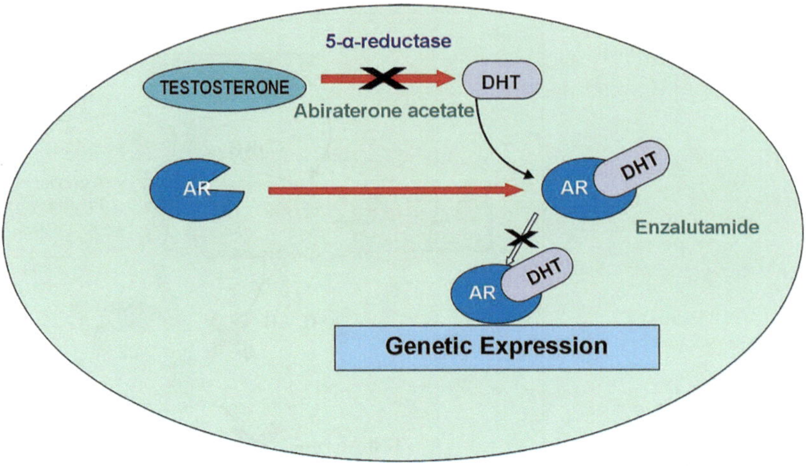

Fig. 6.3 Mechanism of action of antiandrogens and androgen synthesis inhibitor

6.8 Testosterone Synthesis Inhibitors

Abiraterone Acetate It is a selective, irreversible inhibitor of 17α-hydroxylase/C17,20-lyase enzyme (CYP17). This enzyme is expressed in testes, adrenals, and prostate and is required for the synthesis of androgens. Its mechanism of action is illustrated in Fig. 6.3. The dose is 250 mg/day per oral with fatty food or 1000 mg/day after an overnight fast. The lower alternate dose had similar PFS, reduced financial toxicity, and improved adherence [22]. Prednisolone 5 mg is given to prevent mineralocorticoid excess. It needs monitoring of LFT since it causes transaminase elevation [23].

Commonly used drugs for androgen deprivation therapy with their mechanism of action have been summarized in Table 6.6.

6.8.1 Timing of Treatment Initiation

In the case of symptomatic metastases, it is strongly advised to begin androgen-deprivation therapy (ADT) promptly. This not only helps alleviate symptoms but also prevents complications such as pathologic fractures and spinal cord compression. While no randomized trials are demonstrating a survival advantage for early versus deferred ADT in males with symptomatic metastatic disease, the benefits of promptly initiating ADT are evident in terms of improving quality of life and reducing disease-associated progression and morbidity [24]. For patients with asymptomatic metastases, initiating ADT early rather than delaying it is recommended to enhance survival and mitigate the morbidity associated with untreated disease. Potential complications such as ureteral obstruction, spinal cord compression, pathologic fractures and extraskeletal metastases underscore the importance of timely intervention [25].

Table 6.6 Mechanism of action of common drugs used for ADT

Drug	Mechanism of action
Goserelin, leuprolide, Triptorelin	GnRH agonists: they bind to the GnRH receptor on the pituitary leading to the release of FSH and LH. After an initial overstimulation, they downregulate GnRH receptors in the pituitary, leading to reduction in the levels of FSH, LH, and testosterone
Degarelix, Relugolix	GnRH antagonists: they bind to GnRH receptors on the pituitary and suppress the release of LH or FSH, thus lowering testosterone levels
Bicalutamide, enzalutamide, Apalutamide	Antiandrogens: they bind to androgen receptors and inhibit the binding of testosterone to the androgen receptors
Abiraterone acetate	Irreversible inhibitor of 17α-hydroxylase enzyme which is involved in androgen synthesis

6.8.2 Short-Term Combined Androgen Blockade for Disease Flare Prevention

When a GnRH agonist is chosen as the initial therapy, patients may receive a two- to four-week course of concurrent antiandrogen therapy, termed complete androgen blockade (CAB), to prevent flare of disease symptoms. Antiandrogens play a crucial role in managing disseminated prostate cancer during the treatment initiation with a GnRH agonist, preventing a flare-up due to the transient increase in testosterone levels. Typically, antiandrogen therapy is initiated 7 days prior to GnRH agonist commencement to circumvent disease flare due to testosterone surge [26].

6.8.3 Intermittent Versus Continuous ADT

Continuous ADT is generally considered the standard approach for most males with metastatic disease. Intermittent androgen deprivation (IAD) aims to mitigate the side effects of medical castration by discontinuing treatment in patients who have responded to androgen deprivation therapy and then reinstating ADT upon evidence of progressive or recurrent disease [26]. IAD typically involves treatment for a constant time period or until achievement of maximal response based on serum PSA levels. Subsequently, ADT is paused, and patients are monitored for signs of recurrence. As testosterone production resumes, the side effects of ADT diminish, but the risk of disease progression increases. Patients undergo PSA measurements, and ADT is resumed upon reaching a threshold level of serum PSA (often between 10 and 20 ng/mL) or upon new metastatic disease [27].

The rationale for IAD is twofold. Firstly, prolonged ADT may facilitate the transition from androgen dependence to androgen independence. Additionally, many acute and chronic adverse effects of ADT stem from castrate levels of testosterone. Periods of discontinuation of therapy may correlate with reductions in these side effects, potentially improving quality of life.

6.8.4 Management of Adverse Effects of ADT

The recognized negative impacts of ADT are inclusive of hot flashes, gynecomastia, lowered sexual desire, and sexual dysfunction. Other noted effects include bone degradation and reduced bone mineral density, which could potentially increase the risk of fractures; a condition known as sarcopenic obesity that is linked to metabolic syndrome and heightened risk of diabetes and cardiovascular diseases; mood swings and cognitive disruptions; and anemia, reduced size of the testes and penis, as well as testosterone surges associated with LHRH agonists [28]. Managing these adverse side effects involves a short-term administration of a non-steroidal AR inhibitor in conjunction with LHRH agonists to manage testosterone surges. Furthermore, patient education is crucial, alongside the introduction of heart-healthy lifestyle modifications such as increased physical activity and dietary adjustments. Optimizing control over preexisting cardiovascular risk factors is also necessary. Moreover, regular assessments of bone health and protective measures are essential. These measures may include physical activity, calcium intake, vitamin D supplementation, and, if appropriate, bone-supportive therapy such as Denosumab or bisphosphonate. This approach ensures that patients are equipped with the knowledge and tools to manage the adverse effects of ADT effectively [29].

6.9 Double Drug Combination Approach for Low-Volume/Low-Risk Disease

6.9.1 ADT and Docetaxel

Docetaxel marked the first drug to catalyze a paradigm shift in the management of mHSPC. By employing this strategy, the CHAARTED study became the first to showcase a significant improvement in the median overall survival, surpassing 10 months during 50 months. Furthermore, the study revealed that patients with a high tumor volume experienced the most significant benefits. The subsequent STAMPEDE trial, published later, confirmed the CHAARTED trial's overall findings [30]. However, it demonstrated that the benefits were not dependent on the magnitude of the tumor burden. As a result, the German S3-level clinical practice guidelines (S3GLs) recommend the addition of docetaxel to ADT for patients with high tumor volume and suggest it as an option for those with low tumor volume. Adverse events of higher severity (CTC AE $\geq$ G3) were reported in 29% and 52% of patients in the CHAARTED and STAMPEDE trials, respectively. Notably, 6% and 15% of patients experienced potentially life-threatening febrile neutropenia as an adverse event in these trials, respectively. In both studies, the occurrence of peripheral polyneuropathy as a severe adverse event was relatively uncommon, with rates of 1% and 3%, respectively.

6.9.2 ADT and Androgen Receptor Inhibitors

The drugs aimed at the androgen receptor (AR) signaling pathway are engineered to enhance the suppression of androgens' impact on prostate tumor cell proliferation. This enhancement can be attained by impeding the biosynthesis of precursors (such as Abiraterone) or obstructing the AR receptor and its signaling pathway (including drugs like apalutamide, darolutamide, and enzalutamide).

In the LATITUDE trial, Abiraterone was tested in combination with prednisone among patients diagnosed with synchronous mHSPC exhibiting high-risk characteristics [13]. This study demonstrated a significant and clinically meaningful increase in overall survival (OS) through the intensification of therapy. These findings are akin to those previously observed with docetaxel, which were confirmed by the STAMPEDE trial. The latter trial supported the benefits of intensified hormone therapy, though it differed by including patients regardless of the extent of tumor spread and risk profile. Further post-hoc analyses from these trials showed that Abiraterone provided benefits across various subgroups, highlighting its effectiveness beyond the initial high-risk cohort. Despite this broad efficacy, the formal approval of Abiraterone for the treatment of mHSPC was explicitly limited to patients with synchronous metastatic disease who meet the high-risk criteria established by the LATITUDE trial [13]. These trials underscore the importance of tailoring prostate cancer treatment to individual risk profiles and disease stages. They also suggest a potential reevaluation of treatment guidelines to extend the benefits of Abiraterone to a broader range of patients. Such decisions must be backed by further research and discussions within the oncological community to ensure the best outcomes for all patients affected by this condition.

The TITAN trial assessed the effectiveness of Apalutamide along with standard care in patients with mHSPC [31]. This study was inclusive, not discriminating based on the timing of metastasis (synchronous or metachronous), tumor size, or Gleason score. Standard treatment consisted of androgen deprivation therapy (ADT) alone, with 11% of participants in each treatment group also receiving docetaxel prior to randomization. The trial's final analysis revealed a 35% reduction in the risk of death, which increased to 48% after accounting for patients who received Apalutamide post-unblinding and subsequently crossed over to the treatment arm. Parallel studies on enzalutamide, specifically the ARCHES and ENZAMET trials, explored similar populations [32]. The ARCHES trial design closely resembled TITAN's, with nearly 18% of patients receiving docetaxel alongside ADT as the standard treatment [33]. The results showed a 34% improvement in overall survival despite a 31% crossover from the control group, underscoring the benefits of adding enzalutamide to the treatment regimen.

The ENZAMET trial compared the effects of a complete androgen blockade (non-steroidal antiandrogen plus ADT) in the control arm against ADT combined with enzalutamide. Here, 45% of patients in both study arms received concurrent docetaxel. This trial also confirmed a notable enhancement in overall survival across the patient cohort, with a hazard ratio (HR) of 0.67 and a 95% confidence interval of 0.52–0.86 [32]. In the ENZAMET trial, 483 out of 1125 patients (43%) were treated with docetaxel. Notably, ENZAMET was the only study that included a non-steroidal androgen receptor (AR) inhibitor (such as bicalutamide, nilutamide, or flutamide) in combination with ADT, with or without docetaxel in the comparator group. However, the specific benefits of adding docetaxel were less distinct, suggesting that the primary advantage stems from enzalutamide therapy [33].

6.10 Triple Drug Combination Approach for High-Volume/High-Risk Disease

6.10.1 ADT, Docetaxel, and Androgen Receptor Inhibitors

The two randomized, multicenter, phase III trials have started to reshape the landscape of prostate cancer treatment by introducing data on triple combination therapy. Among these, the PEACE-1 study evaluated patients with synchronous mHSPC. This study featured a four-arm design, but the focus was explicitly on the arm that tested the efficacy of combining androgen-deprivation therapy (ADT), docetaxel, and abiraterone/prednisolone. This combination significantly extended radiographic progression-free survival by 2.5 years and reduced the risk of death by 25% compared to the dual therapy of ADT and docetaxel alone. This survival benefit was particularly pronounced in patients with a high tumor burden, showcasing a survival advantage of 1.5 years for the triple therapy group. However, the benefits of this triple combination therapy remain uncertain for patients with low tumor volume [34].

In another pivotal trial, the ARASENS study, the standard hormonal chemotherapy regimen was enhanced with darolutamide. Of 1173 patients, 710 (61%) received docetaxel in the PEACE-1 trial. The study included 710 patients who received ADT combined with docetaxel (with or without radiotherapy) as the standard of care. In this study, the HR for OS was 0.75 (95.1% CI, 0.59–0.95) for Abiraterone in combination with standard of care, compared to standard of care alone [35].

This characteristic contributes to a notably favorable side-effect profile, emphasizing its distinct chemical structure and its targeted effectiveness within the body. These trials are pivotal in demonstrating the potential benefits of intensifying treatment through the addition of new agents to established hormone therapy regimens. However, their optimal application across different patient groups continues to be evaluated.

In the ARASENS study, which involved 1305 patients who all received docetaxel, the HR for OS was 0.68 (95%CI, 0.57–0.80) for darolutamide in combination with ADT and docetaxel compared to placebo with ADT and docetaxel. The trial successfully met its primary endpoint by significantly reducing the risk of death by 32.5% (HR 0.68; 95% CI: [0.57; 0.80]; $p < 0.001$), demonstrating that the addition of darolutamide to standard hormone therapy with docetaxel and ADT provides a consistent survival benefit across all patient subgroups. This finding mirrors the outcomes observed in the PEACE-1 study, where many participants also presented with high-risk cancer at the start of the trial. However, the ARASENS trial has not yet reported how tumor burden might influence treatment outcomes [35].

Regarding safety, the addition of darolutamide did not substantially alter the side effect profile compared to the standard hormonal chemotherapy regimen (adverse side effects ≥ grade 3: triple combination 70.2% vs. hormonal chemotherapy 67.5%). The notable exception was an increase in the incidence of arterial hypertension (6.4% with darolutamide vs. 3.2% without).

Despite these positive results, the ARASENS and PEACE-1 trials have faced criticism for not including a comparison arm that pairs the respective AR signaling pathway-targeted drug with ADT alone, without docetaxel. At the time of design of these studies, such a combination had yet to be established as standard care; hence, it was not included in the trial protocols. This omission makes it challenging to conclusively assess whether the triple combination therapy offers a significant advantage over intensified hormone therapy alone. Further research and comparative studies will be necessary to clarify these benefits more definitively [35].

These trials utilized different comparators, reflecting the evolving treatment landscape for hormone-sensitive prostate cancer (HSPC) over time, particularly in the studies involving triplet therapy. The results of the phase 3 trials demonstrate a gradual improvement in overall survival (OS) when progressing from ADT alone to ADT combined with androgen receptor pathway inhibitors (ARPI) or docetaxel, and finally to ADT combined with ARPI and docetaxel.

Improved treatment with the combination of ADT, ARPI, and docetaxel has been validated through multiple meta-analyses [36]. These analyses indicate that the triple regimen may outperform ADT plus ARPI. However, further evidence is required to confirm the efficacy advantage of ADT plus ARPI plus docetaxel over ADT plus ARPI in prospective head-to-head studies. Regarding doublet therapy, meta-analyses suggest comparable survival benefits between ADT plus ARPI and ADT plus docetaxel [37].

6.11 Metastases-Directed Therapy

Metastasis-directed therapy (MDT) is a targeted approach intended for patients with limited metastatic lesions. This treatment aims to address all visible lesions detected through imaging, utilizing radiotherapeutic or surgical interventions. To date, the evidence supporting MDT primarily comes from randomized phase II trials. For example, in the STOMP trial, metastasis-directed therapy led to a 26% increase in the 5-year androgen-deprivation therapy (ADT) free survival compared to surveillance alone. However, this result approached but did not reach statistical significance ($p = 0.06$) [38]. Similarly, the ORIOLE study demonstrated the effectiveness of stereotactic ablative radiotherapy in significantly reducing the risk of progression at 6 months—from 61% in the control group to 19% in the treatment group ($p = 0.005$) [39]. However, a definitive survival benefit from metastasis-directed therapy has not yet been established. Despite the relatively small scale of these studies and the lack of extensive data, metastases-directed therapy has been widely adopted in clinical practice.

6.11.1 Radionuclide Therapy

Radionuclide therapy plays a significant role in the treatment of mHSPC, mainly when bone metastases characterize the disease. This therapeutic approach involves using radioactive substances that target and kill cancer cells, focusing on those that have spread to the bone. Lu-PSMA-617 radioligand therapy is a relatively new and evolving treatment modality that uses a radioactive substance linked to a molecule that specifically binds to the prostate-specific membrane antigen (PSMA) [40]. PSMA is a protein abundantly expressed on the surface of prostate cancer cells, making it a valuable target for therapy. Lu-PSMA-617 combines a PSMA-targeting ligand with Lutetium-177, a radioactive isotope that delivers localized radiation to the tumor cells. While Lu-PSMA-617 has primarily been studied and shown promising results in the treatment of metastatic castration-resistant prostate cancer (mCRPC), its role in hormone-sensitive prostate cancer (HSPC) is still under investigation. The ALSYMPCA trial is a pivotal study that demonstrated the effectiveness of Radium-223. In this trial, Radium-223 significantly improved overall survival compared to placebo. Patients treated with Radium-223 showed a median overall survival of 14.9 months compared to 11.3 months in the placebo group, a statistically significant improvement (HR 0.70; 95% CI: 0.58–0.83; $p < 0.001$) [41]. The eRADicate trial is a phase II study that explores the use of Radium-223 earlier in the disease course with concurrent Abiraterone [42]. Patients had significantly enhanced quality of life and pain relief without adverse side effects. Ongoing Phase III trials combine Ra-223 with new oral hormonal treatments to further assess radiographic progression and overall survival improvements [43].

6.11.2 Role of Bone-Directed Therapy

In hormone-sensitive prostate cancer (HSPC), particularly when metastasized to the bone, bisphosphonates and other bone-directed therapies are integral for managing skeletal-related events (SREs) and improving patient quality of life. These therapies reduce bone resorption, manage pain, and prevent complications such as fractures.

Zoledronic acid is the most studied bisphosphonate in the context of prostate cancer. The pivotal CALGB 90202 trial demonstrated that in men with hormone-sensitive prostate cancer and bone metastases, early administration of zoledronic acid significantly reduced the rate of SREs compared to placebo. This trial highlighted the efficacy of zoledronic acid in delaying SREs such as spinal cord compression, pathological fractures, and the need for radiation or surgery on bone [44].

Denosumab is an alternative to bisphosphonates, which targets the RANKL pathway, which is crucial for osteoclast function and survival, offering another mechanism to inhibit bone resorption. HALT Prostate Cancer Study ('147 trial') compared Denosumab with placebo in men undergoing androgen deprivation therapy for non-metastatic prostate cancer at risk of bone loss [45]. Denosumab increased the bone mineral density significantly and reduced the risk of new vertebral fractures. A subsequent trial focusing on men with bone metastases from prostate cancer found that Denosumab was superior to zoledronic acid in delaying the time to first skeletal-related event [46].

Palliative radiation to bone metastases from dose ranging from 8 Gy single fraction radiation to 20–30 Gy over 1–2 weeks helps to achieve pain control. The role of stereotactic body radiation therapy (SBRT), as demonstrated in the ongoing STOMP trial [38], achieves excellent local control and pain relief with doses ranging from 24 to 30 Gy in one to two fractions; ablative doses in three to five fractions are used in visceral metastases.

6.12 Primary Tumor Management in mHSPC

6.12.1 Role of Radiotherapy in mHSPC

In the past, the primary application of radiotherapy in mHSPC was to alleviate symptoms. However, retrospective investigations have posited a link between controlling the primary tumor and improved overall survival (OS) rates in newly diagnosed mHSPC patients, especially those classified as a low-risk or low-volume disease. This hypothesis was tested in three prospective studies: HORRAD, STAMPEDE, and PEACE-1.

The outcomes of the HORRAD trial did not reveal any OS benefit when combining ADT with radiotherapy to treat the primary tumor compared to using ADT alone in the broader population (hazard ratio [HR], 0.90; 95% CI, 0.70–1.14). However, an encouraging trend (though not statistically meaningful) was observed in patients with less than five bone metastases (HR, 0.68; 95% CI, 0.42–1.10) [47].

The STAMPEDE group H study, which investigated patients newly diagnosed with mHSPC, found that the overall survival hazard ratio (OS HR) was 0.90 (95% CI, 0.81–1.01; $P = 0.08$) for the entire population. Of particular interest was the discovery of a specific advantage for patients with a low load of metastasis (HR, 0.64; 95% CI, 0.52–0.79), but this benefit was not observed in those with a high metastatic count (HR, 1.11; 95% CI, 0.96–1.28) [48].

The PEACE-1 study focused on the role of prostate irradiation in men receiving intensified systemic treatment with ADT and Docetaxel, particularly in low-volume disease. There was favorable radiographic progression-free survival and overall survival in those receiving prostate irradiation [49].

Intriguingly, the most extended survival was seen in those who received radiotherapy alongside an intensified systemic treatment plan (ADT with or without docetaxel, including abiraterone [49]. In line with these results, global clinical guidelines now recommend considering ADT in combination with radiotherapy for newly diagnosed mHSPC patients who present a low metastatic load [48]. Radiation improved failure-free survival, not overall survival, in the STAMPEDE trial;

however, in the subset analysis of low-volume disease according to CHAARTED criteria, there was a significant benefit in failure-free and overall survival. The detailed role of radiation in oligometastatic prostate cancer has been discussed in consecutive chapter.

6.12.2 Cytoreductive Prostatectomy

No one has adequately addressed the role of cytoreductive prostatectomy in mHSPC. Patients diagnosed with de novo mHSPC may benefit substantially from radical prostatectomy, according to extensive retrospective data from US SEER-Medicare and the US National Cancer Data Base [49]. This approach is most effective for patients with lower tumor grade, local stage, metastatic substage, and good general condition. Steuber et al. compared the results of 40 patients who received systemic treatment with those of 43 patients who underwent cytoreductive prostatectomy for small-volume bone metastases (1–3 lesions) caused by prostate cancer [50].

While there were no statistically significant differences in overall survival or castration-resistant-free survival, there were fewer locoregional issues experienced by patients who underwent prostatectomy. Another prospective trial was done by Poelaert et al., in which 17 asymptomatic mHSPC patients underwent surgery, while 29 patients who were ineligible or unwilling for radical prostatectomy got conventional treatment. Patients who underwent radical prostatectomy had improved OS, PSA response, and longer time to ADT failure compared to the control group [51]. However, the patients in the surgery group were younger, had lower PSA levels at diagnosis, and had less significant local and metastatic illness. This suggests a considerable selection bias, affecting the reliability of data. Additional research is necessary to assess the potential advantages of cytoreductive prostatectomy in patients with metastatic hormone-sensitive prostate cancer.

6.13 Response Assessment During Treatment

For males with castration-sensitive prostate cancer (CSPC) who receive systemic therapy, regular evaluations are essential for detecting indications of disease progression. Monitoring revolves primarily around serial measurements of serum prostate-specific antigen (PSA). Guidelines established by the National Comprehensive Cancer Network advocate for PSA testing every 3–6 months throughout the treatment course [52]. Clinicians typically determine the necessity of radiographic assessments based on shifts in PSA levels and/or the emergence of new symptoms.

6.14 Ongoing Trials in mHSPC

The combination of darolutamide and ADT is being assessed in two studies: ARANOTE and ARASEC [53]. The ARANOTE trial is a phase 3 international, multicenter, randomized, double-blind, placebo-controlled trial for patients with conventional imaging evidence of mHSPC [54]. Patients have been randomized into 2:1 to receive darolutamide 600 mg twice daily or placebo with ADT. The primary endpoint is rPFS, with secondary endpoints including OS, CPRC, antineoplastic therapy initiation, PSA progression, undetectable PSA, pain progression, and safety/adverse events.

In the US-based phase 2, open-label, single-arm ARASEC study, patients with mHSPC receive 600 mg of darolutamide twice daily and ADT. The ARASEC control arm is based on 393 mHSPC patients treated with ADT alone in the CHAARTED trial. Baseline characteristics such as age, ECOG performance status, disease severity (low or high volume according to CHAARTED), and presence of bone and visceral metastases have been used to match patients in the active and control arms 1:1. The primary endpoint is PFS, with secondary endpoints including OS, rPFS, time to CPRC, 6-month PSA response rate and safety.

The PSMAddition trial (NCT04720157) is an international, prospective, open-label, randomized, phase 3 trial conducted in adults with metastatic hormone-sensitive prostate cancer (mHSPC) [55]. To meet the eligibility criteria, patients must have PSMA-positive disease as determined by [68Ga]Ga-PSMA-11 PET-CT. Additionally, they should be either treatment-naïve or minimally treated individuals who are suitable candidates for hormonal therapy. The study aims to randomize approximately 1126 patients in a 1:1 ratio. One group will receive Lu-PSMA-617 (7.4 GBq i.v. every 6 weeks, up to six cycles) along with standard of care, while the other group will only receive standard of care (control arm). Within this particular context, the recommended approach is to utilize-second generation antiandrogen therapy in combination with androgen deprivation therapy (ADT).

The study's primary endpoint is radiographic progression-free survival (PFS), which will be evaluated by a blinded, independent, centralized review. Upon the confirmation of radiographic progression by a central authority, participants in the control arm of the study have the option to switch to the Lu-PSMA-617 arm. The primary and secondary endpoint of this study is overall survival. The final analysis for this endpoint will be conducted when approximately 384 deaths have occurred.

TALAPRO-3 (NCT04821622) is a phase III clinical trial that aims to compare the effectiveness of talazoparib plus enzalutamide versus placebo plus enzalutamide in men with mHSPC who have DNA damage repair/homologous recombination repair (DDR/HRR) alterations [56]. The trial is designed as a double-masked, randomized study. The main focus of the study is the measurement of rPFS. Additional measures to be considered are the overall survival rate, safety factors, and patient reported outcomes.

6.15 Cancer Biomarkers and Precision Treatment in mHSPC

Genomic alterations play a crucial role in prognostication and prediction in metastatic hormone-sensitive prostate cancer. Tumor-sequencing data from the STAMPEDE trial has revealed a correlation between increasing copy number burden and the risk of progression and death, regardless of disease volume. Additionally, alterations in key genes, including AR, TP53, PTEN, and RB1, and those involved in the cell cycle and MYC pathways, are associated with shorter time to castration resistance. Detection of AR aberrations in circulating tumor DNA at baseline is linked to reduced overall survival [57]. Conversely, SPOP mutations are linked to prolonged time to progression and death, specifically in patients treated with androgen receptor signaling inhibitors but not with docetaxel for metastatic hormone-sensitive prostate cancer [56].

We are on the brink of exploring the benefits of biomarker-informed clinical trials of precision therapy for mHSPC. With the increasing understanding of personalized and targeted treatments in metastatic castration-resistant prostate cancer (mCRPC), there is a compelling need to investigate these approaches in mHSPC, offering the promise of achieving a better balance between treatment benefits and burdens. The prevalence of germline and somatic BRCA1/2 and homologous recombination–associated gene alterations in metastatic prostate cancer, along with the success of poly (ADP-ribose) polymerase (PARP) inhibitors, has spurred the development of numerous trials investigating PARP inhibitor combinations in mHSPC [58]. Additionally, targeting common PI3K-Akt pathway alterations and cell cycle dysregulation in mCRPC has inspired research in the hormone-sensitive setting, exploring combinations of AKT inhibitors and CDK4/6 inhibitors with hormonal therapy, respectively [59]. The FDA approval of 177Lu-PSMA-617 for the treatment of mCRPC, based on its significant activity and overall survival improvement, heralds a new era of molecular-targeted therapy. Given the widespread expression of PSMA in hormone-sensitive disease, 177Lu-PSMA-617 shows promise in mHSPC. Ongoing trials are investigating combinations of 177Lu-PSMA-617 with chemotherapy and androgen receptor signaling inhibitors (ARSIs) [60]. The rapid advancement of predictive biomarkers is shaping the design of future multiarm umbrella trials in mHSPC, guided by comprehensive molecular, PSA, and imaging characterization both at baseline and during treatment, as well as other individual data levels, to delineate optimal treatment strategies.

6.16 Conclusion

Recent years have witnessed rapid shifts in the paradigm and complexity of therapy for metastatic hormone-sensitive prostate cancer (mHSPC), resulting in significant improvements in overall survival (OS). This progress is particularly noteworthy for individuals with synchronous, high-volume disease, which historically carried a worse prognosis. These advancements have transformed mHSPC to one with the goal of achieving durable control. Contemporary data from clinical trials focusing on mHSPC underscore substantial improvements in patient prognosis across the risk spectrum, necessitating their adoption and implementation in real-world clinical practice [61]. However, numerous unanswered questions persist. As men with metastatic prostate cancer are living longer, it remains crucial that new treatment approaches prioritize personalization to maximize patient benefit while minimizing the burden of treatment-related adverse effects [62].

References

1. Global Cancer Observatory. India Fact Sheet. [Internet]. Lyon, France: International Agency for Research on Cancer; [date unknown] [cited 2024 Jun 2]. Available from: https://gco.iarc.who.int/media/globocan/factsheets/populations/356-india-fact-sheet.pdf.
2. Advanced Centre for Treatment, Research and Education in Cancer. (Year, Month Day). [Internet]. [Cited Year Month Day]. Available from: https://actrec.gov.in/node/5766.
3. SEER Cancer Statistics Review, 1975–2018—Previous Version—SEER Cancer Stat Facts. [cited 2024 Jun 2]. Available from: https://seer.cancer.gov/statfacts/html/prost.html.
4. Thomas TS, Pachynski RK. Treatment of advanced prostate cancer. Mo Med. 2018;115(2):156–61.
5. Ng K, Smith S, Shamash J. Metastatic hormone-sensitive prostate cancer (mHSPC): advances and treatment strategies in the first-line setting. Oncol Ther. 2020;8(2):209–30.
6. Oing C, Bristow RG. Systemic treatment of metastatic hormone-sensitive prostate cancer-upfront triplet versus doublet combination therapy. ESMO Open. 2023;8(2):101194.
7. Crawford ED, Heidenreich A, Lawrentschuk N, Tombal B, Pompeo ACL, Mendoza-Valdes A, et al. Androgen-targeted therapy in men with prostate cancer: evolving practice and future considerations. Prostate Cancer Prostatic Dis. 2019;22(1):24–38.
8. Klusa D, Lohaus F, Furesi G, Rauner M, Benešová M, Krause M, et al. Metastatic spread in prostate cancer patients influencing radiotherapy response. Front Oncol. 2021;10:627379.
9. Jetty S, Loftus JR, Patel A, Gupta A, Puri S, Dogra V. Prostate cancer-PET imaging update. Cancers (Basel). 2023;15(3):796.
10. Fletcher JW, Djulbegovic B, Soares HP, Siegel BA, Lowe VJ, Lyman GH, et al. The role of PET in the management of patients with cancer: clinical recommendations of the PET oncology committee of the society of nuclear medicine. J Nucl Med. 2008;49(3):480–508.
11. Li B, Du Y, Yang H, Huang Y, Meng J, Xiao D. Magnetic resonance imaging for prostate cancer clinical application. Chin J Cancer Res. 2013;25(2):240–9.
12. Sweeney CJ, Chen YH, Carducci M, Liu G, Jarrard DF, Eisenberger M, et al. Chemohormonal therapy in metastatic hormone-sensitive prostate cancer. N Engl J Med. 2015;373(8):737–46.
13. Fizazi K, Tran N, Fein L, Matsubara N, Rodriguez-Antolin A, Alekseev BY, et al. LATITUDE Investigators. Abiraterone plus prednisone in metastatic, castration-sensitive prostate cancer. N Engl J Med 2017;377(4):352–60.
14. Merseburger AS, Krabbe LM, Krause BJ, Böhmer D, Perner S, Amsberg GV. The treatment of metastatic, hormone-sensitive prostatic carcinoma. Dtsch Arztebl Int. 2022;119(37):622–32. https://doi.org/10.3238/arztebl.m2022.0294.
15. Miyoshi Y, Kawahara T, Yao M, Uemura H. Clinical outcome of surgical management for symptomatic metastatic spinal cord compression from prostate cancer. BMC Urol. 2020;20(1):143. https://doi.org/10.1186/s12894-020-00713-3.
16. Marques P, Skorupskaite K, Rozario KS, Anderson RA, George JT. Physiology of GnRH and gonadotropin secretion. In: Huhtaniemi I, editor. Hormone assays in biological fluids. 1st ed. London: Academic; 2018. p. 1–20.
17. Liu Z, Yang C, Zeng X, Ke C, Tian J, Wang Z, Hu Z. Effectiveness of GnRH antagonists and agonists in patients with hormone-sensitive prostate cancer: a retrospective study. Appl Bionics Biomech. 2022;2022:7608428.

18. Perlmutter MA, Lepor H. Androgen deprivation therapy in the treatment of advanced prostate cancer. Rev Urol. 2007;9(Suppl 1):S3–8.
19. Sethi R, Sanfilippo N. Six-month depot formulation of leuprorelin acetate in the treatment of prostate cancer. Clin Interv Aging. 2009;4:259–67.
20. Hoofnagle JH. LiverTox: clinical and research information on drug-induced liver injury. Bethesda: National Institute of Diabetes and Digestive and Kidney Diseases; 2012.
21. Colomba E, Marret G, Baciarello G, Lavaud P, Massard C, Loriot Y, et al. Liver tests increase on abiraterone acetate in men with metastatic prostate cancer: natural history, management and outcome. Eur J Cancer. 2020;129:117–22.
22. Connolly RM, Carducci MA, Antonarakis ES. Use of androgen deprivation therapy in prostate cancer: indications and prevalence. Asian J Androl. 2012;14(2):177–86.
23. Gillessen S, Bossi A, Davis ID, Zapatero A, Zilli T, Omlin A, et al. Management of patients with advanced prostate cancer—metastatic and/or castration-resistant prostate cancer: report of the Advanced Prostate Cancer Consensus Conference (APCCC) 2022. Eur J Cancer. 2023;185:178–215.
24. Kashiwabara T, Suda S. Usefulness of combined androgen blockade therapy with gonadotropin-releasing hormone antagonist for bone metastatic prostate cancer with pretreatment prostate-specific antigen level ≥50 ng/mL. BMC Cancer. 2018;18(1):619.
25. Pokuri VK, Nourkeyhani H, Betsy B, Herbst L, Sikorski M, Spangenthal E, et al. Strategies to circumvent testosterone surge and disease flare in advanced prostate cancer: emerging treatment paradigms. J Natl Compr Cancer Netw. 2015;13(7):e49.
26. Szmulewitz RZ, Peer CJ, ibraheem A, Martinez E, Kozloff MF, Carthon B, et al. Prospective international randomized phase II study of low dose abiraterone with food v/s standar dose abiraterone in CRPC. J Clin Oncol. 2018;36:1389–95.
27. Sciarra A, Abrahamsson PA, Brausi M, Galsky M, Mottet N, Sartor O, et al. Intermittent androgen-deprivation therapy in prostate cancer: a critical review focused on phase 3 trials. Eur Urol. 2013;64(5):722–30.
28. Yu EY, Gulati R, Telesca D, Jiang P, Tam S, Russell KJ, et al. Duration of first off-treatment interval is prognostic for time to castration resistance and death in men with biochemical relapse of prostate cancer treated on a prospective trial of intermittent androgen deprivation. J Clin Oncol. 2010;28(16):2668–73.
29. Yaturu S, Humphrey S, Landry C, Jain SK. Decreased bone mineral density in men with metabolic syndrome alone and with type 2 diabetes. Med Sci Monit. 2009;15(1):CR5.
30. Rhee H, Gunter JH, Heathcote P, Ho K, Stricker P, Corcoran NM, Nelson CC. Adverse effects of androgen-deprivation therapy in prostate cancer and their management. BJU Int. 2015;115(Suppl 5):3–13.
31. Clarke NW, Ali A, Ingleby FC, Hoyle A, Amos CL, Attard G, Brawley CD, Calvert J, Chowdhury S, Cook A, Cross W, et al. Addition of docetaxel to hormonal therapy in low- and high-burden metastatic hormone sensitive prostate cancer: long-term survival results from the STAMPEDE trial. Ann Oncol. 2019;30(12):1992–2003.
32. Merseburger AS, Suttmann H. TITAN-Studie—Evaluation von Apalutamid bei Patienten mit metastasiertem hormonsensitivem Prostatakarzinom [TITAN study: evaluation of apalutamide in patients with metastatic hormone-sensitive prostate cancer—Treatment of metastatic hormone-sensitive prostate cancer (mHSPC)]. Aktuelle Urol. 2021;52(2):155–60. German.
33. Stockler MR, Martin AJ, Davis ID, Dhillon HM, Begbie SD, Chi KN, et al.; ENZAMET Trial Investigators and the Australian and New Zealand Urogenital and Prostate Cancer Trials Group (ANZUP). Health-related quality of life in metastatic, hormone-sensitive prostate cancer: ENZAMET (ANZUP 1304), an international, Randomized phase III trial led by ANZUP. J Clin Oncol. 2022;40(8):837–46.
34. Armstrong AJ, Szmulewitz RZ, Petrylak DP, Holzbeierlein J, Villers A, Azad A, et al. ARCHES: a randomized, phase III study of androgen deprivation therapy with enzalutamide or placebo in men with metastatic hormone-sensitive prostate cancer. J Clin Oncol. 2019;37(32):2974–86.

35. Zattoni F, Rajwa P, Gandaglia G, Young Academic Urologists Prostate Cancer Working Party (YAU-PCa WP). Optimal combination therapy for metastatic hormone-sensitive prostate cancer: new evidence, challenges and unanswered questions. Curr Opin Urol. 2023;33(6):445–51.
36. So AI, Chi K, Danielson B, Fleshner NE, Kinnaird A, Kapoor A, et al. 2022 UPDATE: Canadian Urological Association-Canadian Urologic Oncology Group guideline: metastatic castration-naive and castration-sensitive prostate cancer full-text. Can Urol Assoc J. 2022;16(12):E581–9.
37. Tucci M, Bertaglia V, Vignani F, Buttigliero C, Fiori C, Porpiglia F, et al. Addition of docetaxel to androgen deprivation therapy for patients with hormone-sensitive metastatic prostate cancer: a systematic review and meta-analysis. Eur Urol. 2016;69(4):563–73.
38. Fiorica F, Buttigliero C, Grigolato D, Muraro M, Turco F, Munoz F, et al. Addition of new androgen receptor pathway inhibitors to docetaxel and androgen deprivation therapy in metastatic hormone-sensitive prostate cancer: a systematic review and metanalysis. Curr Oncol. 2022;29(12):9511–24.
39. Zilli T, Ost P. Metastasis-directed therapy: a new standard for oligorecurrent prostate cancer? Oncotarget. 2018;9(76):34196–7.
40. Phillips R, Shi WY, Deek M, Radwan N, Lim SJ, Antonarakis ES, et al. Outcomes of observation vs stereotactic ablative radiation for oligometastatic prostate cancer: the ORIOLE phase 2 randomized clinical trial. JAMA Oncol. 2020;6(5):650–9.
41. Chi KN, Yip SM, Bauman G, Probst S, Emmenegger U, et al. 177Lu-PSMA-617 in metastatic castration-resistant prostate cancer: a review of the evidence and implications for Canadian clinical practice. Curr Oncol. 2024;31(3):1400–15.
42. Parker C, Zhan L, Cislo P, Reuning-Scherer J, Vogelzang NJ, Nilsson S, et al. Effect of radium-223 dichloride (Ra-223) on hospitalisation: an analysis from the phase 3 randomised Alpharadin in Symptomatic Prostate Cancer Patients (ALSYMPCA) trial. Br J Cancer. 2016;114(1):1–5.
43. McDermott RS, Greene J, McCaffrey J, Parker I, Helanova S, Baird AM, et al. Radium-223 in combination with enzalutamide in metastatic castration-resistant prostate cancer: a multi-centre, phase II open-label study. Ther Adv Med Oncol. 2021;13:17588359211042691.
44. Shore ND, Tutrone RF, Mariados NF, Nordquist LT, Mehlhaff BA, Steere KJ, et al. eRADicAte: a prospective evaluation combining Radium-223 dichloride and abiraterone acetate plus prednisone in patients with castration-resistant prostate cancer. Clin Genitourin Cancer. 2018;16(2):149–54.
45. Smith MR, Halabi S, Ryan CJ, Hussain A, Vogelzang N, Stadler W, et al. Randomized controlled trial of early zoledronic acid in men with castration-sensitive prostate cancer and bone metastases: results of CALGB 90202 (alliance). J Clin Oncol. 2014;32(11):1143–50.
46. Smith MR, Egerdie B, Hernández Toriz N, Feldman R, Tammela TL, Saad F, et al.; Denosumab HALT Prostate Cancer Study Group. Denosumab in men receiving androgen-deprivation therapy for prostate cancer. N Engl J Med 2009;361(8):745–55.
47. Boevé LMS, Hulshof MCCM, Vis AN, Zwinderman AH, Twisk JWR, Witjes WPJ, et al. Effect on survival of androgen deprivation therapy alone compared to androgen deprivation therapy combined with concurrent radiation therapy to the prostate in patients with primary bone metastatic prostate cancer in a prospective randomised clinical trial: data from the HORRAD trial. Eur Urol. 2019;75(3):410–8.
48. James ND, Sydes MR, Clarke NW, Mason MD, Dearnaley DP, Spears MR, et al. Addition of docetaxel, zoledronic acid, or both to first-line long-term hormone therapy in prostate cancer (STAMPEDE): survival results from an adaptive, multiarm, multistage, platform randomised controlled trial. Lancet. 2016;387(10024):1163–77. https://doi.org/10.1016/S0140-6736(15)01037-5. PMID: 26719232; PMCID: PMC4787089.
49. Sartor O, Karrison TG, Sandler HM, Gomella LG, Amin MB, Purdy J, et al. Androgen deprivation and radiotherapy with or without docetaxel for localized high-risk prostate cancer: long-term follow-up from the randomized NRG oncology RTOG 0521 trial. Eur Urol. 2023;84(2):156–63.

50. Yanagisawa T, Rajwa P, Kawada T, Bekku K, Laukhtina E, Deimling MV, et al. An updated systematic and comprehensive review of cytoreductive prostatectomy for metastatic prostate cancer. Curr Oncol. 2023;30(2):2194–216.
51. Teuber T, Berg KD, Røder MA, Brasso K, Iversen P, Huland H, et al. Does cytoreductive prostatectomy really have an impact on prognosis in prostate cancer patients with low-volume bone metastasis? Results from a prospective case-control study. Eur Urol Focus. 2017;3(6):646–9.
52. Lee SU, Cho KH, Park W, Cho WK, Kim JS, Wee CW, et al. Clinical outcomes of postoperative radiotherapy following radical prostatectomy in patients with localized prostate cancer: a multicenter retrospective study (KROG 18-01) of a Korean population. Cancer Res Treat. 2020;52(1):167–80.
53. Shore ND, Preston MA, Gregg JR, Salami SS, Ross A, Bruno A, et al. Darolutamide plus androgen-deprivation therapy (ADT) versus ADT in metastatic hormone-sensitive prostate cancer: open-label single-arm study with an external control arm (ARASEC). J Clin Oncol. 2023;41:TPS297.
54. A randomized, double-blind, placebo-controlled phase 3 study of darolutamide in addition to Androgen Deprivation Therapy (ADT) versus placebo plus ADT in men with Metastatic Hormone-sensitive Prostate Cancer (mHSPC).
55. Sartor AO, Tagawa ST, Saad F, De Bono JS, Feng FY, Fizazi K, et al. PSMAddition: a phase 3 trial to compare treatment with 177Lu-PSMA-617 plus standard of care (SOC) versus SOC alone in patients with metastatic hormone-sensitive prostate cancer. J Clin Oncol. 2022;40:TPS210.
56. Agarwal N, Saad F, Azad AA, Mateo J, Matsubara N, Shore ND, et al. TALAPRO-3 clinical trial protocol: phase III study of talazoparib plus enzalutamide in metastatic castration-sensitive prostate cancer. Future Oncol. 2024;20(9):493–505.
57. Tikkinen KAO, Dahm P, Lytvyn L, Heen AF, Vernooij RWM, Siemieniuk RAC, et al. Prostate cancer screening with prostate-specific antigen (PSA) test: a clinical practice guideline. BMJ. 2018;362:k3581.
58. Dorff T, Zengin Z, Henderson N, Ali A, Nguyen C, Hwang C, et al. Clinical implications of AR alterations in advanced prostate cancer: a multi-institutional collaboration. Res Sq [Preprint]. 2023 Aug 10.3.rs-3201150.
59. Kwon WA. PARP inhibitors in the treatment of prostate cancer: from scientific rationale to clinical development. World J Mens Health. 2024;42(2):290–303.
60. Hashemi M, Taheriazam A, Daneii P, Hassanpour A, Kakavand A, Rezaei S, et al. Targeting PI3K/Akt signaling in prostate cancer therapy. J Cell Commun Signal. 2023;17(3):423–43.
61. Jacob A, Raj R, Allison DB, Myint ZW. Androgen receptor signaling in prostate cancer and therapeutic strategies. Cancers (Basel). 2021;13(21):5417.
62. Lu Y, Jiang J, Yang G, Ding H, Zheng Q, Ji L, et al. Comparative effectiveness of multiple androgen receptor signaling inhibitor medicines with androgen deprivation therapy for metastatic hormone-sensitive prostate cancer: a study in the real world. Front Oncol. 2024;14:1324181.

Oligometastatic Prostate Cancer: Current Management Strategies

7

Narendra Kumar, Arun Kumar Yadav, Renu Madan, J. Subalakshmi, and Shikha Goyal

7.1 Introduction

The term oligometastasis was coined by Hellman and Weichselbaum in 1995 to identify patients with limited number of metastases [1]. The concept of oligometastatic disease, where there are a limited number of metastases, was introduced as a potential scenario where localized treatments such as surgery or radiotherapy (RT) might be beneficial.

Oligometastatic prostate cancer (OMPC), a potentially curable disease, is gaining interest in the last few years due to improved imaging modalities and evidence supporting the multimodality and metastatis-directed treatment (MDT). Despite the metastatic disease, the outcomes in patients with OMPC are better compared to the disseminated disease. Few authors consider OMPC as an indolent cancer or cancer with a low metastatic potential [2].

There is no consensus on the definition of OMPC and the commonly used criteria are based on the CHAARTED and LATITUDE trials. Generally, three to five metastatic sites are considered as oligometastatic disease, with considerable variation across clinical trials [3]. Barbato et al. proposed a prostate-specific membrane antigen (PSMA) volume-based criteria to define low-volume and high-volume disease. PSMA low-volume disease (PSMA LVD) is defined as any unifocal, oligometastatic, or disseminated disease <40cm^3, whereas PSMA high-volume disease (PSMA HVD) is defined as oligometastatic or disseminated disease ≥40 cm^3 or

N. Kumar · R. Madan · J. Subalakshmi · S. Goyal
Department of Radiotherapy and Oncology, Postgraduate Institute of Medical Education and Research (PGIMER), Chandigarh, India

A. K. Yadav (✉)
Department of Radiotherapy and Radiation Medicine, Banaras Hindu University, Varanasi, Uttar Pradesh, India

R. Madan, S. Goyal (eds.), *Essentials of Radiotherapy in Uro-Genital Malignancies*, https://doi.org/10.1007/978-981-95-5945-9_7

visceral metastasis [4]. This approach seems more pragmatic and shifting emphasis from simple lesion count to composite metastatic burden.

Broadly, OMPC can be categorized into three types: de novo synchronous oligometastatic hormone-sensitive prostate cancer (HSPC), metachronous oligorecurrent HSPC, and oligoprogressive castration-resistant prostate cancer (CRPC). For standardization of the nomenclature, European Organisation for Research and Treatment of Cancer (EORTC) and European Society of Radiation Therapy and Oncology (ESTRO) have introduced a classification framework, which identifies nine types of OMPC [5].

7.2 Diagnosis of OMPC

Identification of OMPC provides an opportunity for MDT and eradication of all metastatic sites with local therapy. As of now, the definition of OMPC strongly depends on the imaging, and the effectiveness of local therapy will depend on the ability of the imaging to identify the metastatic disease. Key trials guiding the management of OMPC is based on the conventional imaging such as computed tomography (CT) scan and bone scintigraphy, posing a challenge due to adoption of prostate-specific membrane antigen positron emission tomography (PSMA PET) for staging in prostate cancer. PSMA PET is superior to identify bone and lymph nodal metastasis compared to conventional imaging and bone scintigraphy, even at lower prostate-specific antigen (PSA) levels [6]. In a study of CRPC patients with high risk of metastasis, no metastatic disease was identified on conventional imaging, but PSMA PET was able to identify nodal disease and distant metastasis in 44 and 55% patients, respectively, out of which 14% were OMPC [7]. One study showed that SBRT to all PSMA-avid sites improves distant metastasis-free survival, highlighting the importance of metastasis disease identified on PSMA PET [8]. ESTRO-ACROP guidelines recommend PSMA-PET to diagnose metastatic disease and for MDT, until more sensitive imaging tools become available [9]. Once diagnosed with PSMA PET, confirmatory magnetic resonance imaging (MRI) or biopsy should be done in selected cases.

7.3 Management of OMPC

The management of OMPC varies depending on whether the disease is de novo or metachronous HSPC or oligoprogressive CRPC. The treatment options includes systemic therapy and local therapy for primary site along with MDT. ESTRO ACROP guidelines recommend that MDT can be considered for lesions up to 5 in number [9]. Studies have shown that total consolidation of all PSMA-avid sites by MDT is associated with improved outcome [8]. There is a paucity of data on MDT in visceral metastasis, though there is some evidence that MDT improves outcome in carefully selected prostate cancer patients with visceral metastasis [10–12]. As per the latest recommendation, all patients of OMPC irrespective of the age and comorbidities should be considered for MDT. There are no guidelines to decide MDT based on the time interval between primary treatment and oligo recurrent disease.

The rationale for aggressive local therapy in oligometastatic cancer patients stems mostly from surgical experience, where metastasectomies for various tumors have improved outcome. The main concept is that removal of tumor clones that give rise to metastasis will reduce the risk of metastasis and improve OS. Local therapy leads to cytoreduction and reduction in circulating tumor cells [13]. This minimizes the cytokine-mediated interaction between primary and metastatic sites, which may reduce the progression of the metastatic disease. MDT may also produce the abscopal effect by immunomodulation. MDT with stereotactic body radiotherapy (SBRT) can also induce antitumor immunity by immunogenic cell death and release of tumor-associated antigens, the process, responsible for systemic anti-tumor effects or abscopal effect. Total therapy comprising of MDT along with prostatic irradiation and ADT may be a key approach to improve outcome in oligometastatic HSPC patients [14, 15].

7.4 Evidence for Local Therapy to Prostate (Primary Site)

Local treatment for primary tumor may include surgery or radiotherapy (RT). Though the role is not well established, those with fewer than four metastases (none outside vertebral bodies and pelvis) and without visceral metastasis may get benefit from the local treatment to the prostate. Observational studies have shown that local treatment to prostate with either surgery or radiotherapy in addition to androgen-deprivation therapy (ADT) improves overall survival (OS) compared to ADT alone [16, 17].

Radiotherapy as local therapy Radiotherapy is one of the most important local therapeutic strategies for management of OMPC, though there are variations in the RT dose/fractionation and combination with systemic therapy. Investigators from HORRAD trial reported that prostate RT, in addition to ADT, in patients with metastatic prostate cancer improved median time to progression but not the overall survival (OS) [18]. Later in an unplanned analysis, a non-significant improvement in median OS was observed in those with fewer than five metastases. There was an increase in urinary symptoms and diarrhea after RT, which resolved at 3 months. In STAMPEDE trial, hypofractionated RT to prostate (36Gy/6 fractions weekly or 55 GY/20 fractions daily) improved OS at 61.3 months in low-burden metastatic disease compared to ADT with or without chemotherapy, without detrimental effect on quality of life (QOL), which indicates that prostate RT should be the standard of care (SOC) in low-burden metastatic disease [19]. Prostate RT did not improve OS in high-burden metastatic prostate cancer patients [20]. There was slight increase in acute and late bladder and bowel toxicity with RT (5% vs 1% and 1% vs 0% respectively). STOPCAP meta-analysis showed that addition of RT improved biochemical progression-free survival (PFS) and failure-free survival (FFS), which translated into 10% benefit at 3 years for the entire cohort [21]. Though there was no significant improvement in the survival for the entire cohort, the OS benefit in those with fewer than five metastases resulted in 7% survival benefit at 3 years in this group of the patients. PEACE-1 trial showed that prostate RT significantly improved PFS and delayed castration resistance in low-volume metastatic disease [22].

Surgery as local therapy The role of surgical debulking or radical prostatectomy (RP) is not well established in OMPC patients and is not considered as an SOC. TROMBONE trial showed that RP is safe and should be further investigated in prostate cancer patients with limited metastasis [23]. In total eradication trial, men with fewer than five metastasis received SBRT to all sites, fixed duration ADT, and surgery for the primary [24]. At a median follow-up of 48 months, 3-year biochemical FFS was seen in 67% of the patients. Salvage lymph node dissection (LND) is a less commonly followed approach. In PEACE V STROM trial, only 6% patients underwent salvage LND [25]. Results from ongoing trials such as SWOG S1802 and g-RAMMP are awaited to validate the role of surgery in OMPC patients [26].

Evidence for metastatis-directed therapy MDT is a promising approach in OMPC patients; however, there is no high-quality data to determine its role. The data on how MDT should be integrated with ADT and systemic therapy is also unclear. Several phase 2 trials have suggested that MDT improves PFS in prostate cancer patients with limited metastasis, but long-term data is lacking. MDT alone may improve outcome in selected patients with oligorecurrent disease. STOMP trial compared surveillance versus MDT in patients with oligo-progressive HSPC (up to three metastases diagnosed on choline PET) and found that MDT significantly improved 5-year ADT-free survival compared to surveillance (34% vs 8%), although five-year survival was similar [27]. ORIOLE trial, a phase II randomized controlled trial (RCT), compared SBRT versus observation in one- to three-nodal or bony metastases (diagnosed on conventional imaging) in oligoprogressive HSPC patients [8]. At 6-month follow up, progression occurred in 19% patients in SBRT arm compared to 61% in observation arm. SBRT significantly improved median PFS, 5.8 months versus not reached. The pooled analysis from STOME and ORIOLE suggests that MDT is associated with almost doubling of PFS (11.9 months versus 5.9 months, $p < 0.001$) in oligoprogressive HSPC [28]. Twenty percent patients remained progression free at 4 years. In contrast, one multi-institutional study showed that MDT alone did not provide durable PFS in 90% of the patients [29].

In the EXTEND trial, oligorecurrent HSPCs were randomized to receive intermittent ADT alone versus intermittent ADT and MDT [30]. Addition of MDT significantly improved biochemical PFS at 22 months. Intensification of systemic therapy beyond ADT was delayed in 85% of the patients in MDT arm compared with 53% in the non-MDT arm, at 1 year.

In one meta-analysis consisting of 15 case series, 450 oligoprogressive HSPC patients were identified with PET-CT [31]. Nodal, bone, and visceral metastases were treated in 78%, 21%, and 1% patients, respectively. Patients with nodal metastases were treated with RT or LND. Approximately half of the patients were progression free at 1–3 years after salvage MDT, with most of them receiving adjuvant ADT. Approximately 8–10% patients had RT or surgery-related complications. Another systematic review reported complete biochemical response in 13–80% of the patients after salvage LND [32]. Five-year biochemical FFS rate was observed in 6–31% of the patients.

OLIGOPELVIS GETUG P076 studied the role of high-dose salvage RT (54 Gy at 1.8 Gy/ fraction) with SIB (66 Gy/2.2 Gy/fraction) and short-term ADT (6 months) in 67 oligorecurrent HSPC patients with choline PET-positive isolated recurrence in pelvis [33]. After a median follow-up of 49.4 months, more than half of the patients (58%) remained disease free at 3 years.

SOLAR trial evaluated de novo oligometastatic HSPC patients, staged with PSMA PET and treated with MDT with SBRT along with combination of ADT with androgen receptor pathway inhibitors (ARPI) and local therapy with surgery or RT. [34] The authors found that 83% of the patients achieved the primary end point of undetectable PSA (post RP) or PSA <2 ng/ml (post RT).

In SABR-COMET trial, variety of primary cancer patients with one to five metastases were randomized to palliative SOC alone versus SOC and SBRT [35]. The trial showed that SBRT significantly improved OS compared to SOC alone (42% vs 18%, *p*-0.006).

Ongoing trials such as STAMPEDE 2 SBRT, PLATON trial, TERPS trial, and OLIGO PRESTO trial are evaluating the role of SBRT in addition to SOC in newly diagnosed hormone-sensitive OMPC patients.

The treatment options for CRPC include ARPI, ADT, chemotherapy, and radioisotope therapy, yet the outcome in these patients is less favorable. While systemic therapy is important to eliminate sensitive clones, SBRT could help in the elimination of the resistant clones and delays progression [15]. ARTO trial evaluated the role of SBRT with first-line ARPI in oligometastatic CRPC and found that addition of SBRT significantly improved PFS and freedom from next treatment [36]. A phase II TRAP trial also confirmed that SBRT in oligoprogressive CRPC is safe and improves QoL [37].

Immunomodulation is one of the important advantage of SBRT. In OPeRATIC trial, which studied castration-resistant prostate cancer (CRPC) patients with fewer than three metastases, response to SBRT was correlated with immune cell population [38]. Two-year OS and PSA PFS were 80% and 21%, respectively. The baseline high level of tumor effector T cells and memory cells was associated with superior OS. Post SBRT increase in T cell improved distant and PSA PFS. The study highlights the importance of incorporation of immune-based markers in future SBRT trials particularly in CRPC patients.

The WOLVERINE meta-analysis analyzed 472 patients and compared SOC alone versus SOC with SBRT MDT in OMPC [39]. It was reported that MDT improves PFS across all subgroups, regardless of primary treatment status, staging, castration status, and use of ADT.

The main obstacle in obtaining the favorable outcome is identification of the patients with truly limited number of metastasis and microscopic disease which makes the patient resistant to local and systemic therapy. Unfavorable outcome in some of the MDT trials are because the metastases were identified on the conventional imaging and not on the more sensitive choline-PET or PSMA-PET, which might have missed few of the metastases.

Currently, most centers now adopt an individualized approach to metastatis-directed therapy based on the patient's age, comorbidities, performance status, site and number of metastasis, and PSA doubling time. Metabolic and genomic parameters are emerging as a key determinant for escalating or de-escalating treatment strategies. Those with longer PSA doubling time may get benefitted with MDT alone, while those with shorter PSA doubling time and harboring high-risk mutation (BRCA1 &2, TP53) may require systemic therapy, in addition to MDT.

RT dose and target volume for metastatic disease According to the ESTRO-ACROP consensus guidelines, the bone lesions should be treated when there is PET uptake along with the radiological lesion [9]. Standard guidelines should be followed for target delineation [40–42]. Gross tumor volume (GTV) for spinal lesion consists of the visible lesion, whereas clinical target volume consists of entire vertebral body to avoid marginal failure. Simultaneous integrated boost (SIB) is preferred. For extra-spinal lesion, variable CTV margin (1–5 mm) is recommended based on the location. There is insufficient data to decide the optimal dose for bone metastasis, and studies have shown that biologically effective dose (BED) of >100 Gy improves local control [12]. Spinal lesions can be treated with various dose fractionation regimen including 30–35 Gy/5fractions, 27 Gy/3fractions, and 30 Gy/3fractions. For pelvic nodal metastasis, elective nodal irradiation (ENRT) with a boost to gross node is recommended. There is no consensus for SBRT vs ENRT, though most of the panelists in ESTRO ACROP group agreed for SBRT for 1–3 nodes and ENRT for 4–5 nodes. Earlier guidelines suggest that ENRT may offer better freedom from failure compared with SBRT but at the cost of increased toxicity.

For ENRT, a dose of 45–50 Gy/25fractions is recommended with a SIB to positive lymph nodes (2.2–2.7 Gy/fraction) [9]. It is recommended to include prostate bed in ENRT volume, if high risk (pT3/4 or R1) and if not treated previously. Following pelvic LND, whole pelvic radiotherapy (WPRT) can be given with or without ADT. PEACE V STROM trial is the first randomized controlled trial (RCT) of SBRT (30 Gy/3 fractions) versus ENRT (45/65 Gy in 25 fractions) along with 6 months of ADT in oligorecurrent patients [25]. Despite treating larger volume in ENRT, there was no difference in acute toxicity or patient-reported outcome in both of the trials. At a median follow-up of 4 years, ENRT demonstrated improved metastasis-free survival (MFS) compared with SBRT—76% versus 63%, respectively (*p*-0.06).

Figure 7.1 shows radiotherapy dose color wash of a patient with OMPC, treated simultaneously to the prostate, pelvic lymph nodes, and bony metastasis. Radiotherapy doses were as follows: 44 Gy/20 fractions to pelvic lymph nodes,

48/57.6/60 Gy/20 fractions to prostate and seminal vesicles, and 57.6 Gy in 20 fractions to bone metastasis.

Figure 7.2 depicts a dose color wash of a SBRT treatment plan for an oligorecurrent HSPC patient, treated with 24/28 Gy in two fractions to the bone (humoral) metastasis.

Figure 7.3 shows a dose color wash of oligorecurrent HSPC (pelvic lymph node and bone metastasis). The patient received ENRT 44 Gy/20 fractions with SIB to involved node to a total dose of 56 Gy along with SBRT for vertebral metastasis to a dose of 30/35 Gy in 5 fractions.

Optimal timing of SABR in the course of prostate cancer treatment It's worth noting that the optimal use of SABR in oligo-metastatic prostate cancer, including its timing, is still an area of ongoing research. Future studies may indeed focus on determining the best timing for SABR in the overall treatment strategy for prostate cancer.

Definition of biochemical recurrence after metastasis-directed RT As per ESTRO-ACROP guidelines, biochemical recurrence after MDT is defined as nadir +2 ng/ml (Phoenix definition) and PSA >0.2 ng/ml for those with prostate in place and post-prostatectomy patients, respectively [9]. Few experts recommend that any elevation above the baseline (pre-RT) should be considered as biochemical recurrence.

Systemic therapy Systemic therapy is one of the important modalities in the management of metastatic prostate cancer patients. Combination therapy with ADT and ARPI (Enzalutamide or Abiraterone or Apalutamide or Darolutamide) has significantly improved outcome in these patients, but has a negative impact on QOL. Thus, many men with OMPC can be spared from ADT, the prerequisite for this would be to identify patients with minimal residual disease by advanced imaging.

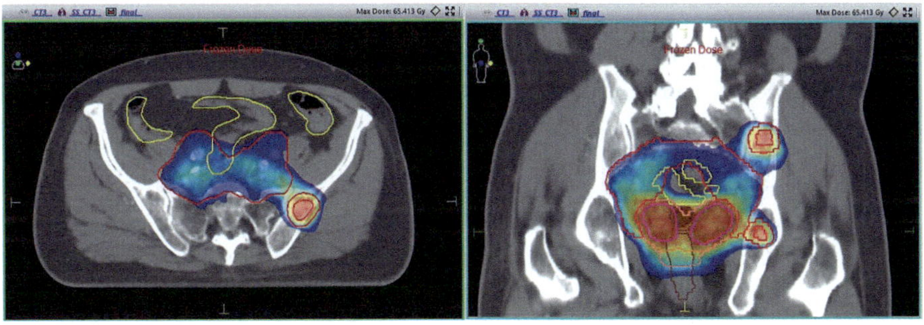

Fig. 7.1 Radiotherapy dose color wash of a patient with OMPC, treated simultaneously to the prostate, pelvic lymph nodes, and bony metastasis. Radiotherapy doses were as follows: 44 Gy/20 fractions to pelvic lymph nodes, 48/57.6/60 Gy/20 fractions to prostate and seminal vesicles, and 57.6 Gy in 20 fractions to bone metastasis

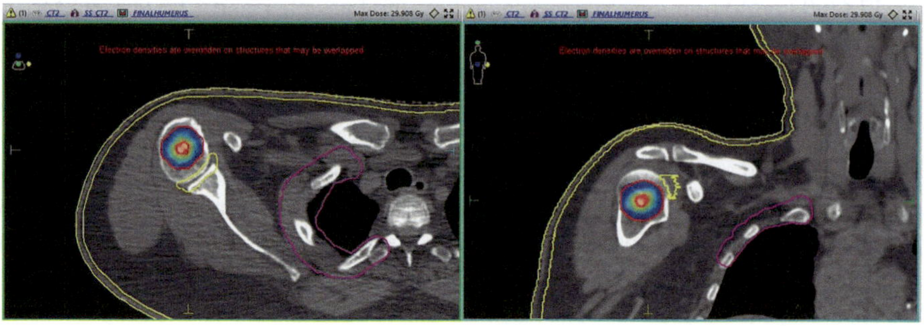

Fig. 7.2 A dose color wash of a SBRT treatment plan for an oligorecurrent HSPC patient, treated with 24/28 Gy in two fractions to the bone (humoral) metastasis

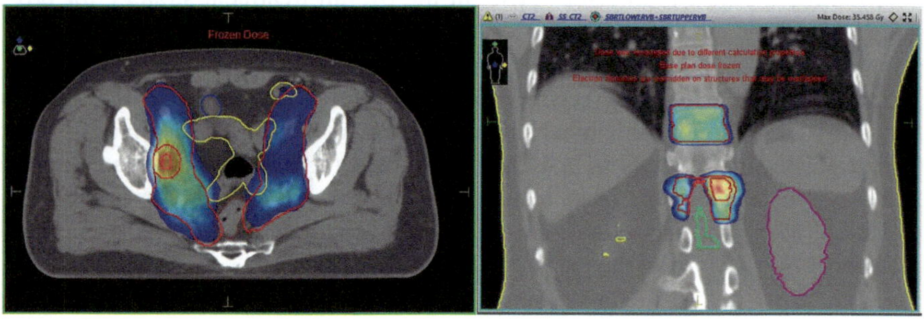

Fig. 7.3 A dose color wash of an oligorecurrent HSPC (pelvic lymph node and bone metastasis). The patient received ENRT 44 Gy/20 fractions with SIB to involved node to a total dose of 56 Gy along with SBRT for vertebral metastasis to a dose of 30/35 Gy in 5 fractions

The proportion of patients receiving systemic therapy in OMPC patients is variable across the clinical trials. None of the patients received systemic therapy in HORRAD trial. In STAMPEDE-H trial, 18% and 0% patients received Docetaxel and Abiraterone, while in PEACE-1 trial, 49% and 52% patients received Docetaxel and Abiraterone, respectively.

RADIOSA trial randomized oligorecurrent HSPC patients to MDT SBRT alone versus MDT SBRT and short-term ADT [43]. At a median follow-up of 27 months, addition of ADT significantly improved biochemical progression-free survival (26.8 months) compared with 12.6 months with SBRT alone.

ESTRO ACROP guidelines recommend a short-course ADT with MDT to all patients, though ADT can be avoided in carefully selected patients with low risk of recurrence. Advanced prostate cancer consortium recommends the duration of systemic therapy for 18–36 months when MDT was given to all sites. The results of ADOPT trial are awaited to define the role of ADT in addition to MDT [44]. Ongoing SPARKLE trial is randomizing PSMA PET-detected hormone-sensitive OMPC patients to SBRT alone versus SBRT and 1 month or 6 months of ADT and Enzalutamide.

Due to the lack of comparative data, the choice of novel hormonal agent is based on patients age, general condition, comorbidities, and preference [45–48].

Radioligant therapy (RLT) is a promising approach to reduce the minimal residual disease following MDT. In BULLSEYE trial, hormone-sensitive prostate cancer patients with one to five metastases were randomized to receive two to four cycles of 177Lu-PSMA-617 versus deferred ADT [49]. At 6 months, 177Lu-PSMA-617 therapy significantly improved PFS. Based on this, LUNAR trial is evaluating the role of RLT in addition to MDT in oligorecurrent HSPC.

7.5 Conclusion

While awaiting the results of phase III clinical trials, current evidence suggest that MDT should be integrated in the management of patients with OMPC, though additional data is required to determine how MDT and ADT should be integrated. Careful patient selection is crucial for treatment escalation or de-escalation for achieving optimal outcome and QOL.

References

1. Hellman S, Weichselbaum RR. Oligometastases. J Clin Oncol Off J Am Soc Clin Oncol. 1995;13(1):8–10.
2. Sridharan S, Steigler A, Spry NA, Joseph D, Lamb DS, Matthews JH, et al. Oligometastatic bone disease in prostate cancer patients treated on the TROG 03.04 RADAR trial. Radiother Oncol. 2016;121(1):98–102.
3. Foster CC, Weichselbaum RR, Pitroda SP. Oligometastatic prostate cancer: reality or figment of imagination? Cancer. 2019;125(3):340–52.
4. Barbato F, Fendler WP, Rauscher I, Herrmann K, Wetter A, Ferdinandus J, et al. PSMA-PET for the assessment of metastatic hormone-sensitive prostate cancer volume of disease. J Nucl Med. 2021;62(12):1747–50.
5. Guckenberger M, Lievens Y, Bouma AB, Collette L, Dekker A, deSouza NM, et al. Characterisation and classification of oligometastatic disease: a European Society for Radiotherapy and Oncology and European Organisation for Research and Treatment of Cancer consensus recommendation. Lancet Oncol. 2020;21(1):e18–28.
6. Perera M, Papa N, Roberts M, Williams M, Udovicich C, Vela I, et al. Gallium-68 prostate-specific membrane antigen positron emission tomography in advanced prostate cancer-updated diagnostic utility, sensitivity, specificity, and distribution of prostate-specific membrane antigen-avid lesions: a systematic review and meta-analysis. Eur Urol. 2020;77(4):403–17.
7. Fendler WP, Weber M, Iravani A, Hofman MS, Calais J, Czernin J, et al. Prostate-specific membrane antigen ligand positron emission tomography in men with nonmetastatic castration-resistant prostate cancer. Clin Cancer Res. 2019;25(24):7448–54.
8. Phillips R, Shi WY, Deek M, Radwan N, Lim SJ, Antonarakis ES, et al. Outcomes of observation vs stereotactic ablative radiation for oligometastatic prostate cancer: the ORIOLE phase 2 randomized clinical trial. JAMA Oncol. 2020;6(5):650–9.
9. Zilli T, Achard V, Dal Pra A, Schmidt-Hegemann N, Jereczek-Fossa BA, Lancia A, et al. Recommendations for radiation therapy in oligometastatic prostate cancer: an ESTRO-ACROP Delphi consensus. Radiother Oncol J Eur Soc Ther Radiol Oncol. 2022;176:199–207.

10. Connor MJ, Smith A, Miah S, Shah TT, Winkler M, Khoo V, et al. Targeting oligometastasis with stereotactic ablative radiation therapy or surgery in metastatic hormone-sensitive prostate cancer: a systematic review of prospective clinical trials. Eur Urol Oncol. 2020;3(5):582–93.
11. Battaglia A, Devos G, Decaestecker K, Witters M, Moris L, Van den Broeck T, et al. Metastasectomy for visceral and skeletal oligorecurrent prostate cancer. World J Urol. 2019;37(8):1543–9.
12. Ost P, Jereczek-Fossa BA, As NV, Zilli T, Muacevic A, Olivier K, et al. Progression-free survival following stereotactic body radiotherapy for oligometastatic prostate cancer treatment-naive recurrence: a multi-institutional analysis. Eur Urol. 2016;69(1):9–12.
13. Connor MJ, Shah TT, Horan G, Bevan CL, Winkler M, Ahmed HU. Cytoreductive treatment strategies for de novo metastatic prostate cancer. Nat Rev Clin Oncol. 2020;17(3):168–82.
14. Sutera PA, Shetty AC, Hakansson A, Van der Eecken K, Song Y, Liu Y, et al. Transcriptomic and clinical heterogeneity of metastatic disease timing within metastatic castration-sensitive prostate cancer. Ann Oncol. 2023;34(7):605–14.
15. Singh M, Murthy V, Ost P. Debate 3: metastasis directed therapy in oligometastatic prostate cancer. Semin Radiat Oncol. 2025;35(3):423–32.
16. Rusthoven CG, Jones BL, Flaig TW, Crawford ED, Koshy M, Sher DJ, et al. Improved survival with prostate radiation in addition to androgen deprivation therapy for men with newly diagnosed metastatic prostate cancer. J Clin Oncol Off J Am Soc Clin Oncol. 2016;34(24):2835–42.
17. Löppenberg B, Dalela D, Karabon P, Sood A, Sammon JD, Meyer CP, et al. The impact of local treatment on overall survival in patients with metastatic prostate cancer on diagnosis: a National Cancer Data Base Analysis. Eur Urol. 2017;72(1):14–9.
18. Boevé LMS, Hulshof MCCM, Vis AN, Zwinderman AH, Twisk JWR, Witjes WPJ, et al. Effect on survival of androgen deprivation therapy alone compared to androgen deprivation therapy combined with concurrent radiation therapy to the prostate in patients with primary bone metastatic prostate cancer in a prospective randomised clinical trial: data from the HORRAD trial. Eur Urol. 2019;75(3):410–8.
19. Parker CC, James ND, Brawley CD, Clarke NW, Ali A, Amos CL, et al. Radiotherapy to the prostate for men with metastatic prostate cancer in the UK and Switzerland: long-term results from the STAMPEDE randomised controlled trial. PLoS Med. 2022;19(6):e1003998.
20. Parker CC, James ND, Brawley CD, Clarke NW, Hoyle AP, Ali A, et al. Radiotherapy to the primary tumour for newly diagnosed, metastatic prostate cancer (STAMPEDE): a randomised controlled phase 3 trial. Lancet. 2018;392(10162):2353–66.
21. Burdett S, Boevé LM, Ingleby FC, Fisher DJ, Rydzewska LH, Vale CL, et al. Prostate radiotherapy for metastatic hormone-sensitive prostate cancer: a STOPCAP systematic review and meta-analysis. Eur Urol. 2019;76(1):115–24.
22. Bossi A, Foulon S, Maldonado X, Sargos P, MacDermott R, Kelly P, et al. Efficacy and safety of prostate radiotherapy in de novo metastatic castration-sensitive prostate cancer (PEACE-1): a multicentre, open-label, randomised, phase 3 study with a 2 × 2 factorial design. Lancet. 2024;404(10467):2065–76.
23. Sooriakumaran P, Wilson C, Rombach I, Hassanali N, Aning J, D Lamb A, et al. Feasibility and safety of radical prostatectomy for oligo-metastatic prostate cancer: the Testing Radical prostatectomy in men with prostate cancer and oligo-Metastases to the bone (TRoMbone) trial. BJU Int. 2022;130(1):43–53.
24. Reyes DK, Trock BJ, Tran PT, Pavlovich CP, Deville C, Allaf ME, et al. Interim analysis of companion, prospective, phase II, clinical trials assessing the efficacy and safety of multimodal total eradication therapy in men with synchronous oligometastatic prostate cancer. Med Oncol. 2022;39(5):63.
25. Ost P, Siva S, Brabrand S, Dirix P, Liefhooghe N, Otte FX, et al. PEACE V-Salvage Treatment of OligoRecurrent nodal prostate cancer Metastases (STORM): acute toxicity of a randomized phase 2 trial. Eur Urol Oncol. 2024;7(3):462–8.
26. Ranasinghe W, Chapin BF, Kim IY, Sooriakumaran P, Lawrentschuk N. The cytoreductive prostatectomy in metastatic prostate cancer: what the individual trials are hoping to answer. BJU Int. 2020;125(6):792–800.

27. Surveillance or metastasis-directed therapy for oligometastatic prostate cancer recurrence (STOMP): Five-year results of a randomized phase II trial. | J Clin Oncol [Internet]. [cited 2025 Jun 18]. Available from: https://ascopubs.org/doi/10.1200/JCO.2020.38.6_suppl.10.
28. Deek MP, Van der Eecken K, Sutera P, Deek RA, Fonteyne V, Mendes AA, et al. Long-term outcomes and genetic predictors of response to metastasis-directed therapy versus observation in oligometastatic prostate cancer: analysis of STOMP and ORIOLE trials. J Clin Oncol. 2022;40(29):3377–82.
29. Deek MP, Sutera P, Jing Y, Gao R, Rothman E, Day H, et al. Multi-institutional analysis of metastasis-directed therapy with or without androgen deprivation therapy in oligometastatic castration-sensitive prostate cancer. Eur Urol Oncol. 2024;7(6):1403–10.
30. Tang C, Sherry AD, Haymaker C, Bathala T, Liu S, Fellman B, et al. Addition of metastasis-directed therapy to intermittent hormone therapy for oligometastatic prostate cancer: the EXTEND phase 2 randomized clinical trial. JAMA Oncol. 2023;9(6):825–34.
31. Ost P, Bossi A, Decaestecker K, De Meerleer G, Giannarini G, Karnes RJ, et al. Metastasis-directed therapy of regional and distant recurrences after curative treatment of prostate cancer: a systematic review of the literature. Eur Urol. 2015;67(5):852–63.
32. Ploussard G, Gandaglia G, Borgmann H, de Visschere P, Heidegger I, Kretschmer A, et al. Salvage lymph node dissection for nodal recurrent prostate cancer: a systematic review. Eur Urol. 2019;76(4):493–504.
33. Supiot S, Vaugier L, Pasquier D, Buthaud X, Magné N, Peiffert D, et al. OLIGOPELVIS GETUG P07, a multicenter phase II trial of combined high-dose salvage radiotherapy and hormone therapy in oligorecurrent pelvic node relapses in prostate cancer. Eur Urol. 2021;80(4):405–14.
34. Nickols NG, Tsai S, Kane N, Tran S, Ghayouri L, Diaz-Perez S, et al. Systemic and tumor-directed therapy for oligometastatic prostate cancer: the SOLAR phase 2 trial in De Novo oligometastatic prostate cancer. Eur Urol. 2024;86(2):190–3.
35. Palma DA, Olson R, Harrow S, Gaede S, Louie AV, Haasbeek C, et al. Stereotactic ablative radiotherapy for the comprehensive treatment of oligometastatic cancers: long-term results of the SABR-COMET phase II randomized trial. J Clin Oncol Off J Am Soc Clin Oncol. 2020;38(25):2830–8.
36. Francolini G, Allegra AG, Detti B, Di Cataldo V, Caini S, Bruni A, et al. Stereotactic body radiation therapy and abiraterone acetate for patients affected by oligometastatic castrate-resistant prostate cancer: a randomized phase II trial (ARTO). J Clin Oncol Off J Am Soc Clin Oncol. 2023;41(36):5561–8.
37. Patel PH, Dreibe S, Reid A, Parker C, Murray J, Pathmanathan A, et al. Stereotactic body radiotherapy for oligoprogression in castration-resistant prostate cancer: early toxicity analysis of the TRAP trial. Clin Oncol R Coll Radiol G B. 2024;36(9):585–92.
38. Zhang H, Orme JJ, Abraha F, Stish BJ, Lowe VJ, Lucien F, et al. Phase II evaluation of stereotactic ablative radiotherapy (SABR) and immunity in 11C-choline-PET/CT-identified oligometastatic castration-resistant prostate cancer. Clin Cancer Res. 2021;27(23):6376–83.
39. World-wide oligometastatic prostate cancer (omPC) meta-analysis leveraging individual patient data (IPD) from randomized trials (WOLVERINE): An analysis from the X-MET collaboration. | Journal of Clinical Oncology [Internet]. [cited 2025 Jul 1]. Available from: https://ascopubs.org/doi/10.1200/JCO.2025.43.5_suppl.15
40. Cox BW, Spratt DE, Lovelock M, Bilsky MH, Lis E, Ryu S, et al. International Spine Radiosurgery Consortium consensus guidelines for target volume definition in spinal stereotactic radiosurgery. Int J Radiat Oncol Biol Phys. 2012;83(5):e597–605.
41. Dunne EM, Sahgal A, Lo SS, Bergman A, Kosztyla R, Dea N, et al. International consensus recommendations for target volume delineation specific to sacral metastases and spinal stereotactic body radiation therapy (SBRT). Radiother Oncol J Eur Soc Ther Radiol Oncol. 2020;145:21–9.
42. Nguyen TK, Chin L, Sahgal A, Dagan R, Eppinga W, Guckenberger M, et al. International multi-institutional patterns of contouring practice and clinical target volume recommendations

for stereotactic body radiation therapy for non-spine bone metastases. Int J Radiat Oncol Biol Phys. 2022;112(2):351–60.
43. Marvaso G, Corrao G, Zaffaroni M, Vincini MG, Lorubbio C, Gandini S, et al. ADT with SBRT versus SBRT alone for hormone-sensitive oligorecurrent prostate cancer (RADIOSA): a randomised, open-label, phase 2 clinical trial. Lancet Oncol. 2025;26(3):300–11.
44. Janssen J, Staal FHE, Brouwer CL, Langendijk JA, de Jong IJ, van Moorselaar RJA, et al. Androgen deprivation therapy for oligo-recurrent prostate cancer in addition to radioTherapy (ADOPT): study protocol for a randomised phase III trial. BMC Cancer. 2022;22(1):482.
45. Fizazi K, Tran N, Fein L, Matsubara N, Rodriguez-Antolin A, Alekseev BY, et al. Abiraterone plus prednisone in metastatic, castration-sensitive prostate cancer. N Engl J Med. 2017;377(4):352–60.
46. Chi KN, Protheroe A, Rodríguez-Antolín A, Facchini G, Suttman H, Matsubara N, et al. Patient-reported outcomes following abiraterone acetate plus prednisone added to androgen deprivation therapy in patients with newly diagnosed metastatic castration-naive prostate cancer (LATITUDE): an international, randomised phase 3 trial. Lancet Oncol. 2018;19(2):194–206.
47. Sathianathen NJ, Koschel S, Thangasamy IA, Teh J, Alghazo O, Butcher G, et al. Indirect comparisons of efficacy between combination approaches in metastatic hormone-sensitive prostate cancer: a systematic review and network meta-analysis. Eur Urol. 2020;77(3):365–72.
48. Attard G, Murphy L, Clarke NW, Sachdeva A, Jones C, Hoyle A, et al. Abiraterone acetate plus prednisolone with or without enzalutamide for patients with metastatic prostate cancer starting androgen deprivation therapy: final results from two randomised phase 3 trials of the STAMPEDE platform protocol. Lancet Oncol. 2023;24(5):443–56.
49. Privé BM, Janssen MJR, van Oort IM, Muselaers CHJ, Jonker MA, van Gemert WA, et al. Update to a randomized controlled trial of lutetium-177-PSMA in oligo-metastatic hormone-sensitive prostate cancer: the BULLSEYE trial. Trials. 2021;22(1):768.

Management of CRPC (Metastatic and Non-metastatic)

8

Lakhan Kashyap

Prostate cancer is an androgen-driven tumor. In castration-resistant prostate cancer (CRPC), there is continued androgen pathway signaling despite low circulating androgens and androgen receptor blockade. CRPC is an aggressive disease with median survival ranging from 12 to 24 months.

8.1 Definition

The biochemical (PSA) and/or clinicoradiological progression of prostate cancer in the background of castrate level of testosterone (less than 50 ng/mL) heralds CRPC [1].

CRPC is a heterogeneous group that includes:

1. Non-metastatic CRPC: Prostate cancer characterized by rising PSA levels without loco-regional or metastatic progression.
2. Metastatic CRPC: There is progression in the metastatic site. This may occur in de novo metastatic disease wherein the patients may have received taxane or androgen receptor pathway inhibitors (ARPi). This subgroup will have a different prognosis than those who develop CRPC after loco-regional treatment of limited prostate cancer.

8.2 Molecular Mechanism of Androgen Resistance

Mechanism underpinning CRPC can be divided into androgen receptor (AR)-driven and AR-indifferent resistance.

L. Kashyap (✉)
Department of Medical Oncology, Manipal Hospitals, Pune, Maharashtra, India

R. Madan, S. Goyal (eds.), *Essentials of Radiotherapy in Uro-Genital Malignancies*, https://doi.org/10.1007/978-981-95-5945-9_8

1. AR-driven resistance: The most common mechanism of AR-driven resistance is through the amplification of androgen receptors. Mutations in the AR ligand-binding domain (W742C, H875Y, T878A, and F877L) are seen in 15–20% of CRPC patients. These mutations prevent androgens from binding to AR and, in some cases, can paradoxically lead to activation by an AR antagonist [2]. Alternative splicing of AR transcripts can generate AR splice variants. They exhibit truncation of the carboxy terminal ligand-binding domain while retaining the amino terminal transactivation domain and DNA-binding domain. AR-V7 is the best characterized splice variant. It leads to metabolic rewiring to produce a more bioenergetic state, which supports the progression of CRPC in a hypoxic environment [3].
2. AR-indifferent resistance: This occurs through the activation of non-androgen signaling pathways, including FGF signaling, TGFβ pathway, and RAS/RAF/MAPK pathway [4]. An important androgen-independent mechanism is the lineage plasticity of prostate adenocarcinoma. There are underlying genetic and epigenetic changes (RB1 loss and TP53 mutation and overexpression of histone methyltransferase *EZH2* gene) that promote neuroendocrine differentiation [5].

8.3 Evaluation of the CRPC

1. Imaging: Trials evaluating patients with CRPC have used conventional imaging, which includes CECT thorax, abdomen, and pelvis and Tc-99m methyl diphosphonate scintigraphy (bone scan). Prostate-specific radionuclide ligand-based PET CT has higher sensitivity than conventional imaging; however, its clinical impact is still evolving. The decision for PET-CT should be individualized and considered where it can impact clinical decision.
2. PSA progression: As per the Prostate Cancer Working Group 3, it is defined as a 25% increase in value from the nadir along with a minimum rise of 2 ng/mL. Apart from the absolute value of PSA, the kinetics of PSA rise has also been used in some nmCRPC trials (PSA doubling time <10 months).
3. Molecular testing:
   (a) HRR deficiency: Germline or somatic mutations in HRR pathway genes help identify patients who may respond to PARP inhibitors. Apart from *BRCA1/2*, pathogenic variants can be observed in *ATM, CHEK2, PALB2, FANCA, RAD51B/C/D,* and *BRIP1* [6]. Both somatic and germline testing should be considered. Germline testing alone may miss 50% of somatic *BRCA,* whereas somatic testing by tumor sequencing alone may miss pathogenic germline variants [7, 8].
   (b) NGS: This may identify targetable mutations such as NTRK fusion where specific TKI is available and high MSI tumors where immune checkpoint inhibitors can be administered.

8.4 Prognostic Factors

1. Clinical parameters: PSA kinetics with shorter PSA doubling time have been associated with poor prognosis [9]. Poor performance status (ECOG PS ≥ 2), visceral metastases, elevated LDH or ALP, low serum albumin and hemoglobin, and use of opioid analgesics portend poor survival in CRPC [10]. Prior treatment such as ADT alone or doublet (ADT+ APRi/taxane) or triplet (ADT+ARPi+taxane) also impacts prognosis.
2. Circulating tumor cells: Presence of ≥5 CTCs per 7.5 mL has been shown to be associated with poor survival [11, 12]. Similarly, a change in the number of CTCs is associated with response to treatment [13].
3. Neuroendocrine differentiation: Although de novo neuroendocrine carcinoma of the prostate is rare, previous ADT for adenocarcinoma may lead to the emergence of neuroendocrine differentiation. This subtype shows androgen receptor negativity, small cell morphology, and neuroendocrine markers and is associated with low serum PSA levels and an aggressive clinical course [14].
4. Biomarkers of bone turnover: High levels of bone resorption markers (N-telopeptide and pyridinoline) and high levels of bone formation markers (C-terminal collagen propeptide, bone ALP) have been associated with shorter survival [15].

8.5 Treatment of Metastatic CRPC

8.5.1 Androgen Receptor Pathway Inhibitors (ARPi)

Two ARPis, abiraterone acetate and enzalutamide, have been approved for use in CRPC. The other newer anti-androgens (apalutamide and darulatamide) have not been studied in this population.

1. *Abiraterone acetate*: Abiraterone irreversibly inhibits products of the cytochrome P450 17-alpha hydroxysteroid dehydrogenase gene, i.e., 17,20 lyase and 17-alpha hydroxylase. This results in the inhibition of the synthesis of androgens in tumor tissue, adrenal glands, and testes, thus blocking autocrine, paracrine, and endocrine stimulation of prostate cancer.
   (a) No Prior Chemotherapy: In the COU-AA-302 phase III trial, 1088 asymptomatic or minimally symptomatic mCRCP patients were randomized to receive either abiraterone acetate and prednisolone or placebo plus prednisolone. Abiratrone and prednisolone were associated with OS benefit (median OS 34.7 vs. 30.3 months, HR = 0.81; 95% CI, 0.70–0.93; $p = 0.0033$) as well as radiological PFS benefit (median PFS 16.5 vs. 8.2 months, HR = 0.52; 95% CI, 0.45–0.61; $p < 0.0001$). There was also delay in PSA progression, deterioration in performance status, and use of cytotoxic chemotherapy [16–18].

(b) Prior Chemotherapy: In the phase 3 COU-AA-301 trial, 1195 patients with CRPC who had received docetaxel, were randomized to abiraterone plus prednisolone or placebo plus prednisolone. The median OS was 15.8 vs. 11.2 months (HR = 0.74; 95% CI, 0.64–0.86; $p < 0.0001$) and median PFS was 5.6 vs. 3.6 months (HR = 0.66; 95% CI, 0.58–0.76; $p < 0.0001$). There was improvement in the time to PSA progression, PSA relapse, and control of pain due to bone metastases [19, 20].

(c) Tolerance: Adverse effects commonly associated with abiraterone include hypertension, hypokalemia, fluid retention, nonspecific cardiac abnormality, and abnormal liver function. Some of these adverse effects (hypertension and hypokalemia) are due to mineralocorticoid excess, which can be treated with low-dose concomitant prednisolone.

(d) Abiraterone dosing: The recommended dose of abiraterone in CRPC is 1000 mg in empty stomach along with 5 mg prednisolone twice daily. However, dosing of 250 mg with low-fat breakfast along with prednisolone has shown similar PSA response, PFS, and pharmacodynamics effects.

2. *Enzalutamide*: It binds to androgen receptors (AR) expressed on prostate cancer cells and prevents the translocation of AR into the nucleus and association of AR with DNA. This results in the inhibition of androgen signaling driving the growth of prostate cancer.

   (a) No prior chemotherapy: This was studied in the phase 3 PREVAIL trial, in which, 1717 chemotherapy-naïve CRPC patients were randomized to enzalutamide or placebo. The median OS was 32.4 vs. 30.2 months (HR = 0.71; 95% CI, 0.60–0.84; $p < 0.001$) and radiological PFS was 20 vs. 5.4 months (HR = 0.32; 95% CI, 0.28–0.36; $p < 0.0001$) [21, 22]. In the TERRAIN and STRIVE trials, enzalutamide was compared with the first-generation anti-androgen bicalutamide. Enzalutamide showed a significant PFS benefit [23, 24].

   (b) Prior chemotherapy: This was studied in the phase 3 AFFIRM trial, where 1199 CRPC patients who had received docetaxel were randomized to enzalutamide or placebo. The median OS was 18.4 vs. 13.6 months (HR = 0.63; 95% CI, 0.53–0.75; $p < 0.001$). There was improvement in PSA response, soft tissue response, time to PSA progression, and radiological PFS [25].

   (c) Tolerance: Enzalutamide is fairly well tolerated. It is associated with fatigue, diarrhea, hot flashes, headache, and musculoskeletal pain. Seizures are an important but infrequent side effect [25].

   (d) Switching of ARPI: Abiraterone and enzalutamide interfere with androgen signaling; thus, progression on one ARPi may limit tumor responsiveness to other ARPis. There is no apparent activity of abiraterone post enzalutamide progression as was evident in a subset of patients in the control arm of the CARD trial [26]. Although, there is some activity of enzalutamide post abiraterone progression, the clinical benefit is less. Therefore, in routine practice, switching of ARPI is not recommended [27, 28].

(e) Combination of abiraterone and enzalutamide: In the ALLIANCE study, the combination of abiraterone plus prednisolone and enzalutamide was compared with enzalutamide alone, whereas the combination of abiraterone plus prednisolone and apalutamide was compared with abiraterone plus prednisolone alone in the ACIS study. Both studies showed higher PSA response and some PFS benefit; however, the combination did not result in OS benefit. Considering the increase in toxicity of the combination, there is limited benefit of this strategy in mCRPC patients [29, 30].

8.5.2 Metastatic CRPC with HRR Alteration

1. Pathogenic HRR alteration: In metastatic CRPC, approximately 11.8% harbor germline and 23% harbor somatic pathogenic variants in HRR genes. Commonly altered genes with decreasing frequency are *BRCA2>CHEK2>ATM>BRCA1* [7, 31]. The frequency of combined germline and somatic *BRCA1/2* and *ATM* pathogenic variants is 8% [32]. *BRCA2* alteration is associated with the greatest benefit from PARP inhibitors [33–35].
2. *mCRPC with prior ARPi*:
   - *Olaparib*: In the PROfound trial, 387 mCRPC patients (post ARPi progression) with HRR gene mutation were randomized to Olaparib 300 mg BD vs. abiraterone or enzalutamide. Approximately 65% of patients had received prior taxane. In cohort A (*BRCA1/2 & ATM*), radiological PFS (rPFS) was 7.4 vs. 3.6 months (HR = 0.34; 95% CI, 0.25–0.47; $p < 0.001$). In cohort B, the rPFS benefit was less prominent (5.8 vs. 3.5 months). There was improvement in OS in both cohorts, although the benefit was less in cohort B. Median OS was 19.1 vs. 14.7 months (HR = 0.69; 95% CI, 0.50–0.97; $p = 0.02$) in cohort A while it was 14.1 vs. 11.5 months (HR = 0.96; 95% CI 0.63–1.49) in cohort B [36, 37].
   - *Rucaparib*: In the TRITON-3 trial, 405 mCRPC patients (post ARPi progression) with *BRCA1/2* (75%) and *ATM* (25%) pathogenic variants were randomized to Rucaparib 600 mg BD vs. physician choice of therapy (Docetaxel = 56%, Abiraterone = 21%, and Enzalutamide = 24%). Median rPFS in *BRCA1/2* altered subset was 11.2 vs. 6.4 months (HR = 0.50; 95% CI, 0.36–0.69; $p < 0.001$), whereas in the ATM altered subset, the difference in rPFS was not significant (8.1 vs. 6.8 months). The overall survival data of the trial is still immature. Of note, the trial has shown a PFS benefit of rucaparib against taxane (56% of control arm patients received docetaxel). In phase 2 single-arm TRITON-2 trial, rucaparib showed a median PFS of 9 months and a response rate of 44% in *BRCA1/2* altered mCRPC patients who had received prior taxane [32, 38].
3. *mCRPC with no prior ARPi*:
   - *Olaparib and Abiraterone*: In the PROpel trial, 796 mCRPC (irrespective of HRR status) patients in first-line treatment were randomized to abiraterone plus prednisolone with either olaparib or placebo. There were 28% patients

with HRR mutations, including 12% with *BRCA1/2* pathogenic variants. Approximately one-fourth of patients had received docetaxel in castration-sensitive disease. In all patients, rPFS was 24.8 vs. 16.6 months; HR = 0.66; 95% CI, 0.54–0.81; $p < 0.001$. Hazard ratio for rPFS favored combination in both mHRR and non-mutant HRR subsets. No OS benefit was observed at median follow-up of 3 years. However, exploratory analysis in the *BRCA1/2* subset showed median OS not reached vs. 23 months (HR = 0.30; 95% CI, 0.15–0.59) [39, 40].

- *Talazoparib and enzalutamide*: In the TALAPRO-2 trial, 805 mCRPC patients (HRR mutation = 169) in the first line were randomized to enazolutamide with either talazoparib or placebo. At median follow-up of 24 months, median rPFS was not reached vs. 21.9 months (HR = 0.63; 95% CI, 0.51–0.78; $p < 0.0001$) favoring the combination arm. In the HRR-mutated subset ($n = 169$) at a median follow-up of 17 months, rPFS favored the combination (not reached vs. 13.8 months; HR = 0.45; 95% CI, 0.33–0.50). Overall survival data is still immature [41, 42].
- *Niraparib and abirateone*: In the MAGNITUDE trial, 423 mCRPC patients with HRR alteration in the first line were randomized to abiraterone plus prednisolone with either niraparib or placebo. At planned interim analysis, there was improvement in rPFS, median 16.7 vs. 13.7 months (HR = 0.76; 95% CI, 0.60–0.97; $p = 0.0280$). The rPFS benefit was greater in *BRCA1/2* subset, median 19.5 vs. 10.9 months (HR = 0.55; 95% CI, 0.39–0.78; $p = 0.0007$) [43].
- The above-mentioned trials have shown consistent PFS benefits for the combination of ARPi with PARP inhibitors in the HRR-altered subset of mCRPC patients. The improvement in PFS is greater in the *BRCA 1/2* altered subset. However, overall survival data is still immature and inconsistent. In addition, the PFS benefit appears to be less in patients with symptomatic disease burden and prior chemotherapy.

4. Tolerance of PARP inhibitors: Common adverse events associated with PARPi or the combination of PARPi and ARPi are anemia, nausea, and asthenia. Across the trials, approximately 10–15% patients required PARPi discontinuation due to adverse events. There is a small risk of developing myelodysplastic syndrome or acute myeloid leukemia with PARPi [37–39, 43].

8.5.3 Chemotherapy for Metastatic CRPC

1. *Chemotherapy-naïve patients*: In mCRPC patients progressing on ADT +/– ARPi who are fit for chemotherapy, chemotherapy should be considered while continuing ADT. Docetaxel at 3 weekly interval is the preferred chemotherapy; however, in frail and older patients, docetaxel 2 weekly or cabazitaxel (20 mg/m^2 every 3 weeks) can also be considered.

(a) *Docetaxel*: In the TAX 327 trial, 1006 mCRPC chemotherapy-naïve patients were randomized to docetaxel 75 mg/m^2 every 3 weeks vs. docetaxel 30 mg/m^2 every week vs. mitoxantrone 12 mg/m^2 every 3 weeks. All patients received prednisolone 5 mg BD. Median OS was 19.2 months (Doce 75) vs. 16.3 months (Mitoxantrone) (HR = 0.79; 95% CI, 0.67–0.93; $p = 0.004$) and 17.8 months (Doce 30) vs. 16.3 months (Mitoxantrone) (HR = 0.87; 95% CI, 0.74–1.02; 0.086). There was a higher PSA response rate in the docetaxel arms: 45% (Doce 75) and 48% (Doce 30) vs. 32% [44].

(b) *Docetaxel (50 mg/m^2)*—In a phase 3 randomized trial, 347 chemo-naïve mCRPC patients were randomized to docetaxel 50 mg/m^2 every 2 weeks vs. docetaxel 75 mg/m^2 every 3 weeks along with prednisolone 10 mg daily. Time to treatment failure and overall survival were 5.6 vs. 4.9 months and 19.5 vs. 17.0 months, respectively. There was no significant difference in the time to treatment failure, time to progression, and OS. The incidence of grade 3 or 4 neutropenia and febrile neutropenia were 36% vs. 53% and 4% vs. 14%, respectively. This schedule can be considered in frail patients and those at risk of febrile neutropenia [45].

(c) *Cabazitaxel*—In phase 3 FIRSTANA trial, 1168 chemo-naïve mCRPC patients were randomized to cabazitaxel 20 mg/m^2 vs. cabazitaxel 25 mg/m^2 vs. docetaxel 75 mg/m^2. Chemotherapy was administered every 3 weeks, and all patients received prednisolone. There was no statistically significant difference in OS among the three arms (cabazitaxel 20: 24.5 months, cabazitaxel 25: 25.2 months, and docetaxel: 24.3 months). Median PFS did not differ among the three arms. There were numerically higher tumor responses in the cabazitaxel 25 arm (42% vs. 31%). The incidence of febrile neutropenia were 2.4% (cabazitaxel 20), 12% (cabazitaxel 25), and 8.3% (docetaxel). The incidence of grade 3 or 4 adverse events was lower in the cabazitaxel 20 arm [46].

2. *Prior Chemotherapy.*

(a) *Cabazitaxel*: cabazitaxel in mCRPC patients after docetaxel progression has been compared with chemotherapy as well as with ARPi.

- In the phase 3 tropic trial, 755 mCRPC patients who progressed on docetaxel were randomized to cabazitaxel (25 mg/m^2) plus prednisolone vs. mitoxantrone plus prednisolone. Around 78% patients in the cabazitaxel arm and 72% patients in the mitoxantrone arm had progressed within 3 months of docetaxel exposure. Median OS was 15.1 vs. 12.7 months (HR = 0.70; 95% CI, 0.59–0.83; $p < 0.0001$). Median PFS was better with cabazitaxel (2.8 vs. 1.4 months). Routine GCSF prophylaxis was not given. The incidence of grade 3 or 4 neutropenia was 82% vs. 58%, and that of febrile neutropenia was 8% vs. 1%. Treatment-related deaths were 4.9% vs. 2.4% [47].
- In the phase 3 CARD trial, 255 mCRPC patients with prior docetaxel exposure who progressed within 12 months of ARPi (abiraterone or enzalutamide) were randomized to cabazitaxel (25 mg/m^2) vs. either enzalutamide or abiraterone. There was improvement in median OS (13.6

vs. 11 months; HR =0.64; 95% CI, 0.46–0.89; $p = 0.008$) and median rPFS (8 vs. 3.7 months, HR = 0.54; 95% CI, 0.40–0.73; $p < 0.001$) with cabazitaxel. Diarrhea, fatigue, and febrile neutropenia were more common with cabazitaxel [26].

- Among the mCRPC patients, approximately 40% patients receive ≥2 lines of therapy. Therefore, considering the risk of life-threatening toxicity, patients should be carefully selected for chemotherapy in this setting, and prophylactic G-CSF should be considered in patients >65 years and those with risk factors for febrile neutropenia (prior pelvic RT and comorbidities) [48].

(b) *Cabazitaxel dose*: In the PROSELICA trial, cabazitaxel 20 mg/m^2 every 3 weeks was found to be non-inferior to cabazitaxel 25 mg/m^2 in mCRPC patients who had progressed on docetaxel. This schedule was associated with lower toxicity. In patients with concern for toxicity, cabazitaxel administered every 2 weekly at 16 mg/m^2 dose was associated with comparable survival outcomes and less grade 3 or 4 neutropenia (5.1% vs. 62.5%) than cabazitaxel 25 mg/m^2 every 3 weeks [49, 50].

(c) *Docetaxel rechallenge*: In mCRPC patients who have been exposed to docetaxel, it is preferable to use cabazitaxel. However, in patients with a treatment-free interval >3 months, docetaxel rechallenge may provide some benefit, albeit with an increase in the risk of neuropathy [51].

3. *Platinum-Based Chemotherapy for mCRPC.*

(a) Aggressive prostate cancer variants: CRPC with small cell variant has an aggressive disease course with poor prognosis. ARPi does not have clinically meaningful activity in this subset. They are treated in a similar line as small cell lung cancer. There is activity of combination chemotherapy of platinum with either taxanes or etoposide. Immunotherapy (Atezolizumab or Durvalumab) can also be integrated as done in extensive-stage small-cell carcinoma [52–55].

(b) mCRPC patients with HRR alteration: Tumors with HRR alteration, particularly BRCA1/2 mutant, are sensitive to platinum-based chemotherapy. Platinum-based chemotherapy increases objective response in mCRPC with HRR alteration, leading to longer PFS without any obvious OS benefit [56, 57].

8.5.4 Radionuclide Therapy for mCRPC

1. *Lu-177-PSMA-617 therapy*: PSMA is a cell membrane protein expressed in prostate cells. Other tissues, such as the salivary gland and kidneys, express it to a lesser extent. Lutetium (Lu-177) vipivotide tetraxetan (Lu-177-PSMA-617) is a PSMA ligand linked to beta emitting radioisotope. It is effective in cases where the tumor expresses PSMA [58].

   - In the phase II ANZUP 1603 trial, Lu-177-PSMA-617 every 6 weeks up to 6 cycles was compared with cabazitaxel 20 mg/m^2 every 3 weeks (up to 10 cycles) in 200 PSMA- expressing mCRPC patients who had progressed on

ARPi and docetaxel. There was ≥50% decline in PSA in 66% vs. 37% patients, and grade 3 or 4 adverse events were observed in 33% vs. 53%. Pain response was also higher in the Lu-177-PSMA-617 arm. Overall survival was similar [59].

- In phase III VISION trial, 831 PSMA-expressing mCRPC patients were randomized to Lu-177-PSMA-617 every 6 weeks for 4 cycles (plus 2 if response was present) along with standard of care vs. standard of care alone (ARPi, steroids, and osteoclast inhibitors). Lu-177-PSMA-617 showed improvement in median rPFS (8.7 vs. 3.4 months, HR = 0.40; 95% CI, 0.29–0.57; $p < 0.001$) and median OS (15.3 vs. 11.3 months, HR = 0.62; 95% CI, 0.52–0.74; $p < 0.001$). There was a higher overall response rate and a longer time to first symptomatic skeletal event. The most common reported all-grade adverse events were fatigue, dry mouth, and nausea, whereas grade 3 or 4 adverse events were anemia (12.9%), thrombocytopenia (7.9%), and leukopenia (2.9%) [60].

2. *Radium-223*: Ra-223 is a bone-seeking calcium mimetic that binds to bone stroma in osteoblastic bone metastases. It is an alpha emitting radioisotope that deposits energy over short ranges <100 μm. It is indicated in mCRPC with symptomatic bone–only metastases.
   - In the phase 3 ALSYMPCA trial, 921 mCRPC patients with multiple bone metastases who had progressed on docetaxel or were ineligible for docetaxel were randomized to Ra-223 (every 4 weeks up to 6 cycles) vs. best supportive care (second-line hormonal therapy and bisphonates). Around 60% of patients had received prior docetaxel. Ra-223 showed a favorable safety profile, and there was a longer time to first symptomatic skeletal event (median 15.6 vs. 9.8 months; HR = 0.66; 95% CI, 0.52–0.83). Median OS was 14.9 vs. 11.3 months (HR = 0.70; 95% CI, 0.58–0.83; $p < 0.001$) [61, 62].
   - Although Ra-223 did not lead to clinically significant hematological toxicity, it can permanently reduce bone marrow reserve. In such a scenario, subsequent treatment with myelosuppressive drugs can be difficult.

8.5.5 Immunotherapy for mCRPC

1. *Immune-checkpoint inhibitors*: These are effective in mCRPC with MSI-high/-deficient MMR status or in high-tumor mutation burden (>10 mutations per megabase). This subset of mCRPC tumors express neo-antigens recognized by CD8+ T-cells [63, 64]. However, MSI-high/-deficient MMR status is relatively uncommon in mCRPC tumors (reported prevalence <1–8%) [65–67].
   - The PD-1 inhibitors Pembrolizumab and Dostarlimab have tissue agnostic approval for refractory tumors with deficient MMR status not having satisfactory treatment alternatives [68]. In a retrospective analysis that included mCRPC patients with deficient MMR status who were treated with pembrolizumab, more than half of the patients (53%) achieved >50% decline in PSA levels [69]. In another analysis that included mCRCP patients, immune-

checkpoint inhibitors led to better outcomes in patients with high tumor mutation burden [64].
2. *Vaccination with Sipuleucal T*: Sipuluecel T is prepared from autologous mononuclear cells obtained from leukepharesis which is then activated ex vivo with the recombinant fusion protein PA2024. PA2024 comprises prostatic acid phosphatase and GM-CSF. It is approved for patients with asymptomatic or minimally symptomatic slowly progressive mCRPC who lack visceral metastases and do not require opioids for cancer. It has shown overall survival benefit compared with placebo in mCRPC patients [70, 71].

8.5.6 Osteoclast Inhibitors in mCRPC

In mCRPC with bone metastases, osteoclast inhibitors can delay or prevent skeletal-related events (SRE). Denosumab (RANKL inhibitor) and zoledronic acid (bisphosphonate) are approved for this indication. Although both have shown benefits, in a phase 3 trial, denosumab led to a longer time to first SRE than zoledronic acid (median 20.7 vs. 17.1 months; HR = 0.82; 95%, 0.71–0.95; $p = 0.008$ for superiority) [72]. Besides, addition of osteoclast inhibitors to contemporary treatment (ARPi) has shown survival benefit in mCRPC patients with bone metastases [73, 74]. It is essential to optimize vitamin D and calcium levels and to complete dental evaluation prior to initiation of osteoclast inhibitors.

8.5.7 Sequencing of Therapy in mCRPC

With the myriad of options available for the treatment of mCRPC patients, it is essential to appropriately sequence them to ensure quality of life and optimize survival. The following factors should be considered while selecting treatment:

1. Patient-related factors: The patient's performance status, preexisting medical condition, organ functions, and bone marrow reserve should be carefully evaluated.
2. Disease burden: Patients with a high disease burden, i.e., symptomatic bony metastases and/or visceral metastases, may benefit more from a relatively quicker response to cytotoxic chemotherapy.
3. Tumor-related factors: mCRPC patients should undergo germline and somatic evaluation to detect HRR alteration. The MSI and TMB status should also be evaluated.
4. Prior treatment: With emerging data of combination therapy in castration-sensitive prostate cancer, CRPC patients are probably already exposed to these agents.

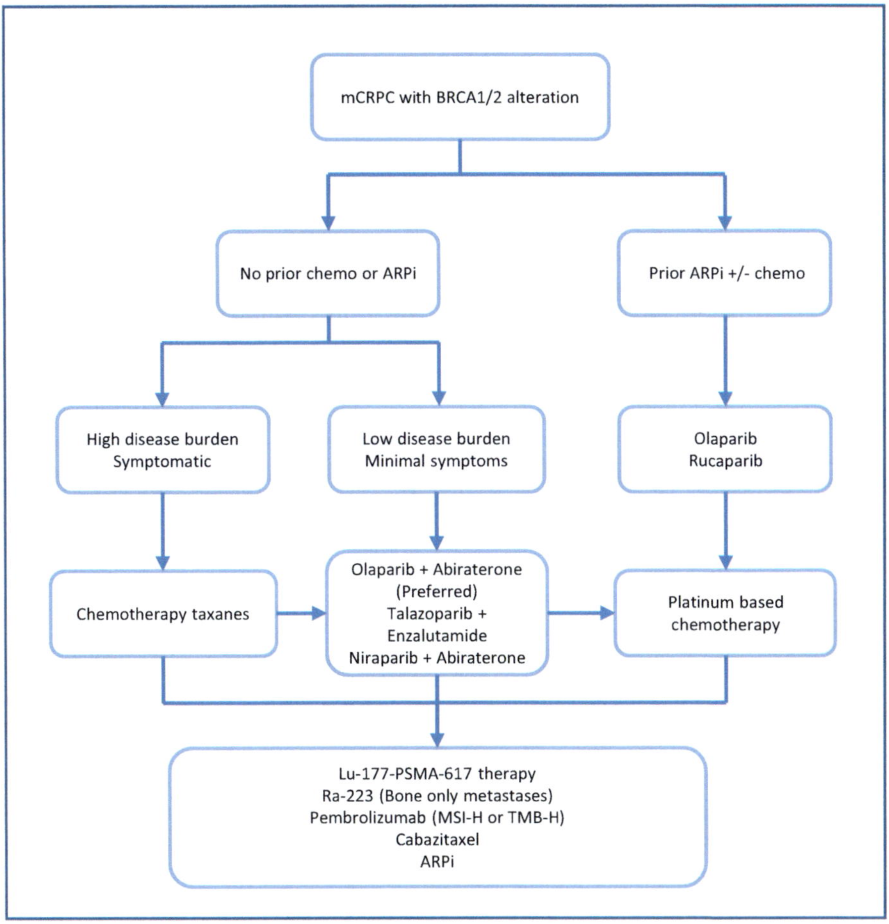

Fig. 8.1 Management of metastatic CRPC patients with BRCA1 or BRCA2 alteration

5. Treatment-related adverse events: The side effect profile of the agent should be considered to balance the benefit of the agent with adverse events. For instance, patients with preexisting liver disease may be at a higher risk of hepatotoxicity from abiraterone acetate [75, 76].

Figures 8.1 and 8.2 show a simplified algorithm for treatment selection in patients with mCRPC.

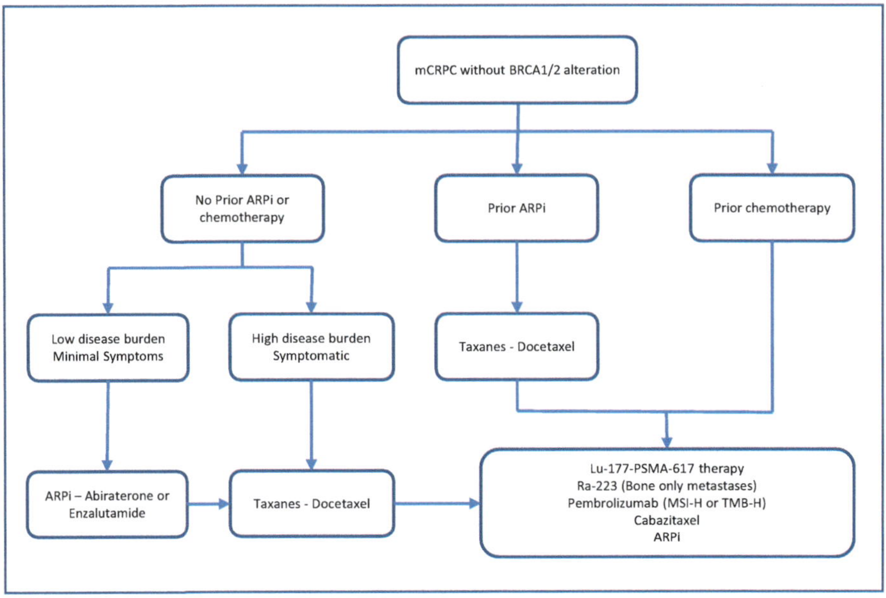

Fig. 8.2 Management of metastatic CRPC patients without BRCA1 or BRCA2 alteration

8.6 Treatment of Non-metastatic CRPC

In nmCRPC, second-generation androgen receptor blockers have shown survival benefits in patients with short PSA doubling time (≤10 months). Table 8.1 summarizes the approved agents and their survival benefit. The trials that evaluated these agents used conventional imaging for staging. More than 90% of these patients, when evaluated with PSMA-PETCT, may demonstrate PSMA-positive disease (44% confined to pelvis and 55% showing metastases) [77]. These subset of patients may require additional treatment beyond systemic therapy (surgery or RT if confined to pelvis).

Table 8.1 Androgen receptor blockers approved for the treatment of nmCRPC

Androgen receptor blocker	Dose	Median MFS	Median OS
Enzalutamide vs. placebo [78, 79]	160 mg OD	36.6 vs. 14.7 months (HR = 0.29; 95% CI, 0.24–0.35; $p < 0.001$)	67 vs. 56.3 months (HR = 0.73; 95% CI, 0.61–0.89; $p = 0.001$)
Apalutamide vs. placebo [80, 81]	240 mg OD	40.5 vs. 16.2 months (HR = 0.28; 95% CI, 0.23–0.35; $p < 0.001$)	73.9 vs. 59.9 months (HR = 0.784; $p = 0.0161$)
Darolutamide vs. placebo [82, 83]	600 mg BD	40.4 vs. 18.4 months (HR = 0.41; 95% CI, 0.34–0.50; $p < 0.001$)	Not reached in both arms (HR = 0.69; 95% CI, 0.53–0.88; $p = 0.003$)

MFS metastasis free survival, *OS* overall survival

References

1. Morote J, Aguilar A, Planas J, Trilla E. Definition of castrate resistant prostate cancer: new insights. Biomedicine. 2022;10(3):689.
2. Watson PA, Arora VK, Sawyers CL. Emerging mechanisms of resistance to androgen receptor inhibitors in prostate cancer. Nat Rev Cancer. 2015;15(12):701–11.
3. Dehm SM, Tindall DJ. Alternatively spliced androgen receptor variants. Endocr Relat Cancer. 2011;18(5):R183–96.
4. Crowley F, Sterpi M, Buckley C, Margetich L, Handa S, Dovey Z. A review of the pathophysiological mechanisms underlying castration-resistant prostate cancer. Res Rep Urol. 2021;13:457–72.
5. Beltran H, Prandi D, Mosquera JM, Benelli M, Puca L, Cyrta J, et al. Divergent clonal evolution of castration-resistant neuroendocrine prostate cancer. Nat Med. 2016;22(3):298–305.
6. Abida W, Campbell D, Patnaik A, Shapiro JD, Sautois B, Vogelzang NJ, et al. Non-BRCA DNA damage repair gene alterations and response to the PARP inhibitor Rucaparib in metastatic castration-resistant prostate cancer: analysis from the phase II TRITON2 study. Clin Cancer Res. 2020;26(11):2487–96.
7. Abida W, Armenia J, Gopalan A, Brennan R, Walsh M, Barron D, et al. Prospective genomic profiling of prostate cancer across disease states reveals germline and somatic alterations that may affect clinical decision making. JCO precis. Oncologia. 2017;2017:PO.17.00029.
8. Lincoln SE, Nussbaum RL, Kurian AW, Nielsen SM, Das K, Michalski S, et al. Yield and utility of germline testing following tumor sequencing in patients with cancer. JAMA Netw Open. 2020;3(10):e2019452.
9. Moreira DM, Howard LE, Sourbeer KN, Amarasekara HS, Chow LC, Cockrell DC, et al. Predictors of time to metastasis in castration-resistant prostate cancer. Urology. 2016;96:171–6.
10. Halabi S, Lin CY, Kelly WK, Fizazi KS, Moul JW, Kaplan EB, et al. Updated prognostic model for predicting overall survival in first-line chemotherapy for patients with metastatic castration-resistant prostate cancer. J Clin Oncol. 2014;32(7):671–7.
11. Goldkorn A, Ely B, Quinn DI, Tangen CM, Fink LM, Xu T, et al. Circulating tumor cell counts are prognostic of overall survival in SWOG S0421: a phase III trial of docetaxel with or without atrasentan for metastatic castration-resistant prostate cancer. J Clin Oncol Off J Am Soc Clin Oncol. 2014;32(11):1136–42.
12. Vogelzang NJ, Fizazi K, Burke JM, De Wit R, Bellmunt J, Hutson TE, et al. Circulating tumor cells in a phase 3 study of docetaxel and prednisone with or without lenalidomide in metastatic castration-resistant prostate cancer. Eur Urol. 2017;71(2):168–71.

13. Heller G, McCormack R, Kheoh T, Molina A, Smith MR, Dreicer R, et al. Circulating tumor cell number as a response measure of prolonged survival for metastatic castration-resistant prostate cancer: a comparison with prostate-specific antigen across five randomized phase III clinical trials. J Clin Oncol. 2018;36(6):572–80.
14. Yamada Y, Beltran H. Clinical and biological features of neuroendocrine prostate cancer. Curr Oncol Rep. 2021;23(2):15.
15. Lara PN, Ely B, Quinn DI, Mack PC, Tangen C, Gertz E, et al. Serum biomarkers of bone metabolism in castration-resistant prostate cancer patients with skeletal metastases: results from SWOG 0421. J Natl Cancer Inst. 2014;106(4):dju013.
16. Ryan CJ, Smith MR, Fizazi K, Saad F, Mulders PFA, Sternberg CN, et al. Abiraterone acetate plus prednisone versus placebo plus prednisone in chemotherapy-naive men with metastatic castration-resistant prostate cancer (COU-AA-302): final overall survival analysis of a randomised, double-blind, placebo-controlled phase 3 study. Lancet Oncol. 2015;16(2):152–60.
17. Rathkopf DE, Smith MR, de Bono JS, Logothetis CJ, Shore ND, de Souza P, et al. Updated interim efficacy analysis and long-term safety of abiraterone acetate in metastatic castration-resistant prostate cancer patients without prior chemotherapy (COU-AA-302). Eur Urol. 2014;66(5):815–25.
18. Basch E, Autio K, Ryan CJ, Mulders P, Shore N, Kheoh T, et al. Abiraterone acetate plus prednisone versus prednisone alone in chemotherapy-naive men with metastatic castration-resistant prostate cancer: patient-reported outcome results of a randomised phase 3 trial. Lancet Oncol. 2013;14(12):1193–9.
19. de Bono JS, Logothetis CJ, Molina A, Fizazi K, North S, Chu L, et al. Abiraterone and increased survival in metastatic prostate cancer. N Engl J Med. 2011;364(21):1995–2005.
20. Fizazi K, Scher HI, Molina A, Logothetis CJ, Chi KN, Jones RJ, et al. Abiraterone acetate for treatment of metastatic castration-resistant prostate cancer: final overall survival analysis of the COU-AA-301 randomised, double-blind, placebo-controlled phase 3 study. Lancet Oncol. 2012;13(10):983–92.
21. Beer TM, Armstrong AJ, Rathkopf DE, Loriot Y, Sternberg CN, Higano CS, et al. Enzalutamide in metastatic prostate cancer before chemotherapy. N Engl J Med. 2014;371(5):424–33.
22. Beer TM, Armstrong AJ, Rathkopf D, Loriot Y, Sternberg CN, Higano CS, et al. Enzalutamide in men with chemotherapy-naïve metastatic castration-resistant prostate cancer: extended analysis of the phase 3 PREVAIL study. Eur Urol. 2017;71(2):151–4.
23. Shore ND, Chowdhury S, Villers A, Klotz L, Siemens DR, Phung D, et al. Efficacy and safety of enzalutamide versus bicalutamide for patients with metastatic prostate cancer (TERRAIN): a randomised, double-blind, phase 2 study. Lancet Oncol. 2016;17(2):153–63.
24. Penson DF, Armstrong AJ, Concepcion R, Agarwal N, Olsson C, Karsh L, et al. Enzalutamide versus bicalutamide in castration-resistant prostate cancer: the STRIVE trial. J Clin Oncol. 2016;34(18):2098–106.
25. Scher HI, Fizazi K, Saad F, Taplin ME, Sternberg CN, Miller K, et al. Increased survival with enzalutamide in prostate cancer after chemotherapy. N Engl J Med. 2012;367(13):1187–97.
26. de Wit R, de Bono J, Sternberg CN, Fizazi K, Tombal B, Wülfing C, et al. Cabazitaxel versus abiraterone or enzalutamide in metastatic prostate cancer. N Engl J Med. 2019;381(26):2506–18.
27. Azad AA, Eigl BJ, Murray RN, Kollmannsberger C, Chi KN. Efficacy of enzalutamide following abiraterone acetate in chemotherapy-naive metastatic castration-resistant prostate cancer patients. Eur Urol. 2015;67(1):23–9.
28. de Bono JS, Chowdhury S, Feyerabend S, Elliott T, Grande E, Melhem-Bertrandt A, et al. Antitumour activity and safety of enzalutamide in patients with metastatic castration-resistant prostate cancer previously treated with abiraterone acetate plus prednisone for ≥24 weeks in Europe. Eur Urol. 2018;74(1):37–45.
29. Saad F, Efstathiou E, Attard G, Flaig TW, Franke F, Goodman OB, et al. Apalutamide plus abiraterone acetate and prednisone versus placebo plus abiraterone and prednisone in metastatic, castration-resistant prostate cancer (ACIS): a randomised, placebo-controlled, double-blind, multinational, phase 3 study. Lancet Oncol. 2021;22(11):1541–59.

30. Morris MJ, Heller G, Hillman DW, Bobek O, Ryan C, Antonarakis ES, et al. Randomized phase III study of enzalutamide compared with enzalutamide plus abiraterone for metastatic castration-resistant prostate cancer (Alliance A031201 trial). J Clin Oncol. 2023;41(18):3352–62.
31. Pritchard CC, Mateo J, Walsh MF, De Sarkar N, Abida W, Beltran H, et al. Inherited DNA-repair gene mutations in men with metastatic prostate cancer. N Engl J Med. 2016;375(5):443–53.
32. Fizazi K, Piulats JM, Reaume MN, Ostler P, McDermott R, Gingerich JR, et al. Rucaparib or physician's choice in metastatic prostate cancer. N Engl J Med. 2023;388(8):719–32.
33. Sandhu SK, Omlin A, Hylands L, Miranda S, Barber LJ, Riisnaes R, et al. Poly (ADP-ribose) polymerase (PARP) inhibitors for the treatment of advanced germline BRCA2 mutant prostate cancer. Ann Oncol. 2013;24(5):1416–8.
34. Marshall CH, Sokolova AO, McNatty AL, Cheng HH, Eisenberger MA, Bryce AH, et al. Differential response to olaparib treatment among men with metastatic castration-resistant prostate cancer harboring BRCA1 or BRCA2 versus ATM mutations. Eur Urol. 2019;76(4):452–8.
35. Taza F, Holler AE, Fu W, Wang H, Adra N, Albany C, et al. Differential activity of PARP inhibitors in BRCA1- versus BRCA2-altered metastatic castration-resistant prostate cancer. JCO precis. Oncologia. 2021;5:PO.21.00070.
36. de Bono J, Mateo J, Fizazi K, Saad F, Shore N, Sandhu S, et al. Olaparib for metastatic castration-resistant prostate cancer. N Engl J Med. 2020;382(22):2091–102.
37. Hussain M, Mateo J, Fizazi K, Saad F, Shore N, Sandhu S, et al. Survival with olaparib in metastatic castration-resistant prostate cancer. N Engl J Med. 2020;383(24):2345–57.
38. Abida W, Patnaik A, Campbell D, Shapiro J, Bryce AH, McDermott R, et al. Rucaparib in men with metastatic castration-resistant prostate cancer harboring a BRCA1 or BRCA2 gene alteration. J Clin Oncol. 2020;38(32):3763–72.
39. Clarke NW, Armstrong AJ, Thiery-Vuillemin A, Oya M, Shore N, Loredo E, et al. Abiraterone and olaparib for metastatic castration-resistant prostate cancer. NEJM Evid. 2022;1(9):EVIDoa2200043.
40. Saad F, Clarke NW, Oya M, Shore N, Procopio G, Guedes JD, et al. Olaparib plus abiraterone versus placebo plus abiraterone in metastatic castration-resistant prostate cancer (PROpel): final prespecified overall survival results of a randomised, double-blind, phase 3 trial. Lancet Oncol. 2023;24(10):1094–108.
41. Agarwal N, Azad AA, Carles J, Fay AP, Matsubara N, Heinrich D, et al. Talazoparib plus enzalutamide in men with first-line metastatic castration-resistant prostate cancer (TALAPRO-2): a randomised, placebo-controlled, phase 3 trial. Lancet. 2023;402(10398):291–303.
42. Fizazi K, Azad AA, Matsubara N, Carles J, Fay AP, De Giorgi U, et al. First-line talazoparib with enzalutamide in HRR-deficient metastatic castration-resistant prostate cancer: the phase 3 TALAPRO-2 trial. Nat Med. 2024;30(1):257–64.
43. Chi KN, Sandhu S, Smith MR, Attard G, Saad M, Olmos D, et al. Niraparib plus abiraterone acetate with prednisone in patients with metastatic castration-resistant prostate cancer and homologous recombination repair gene alterations: second interim analysis of the randomized phase III MAGNITUDE trial. Ann Oncol. 2023;34(9):772–82.
44. Berthold DR, Pond GR, Soban F, de Wit R, Eisenberger M, Tannock IF. Docetaxel plus prednisone or mitoxantrone plus prednisone for advanced prostate cancer: updated survival in the TAX 327 study. J Clin Oncol Off J Am Soc Clin Oncol. 2008;26(2):242–5.
45. Kellokumpu-Lehtinen PL, Harmenberg U, Joensuu T, McDermott R, Hervonen P, Ginman C, et al. 2-weekly versus 3-weekly docetaxel to treat castration-resistant advanced prostate cancer: a randomised, phase 3 trial. Lancet Oncol. 2013;14(2):117–24.
46. Oudard S, Fizazi K, Sengeløv L, Daugaard G, Saad F, Hansen S, et al. Cabazitaxel versus docetaxel as first-line therapy for patients with metastatic castration-resistant prostate cancer: a randomized phase III trial-FIRSTANA. J Clin Oncol. 2017;35(28):3189–97.
47. de Bono JS, Oudard S, Ozguroglu M, Hansen S, Machiels JP, Kocak I, et al. Prednisone plus cabazitaxel or mitoxantrone for metastatic castration-resistant prostate cancer progressing after docetaxel treatment: a randomised open-label trial. Lancet. 2010;376(9747):1147–54.

48. Freedland SJ, Davis M, Epstein AJ, Arondekar B, Ivanova JI. Real-world treatment patterns and overall survival among men with Metastatic Castration-Resistant Prostate Cancer (mCRPC) in the US Medicare population. Prostate Cancer Prostatic Dis. 2024;27(2):327–33.
49. Eisenberger M, Hardy-Bessard AC, Kim CS, Géczi L, Ford D, Mourey L, et al. Phase III study comparing a reduced dose of Cabazitaxel (20 mg/m^2) and the currently approved dose (25 mg/m^2) in Postdocetaxel patients with metastatic castration-resistant prostate cancer-PROSELICA. J Clin Oncol Off J Am Soc Clin Oncol. 2017;35(28):3198–206.
50. Oudard S, Ratta R, Voog E, Barthelemy P, Thiery-Vuillemin A, Bennamoun M, et al. Biweekly vs. triweekly cabazitaxel in older patients with metastatic castration-resistant prostate cancer: the CABASTY phase 3 randomized clinical trial. JAMA Oncol. 2023;9(12):1629–38.
51. Thomas C, Brandt MP, Baldauf S, Tsaur I, Frees S, Borgmann H, et al. Docetaxel-rechallenge in castration-resistant prostate cancer: defining clinical factors for successful treatment response and improvement in overall survival. Int Urol Nephrol. 2018;50(10):1821–7.
52. Aparicio AM, Harzstark AL, Corn PG, Wen S, Araujo JC, Tu SM, et al. Platinum-based chemotherapy for variant castrate-resistant prostate cancer. Clin Cancer Res. 2013;19(13):3621–30.
53. Fléchon A, Pouessel D, Ferlay C, Perol D, Beuzeboc P, Gravis G, et al. Phase II study of carboplatin and etoposide in patients with anaplastic progressive metastatic castration-resistant prostate cancer (mCRPC) with or without neuroendocrine differentiation: results of the French Genito-Urinary Tumor Group (GETUG) P01 trial. Ann Oncol. 2011;22(11):2476–81.
54. Horn L, Mansfield AS, Szczęsna A, Havel L, Krzakowski M, Hochmair MJ, et al. First-line atezolizumab plus chemotherapy in extensive-stage small-cell lung cancer. N Engl J Med. 2018;379(23):2220–9.
55. Paz-Ares L, Dvorkin M, Chen Y, Reinmuth N, Hotta K, Trukhin D, et al. Durvalumab plus platinum-etoposide versus platinum-etoposide in first-line treatment of extensive-stage small-cell lung cancer (CASPIAN): a randomised, controlled, open-label, phase 3 trial. Lancet. 2019;394(10212):1929–39.
56. Corn PG, Heath EI, Zurita A, Ramesh N, Xiao L, Sei E, et al. Cabazitaxel plus carboplatin for the treatment of men with metastatic castration-resistant prostate cancers: a randomised, open-label, phase 1-2 trial. Lancet Oncol. 2019;20(10):1432–43.
57. Ross RW, Beer TM, Jacobus S, Bubley GJ, Taplin ME, Ryan CW, et al. A phase 2 study of carboplatin plus docetaxel in men with metastatic hormone-refractory prostate cancer who are refractory to docetaxel. Cancer. 2008;112(3):521–6.
58. Fendler WP, Rahbar K, Herrmann K, Kratochwil C, Eiber M. 177Lu-PSMA Radioligand therapy for prostate cancer. J Nucl Med. 2017;58(8):1196–200.
59. Hofman MS, Emmett L, Sandhu S, Iravani A, Joshua AM, Goh JC, et al. [177Lu]Lu-PSMA-617 versus cabazitaxel in patients with metastatic castration-resistant prostate cancer (TheraP): a randomised, open-label, phase 2 trial. Lancet. 2021;397(10276):797–804.
60. Sartor O, de Bono J, Chi KN, Fizazi K, Herrmann K, Rahbar K, et al. Lutetium-177-PSMA-617 for metastatic castration-resistant prostate cancer. N Engl J Med. 2021;385(12):1091–103.
61. Parker C, Nilsson S, Heinrich D, Helle SI, O'Sullivan JM, Fosså SD, et al. Alpha emitter radium-223 and survival in metastatic prostate cancer. N Engl J Med. 2013;369(3):213–23.
62. Sartor O, Coleman R, Nilsson S, Heinrich D, Helle SI, O'Sullivan JM, et al. Effect of radium-223 dichloride on symptomatic skeletal events in patients with castration-resistant prostate cancer and bone metastases: results from a phase 3, double-blind, randomised trial. Lancet Oncol. 2014;15(7):738–46.
63. Le DT, Durham JN, Smith KN, Wang H, Bartlett BR, Aulakh LK, et al. Mismatch repair deficiency predicts response of solid tumors to PD-1 blockade. Science [Internet]. 2017 Jul 28 [cited 2024 May 29];357(6349). Available from: https://pubmed.ncbi.nlm.nih.gov/28596308/.
64. Graf RP, Fisher V, Weberpals J, Gjoerup O, Tierno MB, Huang RSP, et al. Comparative effectiveness of immune checkpoint inhibitors vs. chemotherapy by tumor mutational burden in metastatic castration-resistant prostate cancer. JAMA Netw Open. 2022;5(3):e225394.
65. Abida W, Cheng ML, Armenia J, Middha S, Autio KA, Vargas HA, et al. Analysis of the prevalence of microsatellite instability in prostate cancer and response to immune checkpoint blockade. JAMA Oncol. 2019;5(4):471–8.

66. Nava Rodrigues D, Rescigno P, Liu D, Yuan W, Carreira S, Lambros MB, et al. Immunogenomic analyses associate immunological alterations with mismatch repair defects in prostate cancer. J Clin Invest. 2018;128(10):4441–53.
67. Ritch E, Fu SYF, Herberts C, Wang G, Warner EW, Schönlau E, et al. Identification of hypermutation and defective mismatch repair in ctDNA from metastatic prostate cancer. Clin Cancer Res. 2020;26(5):1114–25.
68. Lemery S, Keegan P, Pazdur R. First FDA approval agnostic of cancer site - when a biomarker defines the indication. N Engl J Med. 2017;377(15):1409–12.
69. Graham LS, Montgomery B, Cheng HH, Yu EY, Nelson PS, Pritchard C, et al. Mismatch repair deficiency in metastatic prostate cancer: response to PD-1 blockade and standard therapies. PLoS One. 2020;15(5):e0233260.
70. Kantoff PW, Higano CS, Shore ND, Berger ER, Small EJ, Penson DF, et al. Sipuleucel-T immunotherapy for castration-resistant prostate cancer. N Engl J Med. 2010;363(5):411–22.
71. Sheikh NA, Petrylak D, Kantoff PW, Dela Rosa C, Stewart FP, Kuan LY, et al. Sipuleucel-T immune parameters correlate with survival: an analysis of the randomized phase 3 clinical trials in men with castration-resistant prostate cancer. Cancer Immunol Immunother. 2013;62(1):137–47.
72. Fizazi K, Carducci M, Smith M, Damião R, Brown J, Karsh L, et al. Denosumab versus zoledronic acid for treatment of bone metastases in men with castration-resistant prostate cancer: a randomised, double-blind study. Lancet. 2011;377(9768):813–22.
73. Francini E, Montagnani F, Nuzzo PV, Gonzalez-Velez M, Alimohamed NS, Rosellini P, et al. Association of concomitant bone resorption inhibitors with overall survival among patients with metastatic castration-resistant prostate cancer and bone metastases receiving abiraterone acetate with prednisone as first-line therapy. JAMA Netw Open. 2021;4(7):e2116536.
74. McGregor B, Zhang L, Gray KP, Shaw G, Evan C, Francini E, et al. Bone targeted therapy and skeletal related events in the era of enzalutamide and abiraterone acetate for castration resistant prostate cancer with bone metastases. Prostate Cancer Prostatic Dis. 2021;24(2):341–8.
75. Singh P, Sinha A, Lama Tamang TG, Chandra AB, Huang YJ. Abiraterone-associated fulminant liver failure. Am J Ther. 2018;25(4):e505–6.
76. Akpokavie D, Gubert C, Abdelli I, Stern AO, Zender H. Fatal fulminant hepatitis in a patient taking abiraterone acetate: a case report. Front Med. 2023;10:1143244.
77. Fendler WP, Weber M, Iravani A, Hofman MS, Calais J, Czernin J, et al. Prostate-specific membrane antigen ligand positron emission tomography in men with nonmetastatic castration-resistant prostate cancer. Clin Cancer Res. 2019;25(24):7448–54.
78. Hussain M, Fizazi K, Saad F, Rathenborg P, Shore N, Ferreira U, et al. Enzalutamide in men with nonmetastatic, castration-resistant prostate cancer. N Engl J Med. 2018;378(26):2465–74.
79. Sternberg CN, Fizazi K, Saad F, Shore ND, De Giorgi U, Penson DF, et al. Enzalutamide and survival in nonmetastatic, castration-resistant prostate cancer. N Engl J Med. 2020;382(23):2197–206.
80. Smith MR, Saad F, Chowdhury S, Oudard S, Hadaschik BA, Graff JN, et al. Apalutamide treatment and metastasis-free survival in prostate cancer. N Engl J Med. 2018;378(15):1408–18.
81. Small EJ, Saad F, Chowdhury S, Oudard S, Hadaschik BA, Graff JN, et al. Final survival results from SPARTAN, a phase III study of apalutamide (APA) versus placebo (PBO) in patients (pts) with nonmetastatic castration-resistant prostate cancer (nmCRPC). J Clin Oncol. 2020;38(15_suppl):5516.
82. Karim F, Neal S, Tammela TL, Albertas U, Egils V, Sergey P, et al. Darolutamide in nonmetastatic, castration-resistant prostate cancer. N Engl J Med. 2019;380(13):1235–46.
83. Fizazi K, Shore ND, Tammela T, Ulys A, Vjaters E, Polyakov S, et al. Overall survival (OS) results of phase III ARAMIS study of darolutamide (DARO) added to androgen deprivation therapy (ADT) for nonmetastatic castration-resistant prostate cancer (nmCRPC). J Clin Oncol. 2020;38(15_suppl):5514.

Non-muscle Invasive Bladder Cancer

9

Rohit Chauhan and Aditya Prakash Sharma

9.1 Introduction

Urothelial carcinoma, sometimes referred to as transitional cell carcinoma, is the most common malignancy in the urinary system. It primarily affects the urothelial cells lining the bladder, though it can also impact the lining of the ureters, urethra, and renal pelvis. Globally, bladder cancer ranks seventh in terms of frequency among men and tenth when considering both genders. Urothelial carcinoma stands as the second leading cause of death among all genitourinary tumors [1].

One critical aspect in managing urothelial carcinoma is staging, which helps determine the cancer's extent and guides treatment decisions. The TNM system, representing Tumor, Node, and Metastasis, is the most commonly employed staging system for urothelial carcinoma. Table 9.1 provides an overview of the various stages [2].

The term "non-muscle-invasive bladder cancer" (NMIBC) is commonly used to describe malignant urothelial tumor that has not yet spread to the detrusor muscle of the bladder. This chapter will primarily focus on NMIBC (stages Ta and T1), which encompasses cases where the disease is limited to the mucosa or submucosa. These types of NMIBC account for approximately 70–75% of patients with bladder cancer [3].

Carcinoma in situ (CIS) represents a non-invasive, intra-epithelial, high-grade form of urothelial carcinoma. CIS is sometimes mistakenly labeled as "premalignant," but it is, in fact, a high-grade, noninvasive urothelial carcinoma that is thought to be a precursor to the formation of an invasive high-grade carcinoma. During cystoscopy, it is often overlooked or mistakenly considered as an inflammatory lesion if not subjected to biopsy. CIS is often presented as multifocal and can occur

R. Chauhan · A. P. Sharma (✉)
Department of Urology, PGIMER, Chandigarh, India

R. Madan, S. Goyal (eds.), *Essentials of Radiotherapy in Uro-Genital Malignancies*, https://doi.org/10.1007/978-981-95-5945-9_9

Table 9.1 The TNM classification of carcinoma of the bladder

T—Primary tumor
Tx—Primary tumor cannot be evaluated
T0—Absence of a primary tumor
Ta—Non-invasive papillary tumor
Tis—Carcinoma in situ
T1—Tumor invading subepithelial connective tissue
T2—Tumor invading detrusor muscle T2a Tumor invades superficial muscle (inner half) T2b Tumor invades deep muscle (outer half)
T3—Tumor infiltrating perivesical tissue T3a Microscopic invasion T3b Macroscopic invasion (extravesical mass)
T4—Tumor infiltrating any one of these—prostate stroma, seminal vesicles, uterus, vagina pelvic wall, abdominal wall T4a Tumor infiltrating prostate stroma, seminal vesicles, uterus, or vagina T4b Tumor infiltrating pelvic wall or abdominal wall
N—Regional lymph nodes
NX—Regional lymph nodes cannot be assessed N0—No regional lymph node metastasis N1—Metastasis in a single lymph node in the true pelvis (hypogastric, obturator, external iliac, or presacral) N2—Metastasis in multiple regional lymph nodes in the true pelvis N3—Metastasis in common iliac lymph node(s)
M—Distant metastasis
M0—No distant metastasis M1a—Non-regional lymph nodes M1b—Other distant metastases

not only in the bladder but also in the other parts of urinary tract such as the urethra and upper urinary tracts.

From a clinical perspective, the following categories apply to CIS:

Primary: Isolated CIS without any prior or concurrent papillary tumors and without history of CIS previously.

Secondary: CIS discovered when monitoring individuals who have a history of tumors other than CIS.

Concurrent: When there is another bladder urothelial tumor in addition to CIS.

In untreated cases, muscle invasion can develop in patients with CIS ranging from 40% to 83%, particularly when it is concurrent with papillary growths. Furthermore, among those who were first thought to have CIS without any invasion, up to 20% who undergo cystectomy are subsequently discovered to have invasion upon closer examination of their final pathology [4, 5].

9.2 Risk Factors

Numerous factors and contributors have been identified that can elevate the chances of developing bladder cancer. These factors include:

1. Smoking and Tobacco Use: The leading cause of bladder cancer is tobacco usage, accounting for approximately half of all cases. Smoke from tobacco contains substances like polycyclic aromatic hydrocarbons and aromatic amines, which, since they are eliminated via the kidneys, are thought to contribute to the formation of bladder carcinoma. The longer and more heavily a person smokes, the higher their chance of developing bladder cancer [6, 7].
2. Occupational Exposure: About 10% of instances of bladder cancer are caused by exposure to chlorinated hydrocarbons, polycyclic aromatic hydrocarbons, and aromatic amines at work place. Such exposure is commonly seen in industrial settings where products like paint, dye, metal, and petroleum are manufactured. Additionally, recent research suggests that heightened occupational exposure to diesel exhaust may also make bladder cancer more likely [8, 9].
3. Family History: While there is limited evidence of a direct genetic link to bladder cancer, recent findings indicate that bladder cancer tends to cluster in first- and second-degree relatives. This suggests that genetic predisposition might enhance sensitivity to other risk factors. However, genetic testing for bladder cancer lacks substantial supporting evidence at this time [10].
4. Dietary Habits: The impact of dietary choices on bladder cancer risk appears to be minimal. Some research suggests that flavonoids may offer protective benefits. A Mediterranean diet that emphasizes moderation in protein intake and a high intake of vegetables and unsaturated fats, including olive oil, has been associated with a slight reduction in bladder cancer incidence [11, 12]. On the other hand, a Western diet high in organ meats and saturated fats has been found to be associated with a higher risk of bladder cancer, especially in women [13]. There is also a hypothesis that increasing fruit intake could potentially lower bladder cancer incidence [14]. According to a recent Indian study, urothelial carcinoma patients' serum contained more heavy metals compared to the controls [15].
5. Other Factors: Several other factors may influence bladder cancer risk, though their mechanisms remain unclear. These include metabolic parameters like blood pressure, plasma glucose, cholesterol, and triglycerides [16]. Some evidence suggests that higher levels of vitamin D in the blood may lower the risk of bladder cancer [17]. Bladder cancer can potentially result from a parasite trematode-caused schistosomiasis infection [6]. Additionally, exposure to ionizing radiation in the pelvic region is associated with a higher incidence of bladder cancer [18]. In certain cases, external beam radiation therapy for localized prostate cancer has been independently linked to a second primary bladder cancer [18]. Additionally, there is scant evidence of a tenuous link between bladder cancer and the use of cyclophosphamide and pioglitazone [6].

9.3 Risk Stratification

Extensive efforts have been dedicated to devising clinical tools for classifying the risk in patients with NMIBC. A novel risk classification system emerged following the release of the American Urological Association and Society of Urologic Oncology (AUA/SUO) Guideline for the diagnosis and management of NMIBC (Table 9.2) [19]. These models for risk stratification provide a more detailed evaluation of the likelihood of progression and recurrence in NMIBC patients, allowing for treatment and surveillance plans that are tailored to individual risk profiles.

9.3.1 Histological Grading of NMIBC

In 2004, the World Health Organization (WHO) introduced a histological classification system for urothelial carcinomas. This system encompassed various categories, including papillary urothelial neoplasm of low malignant potential (PUNLMP), low- and high-grade non-invasive papillary carcinoma. This classification system was subsequently retained in the updated WHO classifications of 2016 and 2022 [20, 21]. Interestingly, it differs in how patients are stratified within these groups from the previous 1973 WHO classification, which divided tumors into three grades: grade 1 (G1), grade 2 (G2), and grade 3 (G3) [22, 23].

Nevertheless, in terms of predicting tumor recurrence and progression, a systematic review and meta-analysis did not show that the 2004/2016 categorization outperformed the 1973 classification in terms of predictive ability [24]. It was found

Table 9.2 Risk groups based on the WHO 2004/2016 or the WHO 1973 grading systems

Risk group	
Low	A primary, solitary, TaT1 LG/G1 tumor with a diameter of less than 3 cm and no CIS in a patient younger than 70 years A primary Ta LG/G1 tumor with just ONE of the extra clinical risk factors present and without CIS
Intermediate	Individuals without CIS who do not belong to the very high-, high-, or low-risk categories
High	All T1 HG/G3 without CIS, with the exception of individuals in the extremely high-risk category All CIS patients, with the exception of those in the extremely high-risk category
	Stage, grade with additional clinical risk variables: Ta LG/G2 or T1G1, no CIS with all three risk variables Ta HG/G3 or T1 LG, no CIS with a minimum of 2 risk variables T1G2 no CIS with a minimum of one risk variables
Very High	Stage, grade with additional clinical risk variables: CIS and Ta HG/G3 with all three risk variables T1G2 and CIS with a minimum of two risk variables T1 HG/G3 and CIS with a minimum of one risk variable T1 HG/G3 no CIS with all three risk variables

Tumor diameter greater than 3 cm, age greater than 70, and multiple papillary tumors are additional clinical risk variables that the WHO 1973 and WHO 2004/2016 categories were predictive of illness progression but not recurrence [19].

9.4 Diagnosis

To make an accurate diagnosis, it is crucial to conduct a focused patient history in addition to evaluating signs and symptoms. The most frequent indicator of NMIBC is the presence of hematuria, which can either be visible or non-visible (greater than 3 red blood cells per high-powered field on microscopic urinalysis). It's worth noting that visible hematuria is associated with a higher stage of the disease at the time of presentation compared to non-visible hematuria [25]. Individuals who experience symptoms related to their lower urinary tract, especially irritative voiding, may be suspects of cancer in situ.

Hydronephrosis or filling deficiencies are indicators of papillary tumors in the urinary system, which can be found using imaging techniques like computed tomography (CT) urography [26]. If CT is not accessible, intravenous urography (IVU) can be used as a substitute. However, CT urography offers more detailed information, such as the status of the lymph nodes and surrounding organs, particularly in cases of muscle-invasive bladder cancers and upper tract urothelial carcinomas (UTUCs).

The low likelihood of significant results following the detection of a bladder tumor raises questions about the need for a baseline CT urography [27–29]. In addition to physical examinations, ultrasound (US) may be used to detect a range of anomalies in the urinary tract with a reasonable level of sensitivity. While it does not fully rule out all potential causes of hematuria, it does make it feasible to characterize concurrent renal masses and identify hydronephrosis and intraluminal bladder masses [30, 31].

It is now being investigated how multi-parametric magnetic resonance imaging could be used to diagnose and stage bladder cancer. Recently published, a standardized reporting approach for MRI (Vesical Imaging-Reporting and Data System [VI-RADS]) in patients with bladder cancer needs more validation [32].

Imaging techniques alone cannot be used to diagnose CIS (CT urography, IVU, US, or MRI). In the end, cystoscopic inspection of the bladder and histological evaluation of collected tissue—typically acquired by cold-cup biopsy or resection—are necessary for the diagnosis of papillary bladder cancer. At first, cystoscopy is performed as an outpatient procedure. For better patient compliance, particularly in males, topical intraurethral anesthetic lubricant application and flexible tools are recommended [33, 34].

9.4.1 Urine Cytology

The microscopic analysis of cellular smears from urinary samples is known as urine cytology. Urinary cytology is a subjective laboratory test that depends on a pathologist's assessment of the morphological features of shed urothelial cells, unlike tumor markers. Its most noteworthy characteristic is its high specificity, meaning that most patients have strong indications of malignancy when a test is positive, regardless of cystoscopic/radiographic results. Forty percent of individuals with a negative workup (upper tract imaging, cystoscopy) but continuously positive cytology were found to be diagnosed with genitourinary malignancy within 24 months [35].

Traditionally, cytology has been considered highly sensitive for high-grade cancer, but recent studies suggest that it only identifies 58% of bladder tumors. Its low sensitivity is not restricted to low-grade tumors, as it identifies only 71% of high-grade cancers. Therefore, while cytology exhibits high specificity, its sensitivity for both high-grade and low-grade tumors, including CIS, is limited [36].

9.5 Management

Whenever a bladder tumor is found in a cystoscopy, information is recorded with regard to its location, number, and appearance, as well as any involvement of sites that may indicate the tumor has spread outside of the bladder, such as the prostatic urethra, bladder neck, or ureteral orifices. Additionally, baseline urinary cytology is typically collected to assess the probability of high-grade disease.

The primary treatment for visible lesions is transurethral resection of bladder tumors (TURBT), performed under regional or general anesthesia. This procedure serves both diagnostic and therapeutic purposes by providing tissue samples for pathological evaluation of the stage and grade while also removing or cauterizing all visible tumors. As an alternative, tiny tumors can be removed with just cold-cup biopsy forceps. This is particularly useful for patients whose bladders have weak walls, such as elderly female patients, as typical transurethral resection techniques increase the risk of bladder perforation. If perforation does occur, the biopsy forceps typically result in a smaller perforation than the cutting loop, aiding subsequent healing.

En bloc resection of bladder tumor is another option, involving the excision of the entire tumor along with an underlying segment of muscle. This intact specimen is resected and removed, as opposed to piecemeal removal. This technique reduces cautery artifacts, enabling a more accurate assessment of muscle invasion by pathology. It is most suitable for papillary tumors with a distinct stalk. However, large tumors may pose challenges during specimen extraction, possibly requiring fragmentation for removal through the resectoscope. Despite potential difficulties, en bloc resection offers a viable approach for selected tumors. Given the possibility of a subsequent cystectomy, biopsies of the tumor's base and margins may be done in lieu of a full resection if the tumor looks to have infiltrated the muscle. If invasion is not demonstrated, repeat resection could be necessary unless there are other reasons to proceed with a cystectomy.

Residual tumor risk following the initial transurethral resection of TaT1 lesions is well-documented, underscoring the critical importance of an effective initial procedure for improved oncological outcomes [37]. A second completeness resection is required when the first resection is insufficient because of large tumors or problems during the procedure. Therefore, it is essential to document the completeness of the resection during the initial procedure.

It has been demonstrated that doing a second transurethral resection increases the chance of recurrence-free survival, improves results after BCG therapy, and provides insightful prognostic information. Retrospective assessments have indicated that a second resection conducted 14–42 days after the initial one yields longer recurrence-free and progression-free survival compared to a second resection performed between 43 and 90 days. As a result, the available data is in favor of suggesting a second TURBT in certain instances 2–6 weeks after the first resection [38].

9.5.1 Endoscopic Surgical Management

While transurethral resection of TaT1 tumors can eliminate them completely, these tumors often recur and may progress to muscle-invasive bladder cancer (MIBC). The variability in the 3-month recurrence rate suggests incomplete resection or the provocation of recurrences in many patients [37]. Therefore, considering adjuvant therapy for all patients is essential.

It has been demonstrated that administering intravesical chemotherapy immediately following TURBT can eradicate circulating tumor cells while having an ablative impact on leftover and unnoticed tumor cells [39–41]. Instillation with agents like mitomycin C (MMC), epirubicin, pirarubicin, or gemcitabine has demonstrated a reduction in intravesical recurrence rates [42].

Treatment must be started during the first few hours of TURBT in order to avoid tumor cell implantation, since tumor cells then solidify and get wrapped in extracellular matrix. Flexible procedures should be used to deliver instillation as soon as feasible, particularly during the initial 2 h in the recovery area or perhaps in the operating room, to maximize its efficacy [39].

9.5.2 Additional Adjuvant Intravesical Chemotherapy

Depending on the prognosis, further adjuvant intravesical treatment may be required. In cases of low-risk patients, a single immediate postoperative intravesical instillation (SI) serves as the standard and comprehensive treatment, significantly reducing the risk of recurrence [42, 43]. On the other hand, in cases where there is a significant risk of progression or recurrence, an SI is considered incomplete [19].

Numerous efficacy studies have been published to compare different application schemes, particularly the effect of intravesical Bacillus Calmette-Guérin (BCG) immunotherapy on recurrence and progression. In order to prevent the recurrence of NMIBC, five meta-analyses have consistently confirmed that BCG treatment is preferable to either TURB only or TURB coupled with chemotherapy after transurethral resection of bladder tumors (TURB) [44–47]. Moreover, three randomized controlled trials (RCTs) involving intermediate- and high-risk tumors have corroborated BCG's superiority in preventing tumor recurrence when compared to epirubicin, interferon (INF), or MMC [48–50].

Two meta-analyses have also demonstrated that BCG treatment can postpone tumor development and perhaps lower the probability of progression [51, 52]. Patients receiving BCG maintenance showed 27% decrease in the likelihood of progression when compared to control groups, according to a study by the EORTC GUCG [52]. Additionally, an extended follow-up RCT showed that patients treated with BCG had better overall as well as disease-specific survival and fewer distant metastases than those treated with epirubicin [48]. Contradictory findings have been found in certain studies, albeit this might be because of differences in patient characteristics, length of follow-up, technique, and statistical power. However, most studies showed that using a BCG maintenance plan decreased the probability of progression of high- and even intermediate-risk tumors.

9.5.3 Early Cystectomy

Immediate radical cystectomy (RC), or early cystectomy as it is popularly called, should be considered for specific NMIBC patients for several reasons:

1. Staging accuracy for T1 tumors during transurethral resection of bladder (TURBT) is low, with a substantial percentage (27–51%) being upstaged to muscle-invasive tumors at RC [53].
2. Some NMIBC patients progress to muscle-invasive disease, which carries a worse prognosis than primary muscle-invasive disease [54].

While discussing treatment alternatives with patients as part of a shared process of decision-making, it is critical to balance the possible advantages of RC against its related complications and morbidity. For NMIBC individuals who have a very high chance of the progression of disease, immediate RC may be suggested [55].

For patients with BCG-unresponsive tumors, early RC is strongly recommended, and it should be considered for those with BCG-relapsing high-grade tumors. Delaying RC in such cases may negatively affect disease-specific survival. Before developing muscle-invasive bladder cancer, patients who get RC have a 5-year disease-free survival of more than 80% [56].

9.5.4 Surveillance and Prevention

Surveillance and prevention are crucial aspects of managing bladder cancer, which, because of its chronic nature and requirement of long-term monitoring, incurs significant costs. Traditionally, cystoscopy and urinary cytology have been the gold standard for surveillance, but compliance with standard protocols is low. Various risk stratification models, such as the EORTC risk tables (Table 9.2), help tailor surveillance to individual patients.

Office-based cystoscopy allows for rapid and relatively painless visualization of the bladder's inner lining. It is useful for identifying papillary tumors and classic features of carcinoma in situ (CIS). Cystoscopy is usually done in an outpatient setting using flexible digital cystoscopes, and its positive predictive value for malignancy is high. Its appearance, however, cannot accurately indicate the grade or stage of the tumor.

The recommended surveillance schedule depends on the risk stratification of the tumor, with low-risk tumors possibly requiring annual cystoscopy after the initial 3-month follow-up. Patients with Ta low-grade tumors who remain recurrence-free after 3 months may transition to annual surveillance.

Chemoprevention and lifestyle modifications are examples of secondary prevention techniques. The risk of recurrence may be decreased by quitting smoking, drinking more water, and eating a low-fat diet, especially one that has less cholesterol. In the urothelium, hydration shortens the dwell time and concentration of carcinogens. However, no agents investigated for chemoprevention, including vitamins and retinoids, have proven effective in rigorous trials. High-dose multivitamins may decrease recurrence rates, especially when administered with intravesical BCG therapy, but this finding requires further confirmation.

Balancing surveillance strategies and prevention efforts is crucial for optimizing bladder cancer management and patient outcomes.

References

1. IARC, Cancer Today. Estimated number of new cases in 2020, worldwide, both sexes, all ages. 2021. https://gco.iarc.fr/today/online-analysis-table.
2. American Joint Committee on Cancer. Urinary bladder. In: AJCC cancer staging manual. 8th ed. New York: Springer; 2017. p. 757–65.
3. Aldousari S, Kassouf W. Update on the management of non-muscle invasive bladder cancer. Can Urol Assoc J. 2010;4(1):56–64.
4. Althausen AF, Prout GR Jr, Daly JJ. Non-invasive papillary carcinoma of the bladder associated with carcinoma in situ. J Urol. 1976;116:575–80.
5. Shariat SF, Palapattu GS, Amiel GE, et al. Characteristics and outcomes of patients with carcinoma in situ only at radical cystectomy. Urology. 2006;68(3):538–42.
6. Burger M, et al. Epidemiology and risk factors of urothelial bladder cancer. Eur Urol. 2013;63:234. https://pubmed.ncbi.nlm.nih.gov/22877502/.
7. Teoh JY, et al. Global trends of bladder cancer incidence and mortality, and their associations with tobacco use and gross domestic product per capita. Eur Urol. 2020;78:893. https://pubmed.ncbi.nlm.nih.gov/32972792/.
8. Colt JS, et al. A case-control study of occupational exposure to metalworking fluids and bladder cancer risk among men. Occup Environ Med. 2014;71:667. https://pubmed.ncbi.nlm.nih.gov/25201311/.
9. Pesch B, et al. Screening for bladder cancer with urinary tumor markers in chemical workers with exposure to aromatic amines. Int Arch Occup Environ Health. 2014;87:715. https://pubmed.ncbi.nlm.nih.gov/24129706/.

10. Lenfant L, et al. Genetic variability in 13q33 and 9q34 is linked to aggressiveness patterns and a higher risk of progression of non-muscle-invasive bladder cancer at the time of diagnosis. BJU Int. 2021;127:375. https://pubmed.ncbi.nlm.nih.gov/32975901/.
11. Liu H, et al. Fruit and vegetable consumption and risk of bladder cancer: an updated meta-analysis of observational studies. Eur J Cancer Prev. 2015;24:508. https://pubmed.ncbi.nlm.nih.gov/25642791/.
12. Vieira AR, et al. Fruits, vegetables, and bladder cancer risk: a systematic review and meta-analysis. Cancer Med. 2015;4:136. https://pubmed.ncbi.nlm.nih.gov/25461441/.
13. Dianatinasab M, et al. Dietary fats and their sources in association with the risk of bladder cancer: a pooled analysis of 11 prospective cohort studies. Int J Cancer. 2022;151:44. https://pubmed.ncbi.nlm.nih.gov/35182086/.
14. Jochems SHJ, et al. Fruit consumption and the risk of bladder cancer: a pooled analysis by the bladder cancer epidemiology and nutritional determinants study. Int J Cancer. 2020;147:2091. https://pubmed.ncbi.nlm.nih.gov/32285440/.
15. Panaiyadiyan S, Quadri JA, Nayak B, et al. Association of heavy metals and trace elements in carcinoma urinary bladder: a case-controlled study. Indian J Urol. 2023;39(3):236–40. https://doi.org/10.4103/iju.iju_143_23.
16. Teleka S, et al. Risk of bladder cancer by disease severity in relation to metabolic factors and smoking: a prospective pooled cohort study of 800,000 men and women. Int J Cancer. 2018;143:3071. https://pubmed.ncbi.nlm.nih.gov/29756343/.
17. Hektoen HH, et al. Vitamin D and vitamin D-binding protein and risk of bladder cancer: a nested case-control study in the Norwegian Janus serum Bank cohort. Cancer Med. 2021;10:4107. https://pubmed.ncbi.nlm.nih.gov/34080787/.
18. Moschini M, et al. External beam radiotherapy increases the risk of bladder cancer when compared with radical prostatectomy in patients affected by prostate cancer: a population-based analysis. Eur Urol. 2019;75:319.
19. Sylvester RJ, et al. European Association of Urology (EAU) prognostic factor risk groups for non-muscle-invasive bladder cancer (NMIBC) incorporating the WHO 2004/2016 and WHO 1973 classification systems for grade: an update from the EAU NMIBC guidelines panel. Eur Urol. 2021;79(4):480. https://pubmed.ncbi.nlm.nih.gov/33419683/.
20. Compérat E, et al. What's new in WHO fifth edition—urinary tract. Histopathology. 2022;81:439. https://pubmed.ncbi.nlm.nih.gov/35942645/.
21. WHO Classification of Tumours Editorial Board. WHO classification of tumours of the urinary system and male genital organs. 8th ed. Lyon: IARCC Press; 2022. https://publications.iarc.fr/610.
22. Moch H, et al. WHO classification of Tumours of the urinary system and male genital organs. 4th ed. Lyon: IARCC Press; 2016. https://publications.iarc.fr/Book-And-Report-Series/Who-Classification-Of-Tumours/WHOClassification-Of-Tumours-Of-The-Urinary-System-And-Male-Genital-Organs.
23. Sauter G, et al. Tumours of the urinary system: non-invasive urothelial neoplasias. In: WHO classification of classification of tumours of the urinary system and male genital organs. Lyon: IARCC Press; 2004. https://publications.iarc.fr/Book-And-Report-Series/Who-Classification-Of-Tumours/WHOClassification-Of-Tumours-Of-The-Urinary-System-And-Male-Genital-Organ.
24. Soukup V, et al. Prognostic performance and reproducibility of the 1973 and 2004/2016 World Health Organization grading classification Systems in non-muscle-invasive Bladder Cancer: a European Association of Urology non-muscle invasive bladder cancer guidelines panel systematic review. Eur Urol. 2017;72:801. https://pubmed.ncbi.nlm.nih.gov/28457661/.
25. Ramirez D, et al. Microscopic haematuria at time of diagnosis is associated with lower disease stage in patients with newly diagnosed bladder cancer. BJU Int. 2016;117:783. https://pubmed.ncbi.nlm.nih.gov/26435378/.
26. Trinh TW, et al. Bladder cancer diagnosis with CT urography: test characteristics and reasons for false-positive and false-negative results. Abdom Radiol (NY). 2018;43:663. https://pubmed.ncbi.nlm.nih.gov/28677000/.

27. Goessl C, et al. Is routine excretory urography necessary at first diagnosis of bladder cancer? J Urol. 1997;157:480. https://pubmed.ncbi.nlm.nih.gov/8996338/.
28. Palou J, et al. Multivariate analysis of clinical parameters of synchronous primary superficial bladder cancer and upper urinary tract tumor. J Urol. 2005;174:859. https://pubmed.ncbi.nlm.nih.gov/16093970/.
29. Holmang S, et al. Long-term followup of a bladder carcinoma cohort: routine followup urography is not necessary. J Urol. 1998;160:45. https://pubmed.ncbi.nlm.nih.gov/9628602/.
30. Tan WS, et al. Can renal and bladder ultrasound replace computerized tomography Urogram in patients investigated for microscopic hematuria? J Urol. 2018;200:973. https://pubmed.ncbi.nlm.nih.gov/29702097/.
31. Hilton S, et al. Recent advances in imaging cancer of the kidney and urinary tract. Surg Oncol Clin N Am. 2014;23:863. https://pubmed.ncbi.nlm.nih.gov/25246053/.
32. Panebianco V, et al. Multiparametric magnetic resonance imaging for bladder cancer: development of VI-RADS (vesical imaging-reporting and data system). Eur Urol. 2018;74:294. https://pubmed.ncbi.nlm.nih.gov/29755006/.
33. Krajewski W, et al. How different cystoscopy methods influence patient sexual satisfaction, anxiety, and depression levels: a randomized prospective trial. Qual Life Res. 2017;26:625. https://pubmed.ncbi.nlm.nih.gov/28050795/.
34. Aaronson DS, et al. Meta-analysis: does lidocaine gel before flexible cystoscopy provide pain relief? BJU Int. 2009;104:506. https://pubmed.ncbi.nlm.nih.gov/19239453/.
35. Nabi G, Greene D, O'Donnell MO. Suspicious urinary cytology with negative evaluation for malignancy in the diagnostic investigation of haematuria: how to follow up? J Clin Pathol. 2004;57(4):365–8.
36. Grossman HB, Blute ML, Dinney CP, et al. The use of urine-based biomarkers in bladder cancer. Urology. 2006;67(3 Suppl 1):62–4.
37. Brausi M, et al. Variability in the recurrence rate at first follow-up cystoscopy after TUR in stage ta T1 transitional cell carcinoma of the bladder: a combined analysis of seven EORTC studies. Eur Urol. 2002;41:523. https://pubmed.ncbi.nlm.nih.gov/12074794/.
38. Baltaci S, et al. Significance of the interval between first and second transurethral resection on recurrence and progression rates in patients with high-risk non-muscle-invasive bladder cancer treated with maintenance intravesical bacillus Calmette-Guerin. BJU Int. 2015;116:721. https://pubmed.ncbi.nlm.nih.gov/25715815/.
39. Soloway MS, et al. Urothelial susceptibility to tumor cell implantation: influence of cauterization. Cancer. 1980;46:1158. https://pubmed.ncbi.nlm.nih.gov/7214299/.
40. Pan JS, et al. Inhibition of implantation of murine bladder tumor by thiotepa in cauterized bladder. J Urol. 1989;142:1589. https://pubmed.ncbi.nlm.nih.gov/2511340/.
41. Brocks CP, et al. Inhibition of tumor implantation by intravesical gemcitabine in a murine model of superficial bladder cancer. J Urol. 2005;174:1115. https://pubmed.ncbi.nlm.nih.gov/16094076/.
42. Sylvester RJ, et al. Systematic review and individual patient data meta-analysis of randomized trials comparing a single immediate instillation of chemotherapy after transurethral resection with transurethral resection alone in patients with stage pTa-pT1 urothelial carcinoma of the bladder: which patients benefit from the instillation? Eur Urol. 2016;69:231. https://pubmed.ncbi.nlm.nih.gov/26091833/.
43. Sylvester RJ, et al. A single immediate postoperative instillation of chemotherapy decreases the risk of recurrence in patients with stage ta T1 bladder cancer: a meta-analysis of published results of randomized clinical trials. J Urol. 2004;171:2186. https://pubmed.ncbi.nlm.nih.gov/15126782/.
44. Malmstrom PU, et al. An individual patient data meta-analysis of the long-term outcome of randomised studies comparing intravesical mitomycin C versus bacillus Calmette-Guerin for nonmuscle- invasive bladder cancer. Eur Urol. 2009;56:247. https://pubmed.ncbi.nlm.nih.gov/19409692/.

45. Shelley MD, et al. A systematic review of intravesical bacillus Calmette-Guerin plus transurethral resection vs transurethral resection alone in ta and T1 bladder cancer. BJU Int. 2001;88:209. https://pubmed.ncbi.nlm.nih.gov/11488731/.
46. Han RF, et al. Can intravesical bacillus Calmette-Guerin reduce recurrence in patients with superficial bladder cancer? A meta-analysis of randomized trials. Urology. 2006;67:1216. https://pubmed.ncbi.nlm.nih.gov/16765182/.
47. Shelley MD, et al. Intravesical bacillus Calmette-Guerin is superior to mitomycin C in reducing tumour recurrence in high-risk superficial bladder cancer: a meta-analysis of randomized trials. BJU Int. 2004;93:485. https://pubmed.ncbi.nlm.nih.gov/15008714/.
48. Sylvester RJ, et al. Long-term efficacy results of EORTC genito-urinary group randomized phase 3 study 30911 comparing intravesical instillations of epirubicin, bacillus Calmette-Guerin, and bacillus Calmette-Guerin plus isoniazid in patients with intermediate- and high-risk stage ta T1 urothelial carcinoma of the bladder. Eur Urol. 2010;57:766. https://pubmed.ncbi.nlm.nih.gov/20034729/.
49. Duchek M, et al. Bacillus Calmette-Guerin is superior to a combination of epirubicin and interferonalpha2b in the intravesical treatment of patients with stage T1 urinary bladder cancer. A prospective, randomized, Nordic study. Eur Urol. 2010;57:25. https://pubmed.ncbi.nlm.nih.gov/19819617/.
50. Jarvinen R, et al. Long-term efficacy of maintenance bacillus Calmette-Guerin versus maintenance mitomycin C instillation therapy in frequently recurrent TaT1 tumours without carcinoma in situ: a subgroup analysis of the prospective, randomised FinnBladder I study with a 20-year follow-up. Eur Urol. 2009;56:260. https://pubmed.ncbi.nlm.nih.gov/19395154/.
51. Bohle A, et al. Intravesical bacille Calmette-Guerin versus mitomycin C in superficial bladder cancer: formal meta-analysis of comparative studies on tumor progression. Urology. 2004;63:682. https://pubmed.ncbi.nlm.nih.gov/15072879/.
52. Sylvester RJ, et al. Intravesical bacillus Calmette-Guerin reduces the risk of progression in patients with superficial bladder cancer: a meta-analysis of the published results of randomized clinical trials. J Urol. 2002;168:1964. https://pubmed.ncbi.nlm.nih.gov/12394686/.
53. Huguet J, et al. Cystectomy in patients with high risk superficial bladder tumors who fail intravesical BCG therapy: pre-cystectomy prostate involvement as a prognostic factor. Eur Urol. 2005;48:53. https://pubmed.ncbi.nlm.nih.gov/15967252/.
54. Moschini M, et al. Comparing long-term outcomes of primary and progressive carcinoma invading bladder muscle after radical cystectomy. BJU Int. 2016;117:604. https://pubmed.ncbi.nlm.nih.gov/25851271/.
55. Kamat AM, et al. The case for early cystectomy in the treatment of nonmuscle invasive micropapillary bladder carcinoma. J Urol. 2006;175:881. https://pubmed.ncbi.nlm.nih.gov/16469571/.
56. Raj GV, et al. Treatment paradigm shift may improve survival of patients with high risk superficial bladder cancer. J Urol. 2007;177:1283. https://pubmed.ncbi.nlm.nih.gov/17382713/.

Muscle Invasive Bladder Cancer

10

Anchal Aggarwal and Priyanka Singh

10.1 Introduction

Bladder cancer is the sixth most commonly prevalent cancer among males, but it drops to tenth position when both males and females are considered together [1]. The global age-standardized incidence rate (per 100,000 person/years) is 9.5 for men and 2.4 for women [1]. Most common type of the bladder cancer is urothelial carcinoma, which, on the basis of different management strategies, is further classified as non-muscle-invasive bladder cancer (NMIBC) or muscle-invasive bladder cancer (MIBC). Eighty to ninety percent of MIBCs are diagnosed de novo; however, 10–20% may arise from NMIBC cases that eventually progress. Of the two, MIBC is a more aggressive one, being associated with a 5-year survival rate of 60% and 10% for patients with localized disease and distant metastasis respectively.

10.2 Risk Factors

Smoking, exposure to certain chemicals in specific occupations like aluminium production, rubber production, painting, firefighting, various dyes [e.g. magenta and auramine] or dye intermediates [e.g. 4-aminobiphenyl]), environmental exposures (X radiation or gamma radiation and arsenic), medications (cyclophosphamide and chlornaphazine), opium consumption and Schistosoma parasitic infection common in Africa and Middle East are the most established risk factors [2]. Tobacco smoking alone is related to approximately 50% of cases [3] and is linked with higher grades and stages of tumours, increased chances of disease recurrence, poor

A. Aggarwal (✉)
Patel Multispeciality Hospital, Jalandhar, India

P. Singh
Paras Hospital, Gurugram, India

R. Madan, S. Goyal (eds.), *Essentials of Radiotherapy in Uro-Genital Malignancies*, https://doi.org/10.1007/978-981-95-5945-9_10

surgical outcomes, severe postoperative complications, higher rates of disease progression and tumour recurrence [5]. The risk is found to decrease with time after smoking cessation [4]. Furthermore, there is correlative evidence suggesting specific dietary factors (reduced BC risk with fruits, vegetables and tea intake) [6], imbalance in gut microbiome, interaction of external risk factors with certain genes and exposure to diesel exhaust emission as potential risk factors [7].

10.3 Histology

In accordance with WHO 2022 classification, all MIBC subtypes are to be considered high-grade urothelial carcinomas [11]. However, it is still important to specify the exact percentage of the subtype in the specimen [12] due to its relevance in prognostication and treatment decisions [8–10].

10.4 Clinical Presentation and Examination

Painless visible haematuria is the most common presenting symptom. Other symptoms and signs include non-visible haematuria, urgency, dysuria and increased frequency. Advanced tumours present with symptoms related to urinary tract obstruction and pelvic pain. On physical examination, a palpable pelvic mass can be found in patients with locally advanced disease. It should also include rectal and vaginal bimanual palpation along with general assessment. In addition, bimanual examination under anaesthesia should be carried out before and after transurethral resection of the bladder tumour (TURBT) to assess whether there is a palpable mass or if the tumour is fixed to the pelvic wall [13, 14].

10.5 Diagnosis

A history, physical examination, blood workup (haematology and biochemistry), imaging, cystoscopy, biopsy and/or resection for histological diagnosis and full staging should all be performed on any patient whose bladder shows a mass as detected by diagnostic imaging approach.

Urothelial tumour located anywhere in the urinary tract leads to a positive urinary cytology. However, examining bladder washings for cancer cells is a helpful indicator in situations of high-grade malignancy and has a high sensitivity in high-grade tumours. As per NCCN guidelines, a computed tomography (CT) scan of the abdomen and pelvis without and with contrast, especially in excretory phase (CT urography), should always be done prior to TURBT to evaluate the bladder in patients with suspicion of bladder cancer. It helps in assessing any synchronous upper tract disease, regional lymph nodes and potential metastases [21–23]. In patients with low GFR or iodinated contrast allergy without acute renal failure, MR urography is preferred. Non-contrast MRI-T2 sequences can also be used for urinary tract evaluation if contrast is contraindicated. Retrograde ureteropyelography with renal ultrasound or non-contrast CT and/or ureteroscopy can also be utilized for evaluation of upper urinary tract [15–17].

Better soft tissue contrast resolution of MRI as compared to CT scan helps in evaluation of post-biopsy reaction. This is because enhancement of the tumour occurs earlier than that of the normal bladder wall due to neovascularization [18, 19]. Though CT scan is very useful in detecting the perivesical fat (T3b) and adjacent organ invasion, it has limitations in discriminating between Ta and T3a tumours. Thus, a multiparametric (mp) MRI using the Vesical Imaging Reporting and Data System [VI-RADS] scoring system is suggested to differentiate between T1 vs. T2 bladder tumours, having better diagnostic accuracy [20].

Diagnostic cystoscopy and microscopic analysis of removed tissue are used to diagnose BC. To map the entire image of the bladder, a flexible cystoscopy should be performed as an outpatient procedure. In actual practice, however, diagnostic cystoscopy may be skipped, and the patient might go straight to transurethral resection of bladder tumour (TURBT) if a bladder tumour has been clearly visible by imaging examinations. Obtaining cross-sectional diagnosis and staging for which bladder muscle must be included in the resection material is the aim of TURB. In order to detect any bladder neck tumours during the procedure, a comprehensive examination of the bladder using rigid cystoscopy under anaesthesia is essential [21]. The site, size, number and appearance (solid or papillary) of the tumours, as well as any mucosal abnormalities, must be carefully described in the cystoscopic findings [21, 22]. The pictorial representation of the abnormality is recommended.

Due to FDG excretion in the urine, FDG PET/CT is not very useful for assessing the urinary collecting system, but it is helpful for assessing distant metastases [23, 24].

10.6 Staging and Classification

According to the American Joint Committee on Cancer (AJCC) TNM staging systems, muscle-invasive bladder cancer (MIBC) should be classified into prognosis groups as specified in the manual [25].

10.7 Treatment Recommendations

In MIBC, the aim of the treatment is to decide for bladder preservation or removal and whether local bladder therapy alone or systemic therapy is also to be incorporated. Therefore, multidisciplinary care via tumour board discussions and/or directed consultations with a medical oncologist, radiation oncologist and urologist is recommended for the optimal management.

In patients who undergo radical cystectomy with pelvic lymph node dissection (RC) only, the 5-year survival rate for bladder cancer can be up to 80% for lymph node–negative and organ-limited disease. Survival rate decreases to 40% in patients with extravesical extension of bladder cancer, and it can further go down to 15–35% if lymph node metastases are present [26–29].The primary cause of poor survival rates in patients with locally advanced MIBC may be hidden systemic micrometastatic disease; therefore, the use of neoadjuvant or adjuvant systemic treatment should be considered in most patients with locally advanced MIBC for effective disease management [29, 30].

10.7.1 Radical Cystectomy

Radical cystectomy (RC) with pelvic lymph node dissection (PLND) is the standard treatment of MIBC cT2-T4a, N0 M0 [31]. A continent orthotopic (neobladder), continent cutaneous (catheterizable pouch) or incontinent cutaneous (conduit) reconstruction is chosen based on the patient's general health and choice. A neobladder can be offered to patients lacking any contraindications and who have no tumour in the urethra or at the level of urethral dissection [31]. Dissecting all lymphatic tissues around the common iliac, external iliac, internal iliac and obturator regions up to the crossing of the ureters over the common iliac vessels at a minimum is done in standard PLND [31–33]. In extended lymphadenectomy, lymphatic tissues in the region of the aortic bifurcation, presacral and common iliac vessels above the crossing ureters are also taken out, in addition to the standard PLND region. The optimal extent of PLND is not established till date. In a recently published randomised prospective phase III trial, extended PLND failed to show a significant advantage in absolute improvement of 5-year recurrence-free survival compared with standard PLND, though the study design had a lot of limitations [21, 31, 34].

In females, radical cystectomy involves anterior pelvic exenteration with resection of the bladder, urethra, uterus, ovaries, fallopian tubes and anterior vaginal wall. In males, radical cystectomy involves resection of the bladder, prostate and seminal vesicles [35].

10.7.2 Neoadjuvant Chemotherapy

Several studies have shown the benefit of neoadjuvant chemotherapy prior to cystectomy over cystectomy alone [36–40]. The preferred chemotherapy regimens for non-metastatic muscle-invasive bladder cancer are dose-dense methotrexate, vinblastine, doxorubicin and cisplatin (dose-dense MVAC) or gemcitabine plus cisplatin, depending on patient's age, comorbidities and toxicity profiles [41–47]. For medically fit and cisplatin-eligible patients, either regimen can be used. But for older adults or those with significant comorbidities, gemcitabine plus cisplatin may be preferred due to increased risk of treatment-related adverse effects with toxicity with dose-dense MVAC. For patients with creatinine clearance between 50 and 60 mL/min, gemcitabine plus split-dose cisplatin can be used. It is not advisable to replace it with carboplatin in the absence of sufficient evidence of efficacy. Patients with creatinine clearance <50 mL/min are not eligible for neoadjuvant therapy and may be offered radical cystectomy or trimodality therapy as an alternative.

10.7.3 Adjuvant Chemotherapy

In patients who have not received neoadjuvant chemotherapy before radical cystectomy, high-risk features, including tumours that extend beyond the muscle (pathologic T3 or T4 disease) and/or pathologic node involvement, can be offered adjuvant systemic therapy with the aim of delaying recurrence and improving OS.

The preferred adjuvant chemotherapy regimens for patients who are eligible for cisplatin-based combination chemotherapy are three to four cycles of either MVAC (methotrexate, vinblastine, doxorubicin and cisplatin) or high-dose MVAC with growth factor support, or four cycles of gemcitabine plus cisplatin (GC), or immunotherapy (nivolumab, atezolizumab, pembrolizumab, etc.) [47–52].

10.7.4 Bladder Preservation Therapies

The rationale behind the development of bladder preservation strategies was to improve the patient's quality of life without compromising the oncological outcomes by providing an alternative to radical cystectomy. It is a feasible option for carefully selected patients in those unfit for surgery or for those desirous of retaining their native bladder. Options for bladder preservation include partial cystectomy, TURBT alone, TURBT followed by chemotherapy or radiotherapy and radical radiotherapy. However, none of these stand-alone treatment approaches demonstrated outcomes equivalent to radical cystectomy.

10.7.5 Trimodality Therapy

Trimodality therapy is the standard bladder conservation therapy which incorporates cystoscopy with maximal visible transurethral resection of bladder tumour (TURBT) followed by radiation therapy (RT) with concurrent chemotherapy. Ideal patient for TMT should have the following characteristics which only 6–19% of patients are able to fulfil [53–55]:

1. Urothelial histology.
2. No upper tract (ureter or renal pelvic) involvement on CT or MR scans. This is important to rule out any field cancerization and multifocal disease.
3. Visibly complete maximal TURBT.
4. Stage T2-T4a.
5. Unifocal tumour <6 cm in maximum diameter.
6. Absent extensive CIS.
7. No hydroureteronephrosis or VUJ involvement.

8. Good bladder function and capacity.
9. Adequate kidney function to be eligible for concurrent chemotherapy.
10. Understands the need for long-term surveillance.

10.8 Locally Advanced Disease

It includes unresectable bladder cancer invading nearby structures like rectum, bowel, uterus, vagina, prostate, upper urinary tract, abdominal or pelvic side walls and lymph nodes. Optimal treatment approach is not defined but includes aggressive management with concurrent chemoradiation or neoadjuvant chemotherapy for downstaging before radical cystectomy. It may further require adjuvant chemotherapy for high-risk features for locoregional or distant metastasis. Palliative radiation alone using hypofractionated doses can be offered in case of haematuria, pain or obstruction [56]. Lymph node-positive bladder cancer patients are a unique subset of patients who are potentially curable but are at increased risk of distant metastasis. Therefore, node-positive bladder cancer patients should preferably receive neoadjuvant chemotherapy followed by local treatment [57, 58].

10.9 Principles of Radiation Therapy

CT simulation and advanced radiation techniques like 3D conformal radiotherapy, intensity modulated radiotherapy (IMRT) and volumetric arc therapy (VMAT) or RapidArc (RA) should be used in the treatment of MIBC. The patient is immobilised with simple immobilisation with well- defined bladder filling and rectal emptying protocols. Treatment is usually delivered in either one phase or two phases. Due to the variability in bladder filling on a daily basis, image-guided radiotherapy (IGRT) using cone beam CT scan (CBCT) is to be obtained prior to treatment. Plan and treat phase 1 (and if the entire treatment is in one phase) with an empty bladder, and if two phases are used, treat phase 2 with full bladder [59, 60].

10.10 Treatment Volumes

10.10.1 Radical Radiotherapy [59, 60]

GTV = residual tumour (post-TURB) plus gross extravesical spread (previous site of tumour if complete TURB.

CTV = whole bladder (including GTV) + 0.5 cm margin on gross extravesical extension (EVE). Contour muscle wall of bladder as solid organ and anatomical variants like cystoceles, diverticula, etc. are to be included. Prophylactic regional lymphatics are not routinely irradiated.

Use this CTV for the entire treatment (one phase) unless details of tumour location are available.

Prostatic or vaginal tissue is not usually included unless there is direct micro or macroscopic invasion. If the tumour is multifocal, involving bladder neck or there is extensive carcinoma in situ, then an additional 1.5 cm of prostatic urethra and 1 cm of female urethra can also be included.

CTV for the second phase (boost) of 2-phase technique: GTV, or the site of known tumour, adding a 0.5-cm margin on EVE, if present.

PTV = CTV with anisotropic margin expansion (anteriorly, posteriorly and laterally 1.5–2.0 cm; cranially 2.0–2.5 cm; inferiorly 1–1.5 cm).

10.10.2 Adjuvant Radiotherapy

As per the updated guidelines by IBIS Workgroup, CTV borders in postoperative settings can be contoured as mentioned in Table 10.1 [61].

10.10.3 Radiation Dose

Standard fraction 64 Gy in 32 fractions over 6.5 weeks or hypofractionated radiation using 55 Gy in 20 fractions over 4 weeks.

There is no strong data to show the importance of overall treatment time on MIBC outcomes, and, in general, delays should be avoided.

Radiation Dose Constraints for Conventional Schedule

Rectum V50 < 50%, V60 < 35%.

Femoral head V50 < 30%.

Radiation Dose Constraints for Hypofractionated Schedule

Rectum: Mean dose <40 Gy, V50Gy < 50%.

Small bowel: V50Gy < 98 cc.

Femoral head: V50 < 50%.

Body: Max dose (1 cc) < 105%.

10.10.4 Concurrent Chemotherapy

Cisplatin is the drug of choice as radiosensitizer in patients with adequate kidney function. Other cisplatin-based regimens used are cisplatin with 5FU and cisplatin with paclitaxel [62, 63]. In patients with poor renal function not eligible for cisplatin-based therapies, the various options of concurrent chemotherapy include mitomycin C with 5FU or capecitabine [64, 65], low-dose gemcitabine [66, 67],

Table 10.1 International Bladder Investigator Society updated internal consensus clinical target volume definition

	Superior	Inferior	Anterior	Posterior	Lateral
Presacral nodes	Lumbosacral joint (L5-S1)	Inferior aspect of S3	1–105-cm anterior to sacrum	Sacrum	Right and left common iliac vessels
Iliac nodes	Iliac vessels from bifurcation of the abdominal aorta	External iliac: Superior aspect of femoral heads Internal iliac: Point of exit through greater sciatic notch or no longer visible on CT	7-mm expansion around iliac vessels		
Obturator nodes	Bifurcation of common iliac vessels	Superior aspect of public symphysis	Anterior edge obturator internus muscle	Posterior edge obturator internus muscle	109-cm medial to obturator internus muscle(no cropping to the bowel)
Cystectomy bed	2-cm above superior aspect of public symphysis	Male patients: 2–3 mm superior to penile bulbs. Female Patients: 1 cm below inferior pole of obturator foramen	Posterior aspect of public symphysis and planes extending superiorly and inferiorly from posterior aspect of public symphysis	Anterior one-third aspect of anorectal circumference and plane extending superiorly from anterior border of rectum	Medial border of obturator internus muscle and prostate bed or vaginal wall

Abbreviation: *CT* computed tomography

single-agent paclitaxel [68], single-agent 5FU and single-agent capecitabine. Carboplatin monotherapy is not used due to a lack of sufficient data [69].

10.11 Metastatic Disease

As per the Cancer Genome Atlas ranking, Bladder cancer is the third highest mutated cancer; therefore, genomic or molecular testing should be advised early in the course of diagnosis of advanced bladder cancer. PDL1 and FGFR3 or FGFR2 genetic alterations must be included in the testing for eligibility of corresponding immunotherapy options [70].

For patients eligible for cisplatin-based therapy, the first line of systemic therapy included either GC or ddMVAC with growth factor support. Patients not eligible for cisplatin can receive carboplatin with gemcitabine. If there is no progression on a first-line platinum-containing chemotherapy, avelumab is preferred as the maintenance therapy. For patients with metastatic bladder cancer not eligible for cisplatin-based chemotherapy or who have progression with cisplatin-based first-line therapy, an immune checkpoint inhibitor like pembrolizumab is the treatment of choice. Another option is Atezolizumab in PD-L1-expressing tumours. Enrolment in clinical trials is preferred in subsequent lines of treatment. Some newer drugs demonstrating effectiveness in previously treated metastatic bladder cancer are erdafitinib (FGFR inhibitor), enfortumab vedotin and Sacituzumab govitecan (antibody-drug conjugates).

10.12 Surveillance

Long-term close surveillance and follow-up are critical in bladder cancer due to high risk of recurrences. The recurrence may be local or distant with a short time of progression to death if untreated.

Different follow-up schemes have been advised based on the stage and grade of tumour for both post-cystectomy and post-bladder-preservation patients. It includes regular urine cytology, liver and kidney function tests, electrolyte assessment and imaging of chest, abdomen and pelvis every 3 to 6 months for the first 2 years and annually thereafter. In case of bladder preservation, regular cystoscopies with or without mapping biopsy are a part of routine follow-up.

10.13 Treatment of Recurrences

Management of recurrence of bladder disease after bladder preservation therapy depends on the tumour size, stage and grade at recurrence.

For patients with complete response at TMT with low-grade and non-muscle-invasive recurrences, further preservation of bladder with intravesical therapy is a reasonable approach. They are thus treated with transurethral resection of bladder tumour (TURBT) followed by intravesical therapy with Bacillus Calmette-Guérin (BCG) or mitomycin. However, if there is no response to the intravesical therapy, salvage cystectomy is advised [71, 72].

Patients who fail to have a complete response after TMT or develop a muscle-invasive recurrences are offered salvage cystectomy with urinary diversion. Special concern should be taken in view of delayed bowel healing and risk of urethra neo-bladder anastomosis stricture formation in post-radiation patients.

References

1. IARC. Estimated number of new cases in 2020, worldwide, both sexes, all ages. 2020. https://gco.iarc.fr/today/online-analysis-multi-bars. Access date Dec 2022.
2. International Agency for Research on Cancer. List of classifications by cancer sites with sufficient or limited evidence in humans. IARC monographs volumes 1–132. July 1, 2022. https://monographs.iarc.who.int/wp-content/uploads/2019/07/Classifications_by_cancer_site.pdf.
3. Freedman ND, Silverman DT, et al. Abnet association between smoking and risk of bladder cancer among men and women. JAMA. 2011;306:737–45.
4. Li Y, Tindle HA, et al. Smoking cessation and the risk of bladder cancer among postmenopausal women. Cancer Prev Res. 2019;12(5):305–14.
5. Kumar R, Matulewicz R, et al. Impact of smoking on urologic cancers: a snapshot of current evidence. World J Urol. 2023;41(6):1473–9. https://doi.org/10.1007/s00345-023-04406-y. Epub 2023 Apr 24. PMID: 37093319; PMCID: PMC10241723.26.
6. World Cancer Research Fund/American Institute for Cancer Research. Diet, nutrition, physical activity and bladder cancer. Continuous update project expert report 2015. http://dietandcancerreport.org/.
7. Jubber I, Ong S, et al. Epidemiology of bladder Cancer in 2023: a systematic review of risk factors. Eur Urol. 2023;84(2):176–90. https://doi.org/10.1016/j.eururo.2023.03.029. Epub 2023 May 16.
8. Veskimae E, et al. What is the prognostic and clinical importance of urothelial and non urothelial histological variants of bladder Cancer in predicting oncological outcomes in patients with muscle-invasive and metastatic bladder Cancer? A European Association of Urology muscle invasive and metastatic bladder cancer guidelines panel systematic review. Eur Urol Oncol. 2019;2:625. https://pubmed.ncbi.nlm.nih.gov/31601522/.
9. Sjodahl G, et al. A molecular taxonomy for urothelial carcinoma. Clin Cancer Res. 2012;18:3377. https://pubmed.ncbi.nlm.nih.gov/22553347/.
10. Choi W, et al. Identification of distinct basal and luminal subtypes of muscle-invasive bladder cancer with different sensitivities to frontline chemotherapy. Cancer Cell. 2014;25:152.
11. WHO classification of tumours—urinary and male genital tumours, 2022. IARC, Lyon, France. https://publications.iarc.fr/Book-And-Report-Series/Who-Classification-Of-Tumours/Urinary-AndMale-Genital-Tumours-2022.
12. Willis DL, et al. Clinical outcomes of cT1 micropapillary bladder cancer. J Urol. 2015;193:1129. https://pubmed.ncbi.nlm.nih.gov/25254936/.
13. Fossa SD, et al. Clinical significance of the "palpable mass" in patients with muscle-infiltrating bladder cancer undergoing cystectomy after preoperative radiotherapy. Br J Urol. 1991;67:54. https://pubmed.ncbi.nlm.nih.gov/1993277/.
14. Wijkstrom H, et al. Evaluation of clinical staging before cystectomy in transitional cell bladder carcinoma: a long-term follow-up of 276 consecutive patients. Br J Urol. 1998;81:686.
15. https://www.nccn.org/professionals/physician_gls/pdf/bladder.pdf.
16. Wong VK, Ganeshan D, et al. Imaging and management of bladder cancer. Cancers (Basel). 2021;13(6):1396. https://doi.org/10.3390/cancers13061396.
17. Flaig TW, Spiess PE, et al. Bladder Cancer, version 3.2020, NCCN clinical practice guidelines in oncology. J Natl Compr Cancer Netw. 2020;18:329–54. https://doi.org/10.6004/jnccn.2020.0011.

18. Mallampati GK, et al. MR imaging of the bladder. Magn Reson Imaging Clin N Am. 2004;12:545. https://pubmed.ncbi.nlm.nih.gov/15271370/.
19. Rajesh A, et al. Bladder cancer: evaluation of staging accuracy using dynamic MRI. Clin Radiol. 2011;66:1140.
20. Panebianco V, et al. Multiparametric magnetic resonance imaging for bladder Cancer: development of VI-RADS (vesical imaging-reporting and data system). Eur Urol. 2018;74:294. https://pubmed.ncbi.nlm.nih.gov/29755006/.
21. Alfred Witjes J, et al. European association of urology guidelines on muscle-invasive and metastatic bladder cancer: summary of the 2023 guidelines. Eur Urol. 2024;85(1):17–31. https://doi.org/10.1016/j.eururo.2023.08.016. Epub 2023 Oct 17.PMID: 37858453 Review.
22. Mariappan P, et al. Detrusor muscle in the first, apparently complete transurethral resection of bladder tumour specimen is a surrogate marker of resection quality, predicts risk of early recurrence, and is dependent on operator experience. Eur Urol. 2010;57:843. https://pubmed.ncbi.nlm.nih.gov/19524354/
23. Apolo AB, Riches J, et al. Clinical value of fluorine-18 2-fluoro-2-deoxy-D-glucose positron emission tomography/computed tomography in bladder cancer. J Clin Oncol. 2010;28:3973–8. https://doi.org/10.1200/JCO.2010.28.7052.
24. Voskuilen CS, et al. Staging (18)F-fluorodeoxyglucose positron emission tomography/computed tomography changes treatment recommendation in invasive bladder Cancer. Eur Urol Oncol. 2022;5:366.
25. Amin MB, Edge SB, Greene FL, et al., editors. AJCC Cancer staging manual. 8th ed. New York: Springer; 2017.
26. Stein JP, Lieskovsky G, et al. Radical cystectomy in the treatment of invasive bladder cancer: long-term results in 1,054 patients. J Clin Oncol. 2001;19:666–75.
27. Quek ML, Stein JP, et al. Natural history of surgically treated bladder carcinoma with extravesical tumor extension. Cancer. 2003;98:955–61.
28. Shariat SF, Karakiewicz PI, et al. Outcomes of radical cystectomy for transitional cell carcinoma of the bladder: a contemporary series from the bladder Cancer research consortium. J Urol. 2006;176:2414–22.
29. Kim DK, Lee JY, et al. Role of adjuvant cisplatin-based chemotherapy following radical cystectomy in locally advanced muscle-invasive bladder cancer: systematic review and meta-analysis of randomised trials. Investig Clin Urol. 2019;60(2):64–74. https://doi.org/10.4111/icu.2019.60.2.64.
30. Kim HS, Jeong CW, et al. Adjuvant chemotherapy for muscle-invasive bladder cancer: a systematic review and network meta-analysis of randomised clinical trials. Oncotarget. 2017;8:81204–14.
31. Powles T, Bellmunt J, et al. Bladder cancer: ESMO clinical practice guideline for diagnosis, treatment and follow-up. Ann Oncol. 2022;33(3):244–58. https://doi.org/10.1016/j.annonc.2021.11.012. Epub 2021 Nov 30.
32. Simone G, Papalia R, Ferriero M, et al. Stage-specific impact of extended versus standard pelvic lymph node dissection in radical cystectomy. Int J Urol. 2013;20:390–7.
33. Bruins HM, Veskimae E, Hernandez V, et al. The impact of the extent of lymphadenectomy on oncologic outcomes in patients undergoing radical cystectomy for bladder cancer: a systematic review. Eur Urol. 2014;66:1065–77.
34. Gschwend JE, Heck MM, Lehmann J, et al. Extended versus limited lymph node dissection in bladder cancer patients undergoing radical cystectomy: survival results from a prospective, randomised trial. Eur Urol. 2019;75:604–11.
35. Aragon-Ching JB, Werntz RP, et al. Multidisciplinary management of muscle-invasive bladder cancer: current challenges and future directions. Am Soc Clin Oncol Educ Book. 2018;38:307–18. https://doi.org/10.1200/EDBK_201227.
36. Grossman HB, Natale RB, et al. Neoadjuvant chemotherapy plus cystectomy compared with cystectomy alone for locally advanced bladder cancer. N Engl J Med. 2003;349(9):859–66. https://doi.org/10.1056/NEJMoa022148. Erratum in: N Engl J Med 2003 Nov 6;349(19):1880.

37. International Collaboration of Trialists, Medical Research Council Advanced Bladder Cancer Working Party (now the National Cancer Research Institute Bladder Cancer Clinical Studies Group), European Organisation for Research and Treatment of Cancer Genito-Urinary Tract Cancer Group, Australian Bladder Cancer Study Group, National Cancer Institute of Canada Clinical Trials Group, Finnbladder, Norwegian Bladder Cancer Study Group, Club Urologico Espanol de Tratamiento Oncologico Group, Griffiths G, Hall R, Sylvester R, Raghavan D, Parmar MK. International phase III trial assessing neoadjuvant cisplatin, methotrexate, and vinblastine chemotherapy for muscle-invasive bladder cancer: long-term results of the BA06 30894 trial. J Clin Oncol. 2011;29(16):2171–7. https://doi.org/10.1200/JCO.2010.32.3139. Epub 2011 Apr 18. PMID: 21502557; PMCID: PMC3107740.
38. Advanced Bladder Cancer (ABC) Meta-analysis Collaboration. Neoadjuvant chemotherapy in invasive bladder cancer: update of a systematic review and meta-analysis of individual patient data advanced bladder cancer (ABC) meta-analysis collaboration. Eur Urol 2005;48(2):202–5; discussion 205–6. https://doi.org/10.1016/j.eururo.2005.04.006. Epub 2005 Apr 21.
39. Hamid ARAH, Ridwan FR, et al. Meta- analysis of neoadjuvant chemotherapy compared to radical cystectomy alone in improving overall survival of muscle-invasive bladder cancer patients. BMC Urol. 2020;20(1):158. https://doi.org/10.1186/s12894-020-00733-z. PMID: 33054762; PMCID: PMC7557048.
40. Audenet F, Sfakianos JP, et al. A delay ≥8 weeks to neoadjuvant chemotherapy before radical cystectomy increases the risk of upstaging. Urol Oncol. 2019;37(2):116–22. https://doi.org/10.1016/j.urolonc.2018.11.011. Epub 2018 Dec 1.
41. Soloway MS, Ikard M, et al. Cis-diamminedichloroplatinum (II) in locally advanced and metastatic urothelial cancer. Cancer. 1981;47(3):476–80. https://doi.org/10.1002/1097-0142(19810201)47:3<476::aid-cncr2820470309>3.0.co;2-8.
42. Herr HW, Bajorin DF, et al. Neoadjuvant chemotherapy and bladder-sparing surgery for invasive bladder cancer: ten-year outcome. J Clin Oncol. 1998;16(4):1298–301. https://doi.org/10.1200/JCO.1998.16.4.1298.
43. Sternberg CN, de Mulder P, et al. EORTC Genito-urinary Cancer group. Seven year update of an EORTC phase III trial of high-dose intensity M-VAC chemotherapy and G-CSF versus classic M-VAC in advanced urothelial tract tumours. Eur J Cancer. 2006;42(1):50–4. https://doi.org/10.1016/j.ejca.2005.08.032. Epub 2005 Dec 5.
44. Khaled HM, Shafik HE, et al. Gemcitabine and cisplatin as neoadjuvant chemotherapy for invasive transitional and squamous cell carcinoma of the bladder: effect on survival and bladder preservation. Clin Genitourin Cancer. 2014;12(5):e233–40. https://doi.org/10.1016/j.clgc.2014.04.002. Epub 2014 May 6.
45. Niedersüss-Beke D, Puntus T, et al. Neoadjuvant chemotherapy with gemcitabine plus cisplatin in patients with locally advanced bladder cancer. Oncology. 2017;93(1):36–42. https://doi.org/10.1159/000463389. Epub 2017 Apr 12.
46. Iyer G, Balar AV, et al. Multicenter prospective phase II trial of Neoadjuvant dose-dense gemcitabine plus cisplatin in patients with muscle-invasive bladder Cancer. J Clin Oncol. 2018;36(19):1949–56. https://doi.org/10.1200/JCO.2017.75.0158. Epub 2018 May 9. PMID: 29742009; PMCID: PMC6049398.
47. Pfister C, Gravis G, et al. Perioperative dose-dense methotrexate, vinblastine, doxorubicin, and cisplatin in muscle-invasive bladder cancer (VESPER): survival endpoints at 5 years in an open-label, randomised, phase 3 study. Lancet Oncol. 2024;25(2):255–64. https://doi.org/10.1016/S1470-2045(23)00587-9. Epub 2023 Dec 21. PMID: 38142702.
48. Leow JJ, Martin-Doyle W, et al. Adjuvant chemotherapy for invasive bladder cancer: a 2013 updated systematic review and meta-analysis of randomized trials. Eur Urol. 2014;66(1):42–54. https://doi.org/10.1016/j.eururo.2013.08.033. Epub 2013 Aug 28.
49. Sternberg CN, Skoneczna I et al.; European Organisation for Research and Treatment of Cancer Genito-Urinary Cancers Group; Groupe d' Etude des Tumeurs Urogénitales; National Cancer Research Institute Bladder Cancer Study Group; National Cancer Institute of Canada Clinical Trials Group; German Association of Urologic Oncology. Immediate versus deferred chemotherapy after radical cystectomy in patients with pT3-pT4 or N+ M0 urothelial

carcinoma of the bladder (EORTC 30994): an intergroup, open-label, randomised phase 3 trial. Lancet Oncol. 2015;16(1):76–86. https://doi.org/10.1016/S1470-2045(14)71160-X. Epub 2014 Dec 11.
50. Bajorin DF, Witjes JA, et al. Adjuvant Nivolumab versus placebo in muscle-invasive urothelial carcinoma. N Engl J Med. 2021;384(22):2102–14. https://doi.org/10.1056/NEJMoa2034442. Erratum in: N Engl J Med. 2021;385(9):864. PMID: 34077643; PMCID: PMC8215888.
51. Bellmunt J, Hussain M et al.; IMvigor010 Study Group. Adjuvant atezolizumab versus observation in muscle-invasive urothelial carcinoma (IMvigor010): a multicentre, open-label, randomised, phase 3 trial. Lancet Oncol. 2021;22(4):525–37. https://doi.org/10.1016/S1470-2045(21)00004-8. Epub 2021 Mar 12. PMID: 33721560; PMCID: PMC8495594.
52. https://clinicaltrials.gov/study/NCT03244384.
53. Huddart RA, Birtle A, et al. Clinical and patient-reported outcomes of SPAR E—a randomized feasibility study of selective bladder preservation versus radical cystectomy. BJU Int. 2017;120(5):639–50. https://doi.org/10.1111/bju.13900. Epub 2017 May 29. PMID: 28453896; PMCID: PMC5655733.
54. Mak RH, Hunt D, et al. Long-term outcomes in patients with muscle-invasive bladder cancer after selective bladder-preserving combined-modality therapy: a pooled analysis of Radiation Therapy Oncology Group protocols 8802, 8903, 9506, 9706, 9906, and 0233. J Clin Oncol. 2014;32(34):3801–9. https://doi.org/10.1200/JCO.2014.57.5548. Epub 2014 Nov 3. Erratum in: J Clin Oncol. 2015;33(7):814. PMID: 25366678; PMCID: PMC4239302.
55. Hall E, Hussain SA, et al. BC2001 investigators. Chemoradiotherapy in muscle-invasive bladder cancer: 10-yr follow-up of the phase 3 randomised controlled BC2001 trial. Eur Urol. 2022;82(3):273–9. https://doi.org/10.1016/j.eururo.2022.04.017. Epub 2022 May 14.
56. Duchesne GM, Bolger JJ, et al. A randomised trial of hypofractionated schedules of palliative radiotherapy in the management of bladder carcinoma: results of medical research council trial BA09. Int J Radiat Oncol Biol Phys. 2000;47(2):379–88. https://doi.org/10.1016/s0360-3016(00)00430-2.
57. Galsky MD, Stensland K, et al. Comparative effectiveness of treatment strategies for bladder Cancer with clinical evidence of regional lymph node involvement. J Clin Oncol. 2016;34(22):2627–35. https://doi.org/10.1200/JCO.2016.67.5033. Epub 2016 Jun 6. PMID: 27269939; PMCID: PMC5012691.
58. Hussain MH, Glass TR, et al. Combination cisplatin, 5-fluorouracil and radiation therapy for locally advanced unresectable or medically unfit bladder cancer cases: a southwest oncology group study. J Urol. 2001;165(1):56–60; discussion 60–1. https://doi.org/10.1097/00005392-200101000-00014.
59. Portner R, Bajaj A, et al. A practical approach to bladder preservation with hypofractionated radiotherapy for localised muscle-invasive bladder cancer. Clin Transl Radiat Oncol. 2021;31:1–7. https://doi.org/10.1016/j.ctro.2021.08.003. PMID: 34466667; PMCID: PMC8385113.
60. Hindson BR, Turner SL et al. RANZCR Faculty of Radiation Oncology Genito-Urinary Group (FROGG). Australian & New Zealand Faculty of Radiation Oncology Genito-Urinary Group: 2011 consensus guidelines for curative radiotherapy for urothelial carcinoma of the bladder. J Med Imaging Radiat Oncol. 2012;56(1):18–30. https://doi.org/10.1111/j.1754-9485.2011.02336.x.
61. Verghote F, Sargos P, et al. International consensus guidelines for adjuvant radiation therapy for bladder Cancer after radical cystectomy: update from an IBIS workgroup. Pract Radiat Oncol. 2022;12(6):524–32. https://doi.org/10.1016/j.prro.2022.05.014. Epub 2022 Jun 9.
62. Coppin CM, Gospodarowicz MK, et al. Improved local control of invasive bladder cancer by concurrent cisplatin and preoperative or definitive radiation. The National Cancer Institute of Canada clinical trials group. J Clin Oncol. 1996;14(11):2901–7. https://doi.org/10.1200/JCO.1996.14.11.2901.
63. Mitin T, Hunt D, et al. Transurethral surgery and twice-daily radiation plus paclitaxel-cisplatin or fluorouracil-cisplatin with selective bladder preservation and adjuvant chemotherapy for patients with muscle invasive bladder cancer (RTOG 0233): a randomised multicentre phase

2 trial. Lancet Oncol. 2013;14(9):863–72. https://doi.org/10.1016/S1470-2045(13)70255-9. Epub 2013 Jul 1. PMID: 23823157; PMCID: PMC3955198.
64. James ND, Hussain SA, et al. BC2001 investigators. Radiotherapy with or without chemotherapy in muscle-invasive bladder cancer. N Engl J Med. 2012;366(16):1477–88. https://doi.org/10.1056/NEJMoa1106106.
65. de Haar-Holleman A, van Hoogstraten LMC, et al. Chemoradiation for muscle-invasive bladder cancer using 5-fluorouracil versus capecitabine: a nationwide cohort study. Radiother Oncol. 2023;183:109584. https://doi.org/10.1016/j.radonc.2023.109584. Epub 2023 Mar 1.
66. Kent E, Sandler H, Montie J, et al. Combined- modality therapy with gemcitabine and radiotherapy as a bladder preservation strategy: results of a phase I trial. J Clin Oncol. 2004;22(13):2540–5. https://doi.org/10.1200/JCO.2004.10.070.
67. Choudhury A, Swindell R, et al. Phase II study of conformal hypofractionated radiotherapy with concurrent gemcitabine in muscle- invasive bladder cancer. J Clin Oncol. 2011;29(6):733–8. https://doi.org/10.1200/JCO.2010.31.5721. Epub 2011 Jan 4.
68. Michaelson MD, Hu C, et al. A phase 1/2 trial of a combination of paclitaxel and trastuzumab with daily irradiation or paclitaxel alone with daily irradiation after transurethral surgery for noncystectomy candidates with muscle-invasive bladder cancer (Trial NRG Oncology RTOG 0524). Int J Radiat Oncol Biol Phys. 2017;97(5):995–1001. https://doi.org/10.1016/j.ijrobp.2016.12.018. Epub 2016 Dec 19. PMID: 28333021; PMCID: PMC5536836.
69. Rödel C, Grabenbauer GG, et al. Combined-modality treatment and selective organ preservation in invasive bladder cancer: long-term results. J Clin Oncol. 2002;20(14):3061–71. https://doi.org/10.1200/JCO.2002.11.027.
70. Sanguedolce F, Zanelli M, et al. Are we ready to implement molecular subtyping of bladder cancer in clinical practice? Part 1: general issues and marker expression. Int J Mol Sci. 2022;23(14):7819. https://doi.org/10.3390/ijms23147819. PMID: 35887164; PMCID: PMC9319819.
71. Weiss C, Wittlinger M, et al. Management of superficial recurrences in an irradiated bladder after combined-modality organ- preserving therapy. Int J Radiat Oncol Biol Phys. 2008;70(5):1502–6. https://doi.org/10.1016/j.ijrobp.2007.08.007. Epub 2007 Nov 1.
72. Zietman AL, Grocela J, et al. Selective bladder conservation using transurethral resection, chemotherapy, and radiation: management and consequences of Ta, T1, and Tis recurrence within the retained bladder. Urology. 2001;58(3):380–5. https://doi.org/10.1016/s0090-4295(01)01219-5.

Management of Renal Cancers

11

Animesh Agrawal and M. B. Minu Chandra

11.1 Epidemiology

Renal malignancies form around 2% of all malignancies worldwide (GLOBOCAN 2020). The incidence is the highest in the Baltic countries (~22 and 9 per lakh population for males and females, respectively); in India, the incidence is much lower at ~1 per lakh population (around 17,000 new cases each year), but the mortality is higher (~10,000 deaths/year).

The most commonly cited risk factors for the development of RCC include smoking, obesity, and hypertension. An association with long-term dialysis has also been noted, though this association may be spurious (more imaging leads to higher detection rates).

11.2 Pathology

Histologically RCC is most commonly a *clear cell* carcinoma (ccRCC; 70–80%). These carry the best prognosis and are usually associated with mutations of the VHL gene (at 3p25–26). Other subtypes include *papillary* (previously type 1 and type 2 but now only 1 type is recognized by the WHO); *oncocytic* and *chromophobe* type; *collecting duct* tumors; and a heterogeneous group of tumors collectively classified as *molecularly defined renal cell carcinomas*. For a complete discussion of the various histologies, the reader is referred to the WHO Classification of

A. Agrawal
Apollo Medics Superspecialty Hospital, Lucknow, Uttar Pradesh, India

M. B. M. Chandra (✉)
Department of Medical Oncology, Gujarat Cancer Research Institute, Ahmedabad, India

R. Madan, S. Goyal (eds.), *Essentials of Radiotherapy in Uro-Genital Malignancies*, https://doi.org/10.1007/978-981-95-5945-9_11

Tumors—Urinary and Male Genital Tumors. All carry varying prognoses; however, owing to their rarity, non-ccRCCs lack clear recommendations (and indeed data) to guide management.

Also to be considered to ascertain prognosis (especially in adjuvant setting) is the WHO ISUP (International Society of Urologic Pathologists) grade of the tumor. Based on morphological characteristics, the tumor is assigned a grade (1–4 with 4 carrying the poorest prognosis). ISUP grading is validated for clear cell and papillary histologies only (Table 11.1).

Table 11.1 Histological Subtypes of Renal Tumors

Histological type	Molecular abnormalities	Clinical	Immunohistochemistry[a]
Clear cell RCC (ccRCC) (70–80%)	Mutation/loss at VHL gene locus 3p25 (>90%); VHL syndrome is the familial counterpart	Most common variant; most studied. Prognostication per IMDC risk groups	*Positive*: CAIX, Vimentin, AE1/AE3, AMACR, PAX8 *Negative*: CK7, KIT, GATA3, HMWCK
Papillary (5–10%)	MET (7q31): most common Others: Gain 7, 17 or deletion 9p	Frequently multifocal Prognostication: IMDC risk group May respond to the same regimens as used for ccRCC.	*Positive*: CK7, AMACR, Vimentin, HMWCK *Negative*: CAIX. KIT, GATA3
Chromophobe (<5%)	Loss of multiple chromosomes—1, 2, 6, 10, 13, 17, 21, Y Low somatic mutation rate	6th decade Good prognosis	*Positive*: CK7, AMACR, KIT, MOC31, claudin7, GATA3 (sometimes) *Negative*: CAIX, Vimentin, HMWCK, CD10
Collecting duct (<1%)	Copy number loss or LOH of multiple chromosomes 1p, 6, 8, 9, 14, 22; CDKN2A loss	Poor prognosis Poor response to immunotherapy	*Positive*: HMWCK, PAX8, CK7, CK19 *Negative*: CAIX, Vimentin
Molecularly defined	Includes TFE3 rearranged, TFEB altered, ELOC mutated, fumarate hydratase deficient, HLRCC syndrome associated, SDH deficient, ALK rearranged, SMARCB1 deficient (medullary like/undifferentiated/dedifferentiated), medullary carcinoma		

[a]IHC markers as given in this table may vary considerably based on histological grade and overall tumor heterogeneity

11.3 Approach to an Incidental Renal Mass

Patients presenting with the triad of hematuria, abdominal mass, and flank pain have markedly reduced due to the increased usage of radiological investigations like computerized tomography (CT) and magnetic resonance imaging (MRI), and the incidental detection of renal masses is on a rise. Any solid contrast-enhancing lesion of size more than 4 cm without fat has a 90% chance of being malignant [1].

Investigations in a patient of suspected renal malignancy include complete blood picture, liver function tests including serum albumin and alkaline phosphatase (ALP), kidney function tests, corrected calcium, and lactate dehydrogenase (LDH). A CT scan of the abdomen and thorax is used for staging. Patients with brain and bone metastasis present with clinical symptoms, so a routine staging does not include bone scan or brain imaging. If the patient has a raised ALP or has bone pains, then a bone scan has to be performed. The role of PET-CT scan in the diagnosis and post-treatment follow-up in patients with renal cell cancer is yet to be determined.

In patients found to have an isolated renal mass without any other possible sites of metastasis, an upfront partial nephrectomy or a complete nephrectomy is preferred as it gives the complete tumor (T) and nodal (N) staging. Preoperative biopsy is generally not preferred in a resectable renal mass as it would cause needle track seeding and contamination of the peritoneal cavity. It is reserved for those situations where an alternate etiology is suspected (such as abscess/metastasis) that would alter management, or when the patient is being considered for surveillance/ablative therapy.

Needle biopsy is done in selected patients who may be candidates for strategies like active surveillance, cryosurgery, ablation, radio frequency, etc. [2]. A needle biopsy is also recommended if the lesion is central in location to rule out urothelial carcinoma or if it shows features of homogenous infiltration to rule out lymphoma.

11.4 Partial Nephrectomy vs. Radical Nephrectomy

Partial nephrectomy (also called nephron sparing surgery) was previously indicated only in patients with a single functioning kidney which might render the patient anephric requiring daily dialysis. But recent studies have established that a partial nephrectomy has comparable outcomes to a radical nephrectomy [3–6].

A radical nephrectomy includes a perifascial resection of kidney, peri nephric fat, regional lymph nodes, and the ipsilateral adrenal gland. It is the preferred treatment when the tumor extends to the inferior vena cava. Radical nephrectomy leads to decrease in the number of functional nephrons resulting in chronic kidney disease and associated cardiovascular issues; on the contrary, partial nephrectomy preserves the renal function and decreases the overall mortality. Therefore, a nephron-sparing surgery is preferred whenever possible without compromising the oncologic and functional outcome. Open, laparoscopic, or robotic approaches carry similar oncologic outcomes in skilled hands.

Prophylactic lymph node dissection does not improve the overall survival (OS) or progression-free survival (PFS). Hence, lymph node dissection is done only in patients with palpable or enlarged lymph nodes. Ipsilateral adrenalectomy is considered if the adrenal gland is bulky or in tumors arising from the upper pole of the kidney. Stage is assigned as per the eighth AJCC TNM staging.

11.5 Stage-Wise Management of Renal Cell Carcinoma

11.5.1 Locoregional Therapy

Stage I (T1N0M0): Tumor up to 7 cm in greatest dimension and limited to the kidney is a stage I tumor. Partial nephrectomy by open or laparoscopic routes is the preferred management. If a nephron-sparing approach is not feasible, then a radical nephrectomy is recommended. If the patient is not fit for nephrectomy, conservative approaches such as active surveillance, radiofrequency, ablation, or cryosurgery may be adopted.

Stages II (T2 N0M0) and III (T1-2N1M0, T3Any N M0): A radical nephrectomy is the curative therapy in patients with stage II and III tumors. Nephron-sparing surgeries should be considered wherever technically feasible - especially in specific populations like patients with a solitary kidney, elevated risk of developing progressive CKD due to medical risk factors, etc. Regional Nodal dissection is optional, but should be done for patients with resectable adenopathy on preoperative imaging or intra-operative visualization.

11.5.2 Adjuvant Treatment of Localized Non-metastatic Disease

11.5.2.1 Neoadjuvant Radiation

Two studies have evaluated the role of neoadjuvant radiation in resectable RCC; while there was a small increment in the number of complete resections in patients with locally advanced disease, 5-year survival was similar on both arms of these studies. As of today, it is an obsolete practice.

11.5.2.2 Adjuvant Radiation

Adjuvant treatment with radiation has not shown any benefit, even in disease with nodal involvement or incomplete resections. The few patients who do experience local recurrences can be salvaged by repeat resections. A meta-analysis on this question analyzed 12 studies (10 retrospective, 2 RCTs) including 1624 patients; 37% patients received adjuvant RT and the median follow-up was 49 months. Overall, there was a lower rate of locoregional recurrence with radiation, but no improvement in disease-free survival (DFS) or OS [7].

In modern day practice, the use of radiation is restricted to palliating symptoms of disease at metastatic sites and for local treatment of oligoprogressive disease.

11.5.2.3 Adjuvant Systemic Therapy

The results from adjuvant systemic therapy have been mixed. Both tyrosine kinase inhibitors (TKIs) and checkpoint inhibitors (ICIs) have been assessed in large RCTs. The first of these was ASSURE [8], which randomized 1943 patients with either node-positive or pT1b G3-4 N0 disease in 1:1:1 manner to sunitinib, sorafenib, and placebo for 12 months. There was no difference in disease-free survival (DFS) in the three arms (5.8, 6.1, and 6.6 years, respectively, for sunitinib, sorafenib, and placebo). The S–TRAC trial randomized 615 patients with stage 3 and/or node-positive ccRCC (node positive ~8%) to adjuvant sunitinib and placebo and reported a median DFS of 6.8 years in the sunitinib arm compared to 5.6 years in the placebo arm (HR, 0.76; 95% CI, 0.59–0.98; $P = 0.03$) [9]. Despite the lack of overall survival (OS) benefit, sunitinib was approved in completely resected RCC in the adjuvant setting. Three other trials have evaluated adjuvant TKIs—PROTECT (pazopanib), SORCE (sorafenib), and ATLAS (axitinib) but all failed to find any DFS or OS benefit with adjuvant TKI [10–13]. Of all the TKIs, sunitinib remains the only one to have shown a benefit.

11.5.2.4 Adjuvant Immunotherapy

Four trials have reported results with adjuvant immunotherapy in patients with ccRCC (Table 11.2)—pembrolizumab (Keynote564), atezolizumab (IM Motion 10), nivolumab (PROSPER; EA8143), and nivolumab/ipilimumab (Checkmate 914).

IMMotion 010 [14] randomized 778 patients with T2 G4, T3a G3-4, T3b-4 any grade, node-positive and/or M1 NED disease to receive placebo or adjuvant atezolizumab for 1 year. With a median follow-up of 45 months, the 3-year DFS and OS were nearly identical (59% vs. 59.4% and 89.8% vs. 90.3% for placebo vs. Atezolizumab, respectively), suggesting no benefit for the trial population. Similar results were seen in Checkmate 914 [15], in which 816 patients with T2a G3-4, T2b-4 G(any), and/or node-positive disease were randomized to placebo or adjuvant nivolumab + ipilimumab for 6 months. RFS with a median follow-up of 37 months was 76% vs. 74% for the trial and placebo arms respectively. Keynote 564 [16, 17] had a similar design to the above two trials—994 patients with pT2 G4/sarcomatoid, pT3-4 G(any), node positive, and/or M1 NED disease were randomized to receive placebo or adjuvant pembrolizumab for 1 year. Unlike the previous two studies, however, a significant improvement in RFS was noted at a median follow-up of 30 months (75% vs. 65%, HR 0.63, 95% CI 0.5–0.8). PROSPER [18] was a somewhat similar trial; it randomized patients to surgery alone vs. 1 dose of neoadjuvant Nivolumab and 9 doses of adjuvant treatment. The interim analysis of this study showed no difference in RFS (HR 0.97) and it was closed early for futility.

11.5.2.5 Miscellaneous

Other drugs that have been evaluated in this setting are everolimus (EVEREST) and girentuximab (ARISER). In EVEREST [19], 1545 patients with T1b G3-4, T2-4 G(any), or pN+ disease were randomized to receive 10 mg everolimus or placebo for 1 year. With a median follow-up of 76 months, DFS at 5 years was similar (67% vs. 63%). Notably, 37% patients discontinued everolimus due to adverse

Table 11.2 Adjuvant therapy trials

Trial	Study arms	Dose and duration	Inclusion criteria	Results
Tyrosine kinase inhibitors (TKIs)				
ASSURE [8] (5.8y)	Sunitinib (647) Sorafenib (649) Placebo (647)	50 mg 4/6; 54w 400 mg BD —	pT1b G3-4 N0 T & G (any) N +	70m 73.4m 79.6m
PROTECT [10] (76m)	Pazopanib (769) Placebo (769)	800 ($n = 198$) 600 ($n = 571$)	pT2 G3-4 pT3-4 G (any) pN+	DFS better with 800 mg; no diff in OS
SORCE [12] (6.5y)	Sorafenib 3y (639) Sorafenib 1y (642) Placebo (430)	400 BD 400 BD —	Poor Risk; 84% ccRCC	10y DFS 53% 55% 54%
ATLAS [13]	Axitinib (363) Placebo (361)	5 mg BD —	pT2 pN+	DFS similar HR 0.87, $p = 0.3$
S-TRAC [9] (6.6y)	Sunitinib (309) Placebo (306)	50 mg 4/6; 1yr —	T3 G2+ T4 G (any), N+	Median DFS 6.8y 5.6y
Checkpoint inhibitors (ICIs)				
IM motion 010 [14] (44m)	Atezolizumab (390) Placebo (388)	1200 mg. q3w. 1y —	T2 G4, T3a G3+ T3–4 G (any) N+, M1 NED	mDFS similar 4.7y 4.1y
Checkmate 914 [15] (37m)	Nivolumab (405) Ipilimumab Placebo (411)	240 mg q2w × 6m 1 mg/kg q6w × 6m —	T2a G3+ T2b-4 G(any) pN+	3y DFS ~68% in both arms
PROSPER [18] (16m)	Nivolumab, 1; surgery, 9 Surgery alone	480 mg q4w —	T2+ and/or N+	RFS similar HR 0.97
Keynote 564 [16, 17] (30m)	Pembrolizumab (496) Placebo (498)	200 mg q3w 1y —	Stage 2 G4 / sarcomatoid, Stage 3, N+, M1 NED	DFS (30m) 75% vs. 65% HR 0.63
Misc				
EVEREST [19] (76m)	Everolimus (755) Placebo (744)	10 mg OD; 54 wks —	IB, G3+; Stage II+, G (any); N+	RFS similar (HR 0.85)
ARISER [20] (54m)	Girentuximab (433) Placebo (431)	20 mg weekly; 6m —	T1b-2, G3+; T3+; N+	DFS similar (HR 0.97)

events. Another drug, girentuximab is a monoclonal antibody targeting CAIX (a cell surface glycoprotein expressed in nearly all ccRCCs), and in the ARISER [20] study, 864 patients with pT3-4, pN+, and/or pT1b-2 G3+ disease were randomized to receive weekly doses of the trial drug or placebo for 6 months. Results were reported at a median follow-up of 54 months with similar 5-year DFS (54% vs. 52%).

In summary, only one trial each of a TKI and an ICI in the adjuvant setting has shown any benefit, and pembrolizumab has FDA approval for this indication while NCCN lists sunitinib as a category 3 recommendation. Further follow-up and overall survival results of these trials may shed more light on this question. The authors presently recommend adjuvant pembrolizumab to eligible patients.

11.6 Role of Cytoreductive Nephrectomy (CRN) in Metastatic Setting

Cytoreductive nephrectomy is also called the debulking surgery and is done in patients of metastatic RCC prior to the initiation of systemic therapy. It dates back to the era of interferon immunotherapy. Interferon alfa (IFNα) was used in the treatment of metastatic RCC before the advent of VEGF TKIs.

The South-West Oncology Group (SWOG) included 246 patients with metastatic renal cell carcinoma and assigned them to cytoreductive nephrectomy followed by IFNα or IFNα alone [21]. Patients that underwent cytoreductive nephrectomy followed by IFNα had a longer median OS compared to the IFNα alone group. The survival benefit was more in patients with an ECOG 0 performance status. A similar trial conducted by EORTC also confirmed the survival advantage with cytoreductive nephrectomy compared to interferon alfa (IFNa) alone [22]. A combined analysis of the two studies showed a significant OS improvement with the addition of surgery (13.6m vs. 7.8m, HR 0.69). However, these patients did not receive any VEGF inhibition [23].

With the advent of VEGF TKI for the treatment of metastatic RCC, the question regarding the benefit of cytoreductive nephrectomy resurfaced. CARMENA was a phase 3 study that randomized 450 patients with metastatic ccRCC (MSKCC Intermediate and Poor risk) to assess the non-inferiority of sunitinib alone to cytoreductive nephrectomy followed by sunitinib. With a median follow-up of 51 months, sunitinib alone was non-inferior to the trial arm with a median OS of 18m vs. 14m. This trial suggested that with current VEGF TKI therapy, in patients with MSKCC Intermediate to Poor risk the benefit is limited [24, 25].

SURTIME [26] assessed whether deferred surgery after 16 weeks of sunitinib could allow better selection of patients for cytoreductive nephrectomy based on treatment response. It aimed to enroll 458 patients, but closed recruitment when only 99 patients were enrolled over 5 years. A total of 46 out of 50 patients underwent upfront CRN while the rest received sunitinib followed by reassessment, of which 34 eventually underwent surgery. PFS was similar between the two arms (~7 months) and the OS was 24m vs. 15m for deferred vs. upfront CRN ($p = 0.225$) (Table 11.3).

Patients not fitting into the above criteria should proceed with upfront systemic therapy and may be assessed for cytoreductive nephrectomy if the patient has excellent response to the treatment. There are no prospective data to guide us regarding

Table 11.3 Risk scoring for clear cell renal cell carcinoma (ccRCC)

MSKCC risk score [27]	IMDC risk score [28]
Less than 1 year from diagnosis to treatment KPS < 80 Serum LDH > 1.5 times ULN Corrected serum Ca > ULN Hemoglobin < LLN	Less than 1 year from diagnosis to treatment KPS < 80 Corrected serum Ca > ULN Hemoglobin < LLN ANC > ULN Platelet count > ULN
Low risk: None Intermediate risk: 1–2 factors Poor risk: 3 or more risk factors	Favorable risk: None Intermediate risk: 1–2 factors Poor risk: 3 or more risk factors

KPS Karnofsky Performance Score, *LDH* Lactate Dehydrogenase, *Ca* Calcium, *ULN* Upper Limit of Normal, *LLN* Lower Limit of Normal, *ANC* Absolute Neutrophil Count, *MSKCC* Memorial Sloan Kettering Cancer Center

the benefit of cytoreductive nephrectomy in the era of immunotherapy. Till such evidence becomes available, the above principles can still be applied.

Available evidence would suggest that patients who require systemic therapy should be started on an IO combination (discussed later) with CRN reserved for patients who need local treatment for symptom control. However, based on ad hoc analyses of trials from the TKI era, guidelines suggest that patients with low disease burden, a good PS (ECOG 0-1), and an IMDC/MSKCC risk score of 0-1 may be considered for CRN followed by systemic therapy. Whether these data hold true in the immunotherapy era remains to be seen. Nephrectomy may also be considered as a palliative measure for patients with severe pain or bleeding attributed to the tumor.

Role of Metastasectomy

- Metastasectomy may be done upfront in patients presenting with an oligometastatic (1–3 metastatic sites) prior to systemic therapy.
- Post radical nephrectomy, a metastasectomy may be considered in patients who develop a resectable recurrence after more than 1 year.
- Patients who have resectable persistent disease on systemic therapy.

Disease-free interval of greater than 1 year from nephrectomy to metastasectomy, single metastatic lesion, ECOG PS 0-1 were considered favorable factors to attain greater disease-free survival [29]. Other approaches that have been evaluated include metastasectomy combined with whole brain radiotherapy (WBRT) and/or stereotactic radiosurgery (SRS), which have yielded good results [30–32].

11.7 Systemic Therapy for mRCC—Biologic Rationale

Deeper understanding regarding the tumor microenvironment and molecular aspects has highlighted the importance of the Von Hippel-Lindau (VHL) gene in the pathogenesis of RCC (Fig. 11.1).

VHL is a tumor suppressor gene located on chromosome 3p. In its active state, it keeps a check on hypoxia-inducible transcription factor 1α (HIF1α). HIF1α encodes

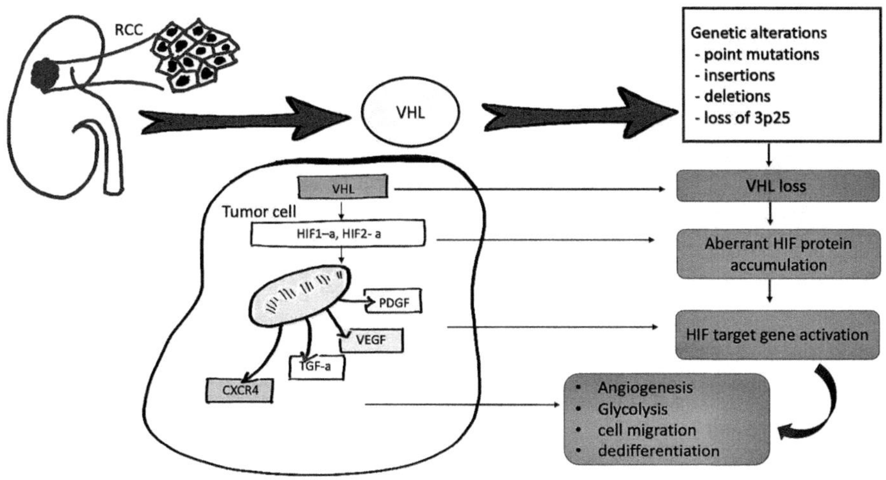

Fig. 11.1 Clear cell renal cell carcinoma showing VHL inactivation and activation of angiogenic genes [33]

the genes responsible for the production of vascular endothelial growth factor (VEGF), platelet-derived growth factor (PDGF), epidermal growth factor (EGF), and transforming growth factor-α (TGF-α) all of which play an essential role in angiogenesis [33].

RCCs are highly vascular tumors. Therefore anti-angiogenic agents such as bevacizumab (anti VEGF-A monoclonal antibody) and tyrosine kinase inhibitors (TKIs) targeting angiogenesis have been evaluated extensively in their management.

As a strategy to overcome this resistance, a new generation of anti-angiogenic drugs such as lenvatinib and cabozantinib which could target many different pathways came into existence. The simultaneous inhibition of VEGFR and accessory pathways was thought to decrease the development of treatment-induced resistance (Fig. 11.2).

The inhibition of MET and AXL with *cabozantinib* has a strong rationale [34]:

- cMET is overexpressed in many ccRCC.
- cMET and AXL are induced by VEGF inhibition.
- Targeting MET and AXL could overcome resistance to anti-VEGF.

Also the combination of *lenvatinib* + *everolimus* has an attractive biological rationale of synergistic activity of VEGFR and mTOR pathways inhibition [35].

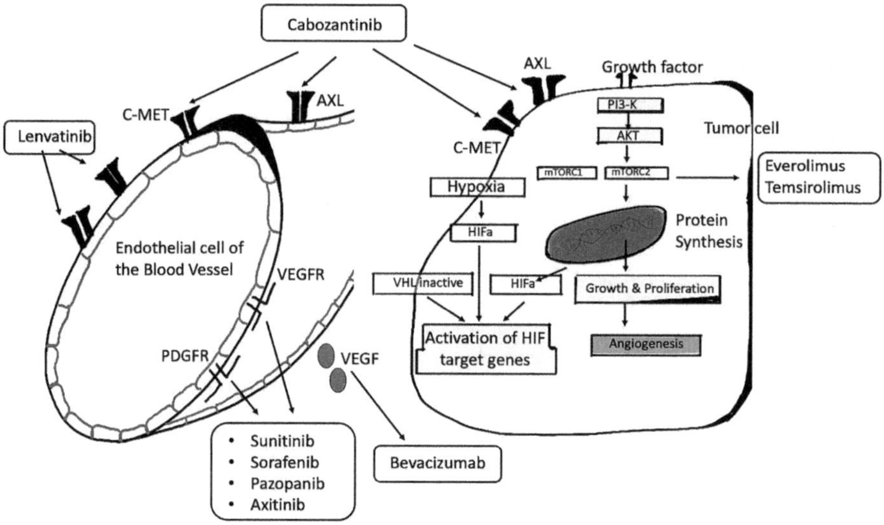

Fig. 11.2 Pathways of signaling and drugs inhibiting them in RCC [63]

11.7.1 Rationale for the Usage of Immunotherapy—The Tumor Microenvironment

Systemic therapy for de novo metastatic RCC has evolved considerably in the last decade. Results with chemotherapy come almost solely from small phase 2 studies. There is significant heterogeneity between studies, but on an average, the ORR is between 15% and 20% and chemotherapy has very little role in present-day management of advanced RCC [36].

However, tales of magical disappearance of the metastatic tumor after local therapy like surgery or radiation therapy have been well documented [37]. This is the *abscopal effect* and is due to the natural anti-tumor immunity due to the presence of high levels of immune infiltrate.

Treatments during 1990s exploited this concept of immune infiltration by using cytokines like IFN-α and high-dose interleukin-2 (IL-2). These were found to result in durable responses in several patients; especially IL-2 provided complete responses in 5–10% of all treated patients, with a median PFS of around 5 months [38–42]. This remained the standard of care (SoC) until the emergence of the TKIs.

The first study to demonstrate a significant benefit of a TKI over cytokine-based treatment was reported by Motzer et al. [43], who reported a significant PFS improvement with first-line sunitinib (the improvement in OS was not statistically significant). Subsequently other TKIs such as pazopanib (COMPARZ), sorafenib (TARGET), axitinib (AXIS) and cabozantinib (METEOR) were demonstrated to have clinical activity, and VEGF inhibitors as a class became the SoC for these patients [44–52]. The median PFS with these drugs in the first line is around 9–12 months and in subsequent lines between 4 and 6 months. They are generally well tolerated with discontinuation rates ranging between 5% and 15%. Adverse drug reactions (ADRs) tend to be dose dependent, with hypertension being the most common. Other common ADRs include fatigue, hand foot syndrome, mucositis, diarrhea, and rashes, which are experienced by ~20–75% of all patients. The potential for cardiotoxicity with TKIs also needs to be kept in mind for patients with preexisting heart disease.

Everolimus, an mTOR inhibitor, has also shown efficacy in second-line treatment in several studies with a median PFS of 6–8 months. In combination with Lenvatinib, the PFS in second-line treatment is around 12 months. However, this combination is associated with a higher rate of adverse events with ~25% discontinuation rates, and 60–70% patients require dose reductions because of grade 3/4 adverse events [53–55].

Revisiting the concept of treating RCC by using the immune infiltrate was possible with the advent of immune checkpoint inhibitors (ICI), which were more efficacious than the cytokines and had a better toxicity profile. These drugs (specifically anti-PD-1, PDL1, and CTLA4 monoclonal antibodies) now form the principal treatment modality for patients with advanced RCC. Dual ICI or an ICI/TKI combination is now the first line of therapy for these patients based on data from multiple randomized studies (Table 11.4). There are, however, certain facts to be kept in mind. *Firstly*, these regimens have not been compared to each other. Choosing one over the other is largely an exercise in cross-trial comparison, which introduces physician biases into the decision-making process. *Secondly*, post-progression therapy in these studies is off protocol, meaning that around half of all patients on control arms do not receive ICIs upon progression. While this allows a better understanding of the impact of ICI, it does not reflect SoC; therefore, the OS benefit as noted in these trials might be exaggerated. *Thirdly*, in a Low and Middle Income Country (LMIC) like India, these agents are beyond the reach of most patients as long as the patents are in place.

With the above in mind, a general pattern does emerge:

- ICI and TKI combination is a valid treatment option for nearly all patients.
- For intermediate to poor-risk patients, dual ICI is a reasonable option with durable responses.
- For selected patients with low burden, favorable risk disease, even TKI alone might be a reasonable option, with immunotherapy reserved for later lines.
- Cytoreductive nephrectomy may be considered in carefully selected patients. This could be either upfront or delayed based on symptoms and response to systemic therapy.

11.7.2 Second-Line Systemic Therapy

Second-line therapy was typically an ICI-based regimen before modern trials firmly pushed them into the first line. In the current era after treatment failure with an ICI combination, a TKI (alone or in combination) will be the most appropriate therapy.

Table 11.4 First-line management of advanced RCC

	CM 214	CM 9ER	KN 426	CLEAR	Javelin 101
1^0 end point	OS, PFS, ORR	PFS	PFS, OS	PFS	PFS, OS (in PDL1+)
Trial	Nivolumab Ipilimumab	Nivolumab Cabozantinib	Pembrolizumab Axitinib	Pembrolizumab Lenvatinib	Avelumab Axitinib
Control	Sunitinib				
N	1096	651	861	712	886
IMDC Risk F/I/P	23/60/17	23/53/19	32/55/13	31/60/9	21/61/9
Follow-up	Min 5y	Median 44m	Min 5y	Median 4y	Median 34m
ORR	39%	56%	60%	71%	53%
PR	28%	43%	50%	54%	49%
CR	12%	12%	10%	17%	4%
PD	18%	6%	11%	5%	12%
PFS HR	12m vs. 12m 0.86 (ns)	16m vs. 8m 0.56	15m vs. 11m 0.71	23m vs. 9m 0.42	13m vs. 8m 0.69
OS HR	47m vs. 27m 0.68 (IR/PR)	50m vs. 36m 0.7	47m vs. 41m 0.84	54m vs. 54m 0.79	NR vs 38m 0.79
ADR: Grade 3+	48% vs. 64%	65% vs. 54%	68% vs. 64%	82% vs. 72%	81% vs. 77%
Discontinuation	23% vs. 13%	27% vs. 10%	21% vs. 12%	37% vs. 14%	19% vs. 14%

Everolimus was first evaluated against a placebo in the RECORD 1 trial in 410 patients who had progressive disease after a first-line TKI. This study showed that everolimus improved the PFS to 4.9m vs. 1.9m with placebo in this setting [56, 57]. Subsequently, cabozantinib was pitted against everolimus in the METEOR trial and shown to result in a better PFS (7.4m vs. 3.8m, HR 0.51) and OS (21.4m vs. 17.1m, HR 0.7). However, less than a quarter of these patients received ICI in a later line [50–52]. Other drugs to have been evaluated include axitinib, which was compared to sorafenib in the AXIS trial, and a better PFS (8.3m vs. 5.7m, HR 0.66) but similar OS (20.1m vs. 19.2m, ns) was reported. This trial predated the ICI era [48, 49]. The TKI-mTOR inhibitor combination of lenvatinib and everolimus [53, 58] was then evaluated in a phase II trial, and the combination, while associated with high rates of ADRs and discontinuation, had a marked improvement in PFS (14.6 months with the combination vs. 6–8m with either drug alone).

It would seem that a VEGF TKI is the best treatment option for a patient who has treatment failure after an ICI-based regimen. The options include cabozantinib, lenvatinib with or without everolimus, and axitinib. At an individual patient level, this decision should be made on the basis of prior treatment received and toxicity profile of the planned regimen. For a patient who has not received an ICI previously, a survival improvement has been seen with their use. Checkmate 025 [59, 60] demonstrated an OS of 25m vs. 19.6m with everolimus with a more favorable adverse event profile. Checkmate 016 showed that dual ICI combination had good activity in the setting with an ORR of 46% and median PFS of 7.7 months [61]. Keynote 146 evaluated the combination of lenvatinib and pembrolizumab; 145 patients were enrolled on the RCC cohort and the ORR was ~41% with a median PFS of 12 months [62]. Where feasible, a patient should be offered a checkpoint inhibitor in the first line or the next.

11.7.3 What's Ahead?

Much work is still needed for patients with RCC. Challenges include optimizing outcomes for patients with less common histologies, identifying patients with the highest risk of relapse and treating them accordingly, improving outcomes for patients with metastatic disease (especially IMDC IR/PR disease), and better understanding the molecular pathways implicated in carcinogenesis to develop ever more accurate targeted drug delivery. Several trials involving ICIs, new combinations, and newer TKIs are ongoing in various disease settings. Their results will continue to guide treatment for the next few years.

References

1. Frank I, Blute ML, Cheville JC, Lohse CM, Weaver AL, Zincke H. Solid renal tumors: an analysis of pathological features related to tumor size. J Urol. 2003;170(6):2217–20.

2. Shannon BA, Cohen RJ, de Bruto H, Davies RJ. The value of preoperative needle core biopsy for diagnosing benign lesions among small, incidentally detected renal masses. J Urol. 2008;180(4):1257–61.
3. Dash A, Vickers AJ, Schachter LR, et al. Comparison of outcomes in elective partial vs. radical nephrectomy for clear cell renal cell carcinoma of 4–7 cm. BJU Int. 2006;97(5):939–45.
4. Lee CT, Katz J, Shi W, et al. Surgical management of renal tumors 4 cm. or less in a contemporary cohort. J Urol. 2000;163(3):730–6.
5. Zini L, Perrotte P, Capitanio U, et al. Radical versus partial nephrectomy: effect on overall and noncancer mortality. Cancer. 2009;115(7):1465–71.
6. Lee HJ, Liss MA, Derweesh IH, et al. Outcomes of partial nephrectomy for clinical T1b and T2 renal tumors. Curr Opin Urol. 2014;24(5):448–52.
7. Rodríguez-Fernández IA, et al. Adjuvant radiation therapy after radical nephrectomy in patients with localized renal cell carcinoma: a systematic review and meta-analysis. Eur Urol Oncol. 2019;2:448.
8. Haas NB, Manola J, Uzzo RG, et al. Adjuvant sunitinib or sorafenib for high-risk, non-metastatic renal-cell carcinoma (ECOG-ACRIN E2805): a double-blind, placebo-controlled, randomised, phase 3 trial. Lancet. 2016;387(10032):2008–16.
9. Ravaud A, Motzer RJ, Pandha HS, et al. Adjuvant sunitinib in high-risk renal-cell carcinoma after nephrectomy. N Engl J Med. 2016;375(23):2246–54.
10. Motzer RJ, Haas NB, Donskov F, et al. Randomized phase III trial of adjuvant pazopanib versus placebo after nephrectomy in patients with localized or locally advanced renal cell carcinoma. J Clin Oncol. 2017;35(35):3916–23.
11. Motzer R, Russo P, Haas NB, et al. Adjuvant pazopanib versus placebo after nephrectomy in patients with localized or locally advanced renal cell carcinoma: final overall survival analysis of the phase 3 PROTECT trial. Eur Urol. 2021;79(3):334–8.
12. Eisen T, Frangou E, Oza B, et al. Adjuvant sorafenib for renal cell carcinoma at intermediate or high risk of relapse: results from the SORCE randomized phase III intergroup trial. J Clin Oncol. 2020;38(34):4064–75.
13. Gross-Goupil M, Kwon TG, Eto M, et al. Axitinib versus placebo as an adjuvant treatment of renal cell carcinoma: results from the phase III, randomized ATLAS trial. Ann Oncol. 2018;29(12):2371–8.
14. Pal SK, Uzzo R, Karam JA, et al. Adjuvant atezolizumab versus placebo for patients with renal cell carcinoma at increased risk of recurrence following resection (IMmotion010): a multicentre, randomised, double-blind, phase 3 trial. Lancet. 2022;400(10358):1103–16.
15. Motzer RJ, Russo P, Grünwald V, et al. Adjuvant nivolumab plus ipilimumab versus placebo for localised renal cell carcinoma after nephrectomy (CheckMate 914): a double-blind, randomised, phase 3 trial. Lancet. 2023;401(10379):821–32.
16. Choueiri TK, Tomczak P, Park SE, et al. Adjuvant pembrolizumab after nephrectomy in renal-cell carcinoma. N Engl J Med. 2021;385(8):683–94.
17. Powles T, Tomczak P, Park SE, et al. Pembrolizumab versus placebo as post-nephrectomy adjuvant therapy for clear cell renal cell carcinoma (KEYNOTE-564): 30-month follow-up analysis of a multicentre, randomised, double-blind, placebo-controlled, phase 3 trial. Lancet Oncol. 2022;23(9):1133–44.
18. Allaf M, Kim S, Harshman L, et al. LBA67 Phase III randomized study comparing perioperative nivolumab (nivo) versus observation in patients (Pts) with renal cell carcinoma (RCC) undergoing nephrectomy (PROSPER, ECOG-ACRIN EA8143), a National Clinical Trials Network trial. Ann Oncol. 2022;33:S1432–3.
19. Ryan CW, Tangen CM, Heath EI, et al. Adjuvant everolimus after surgery for renal cell carcinoma (EVEREST): a double-blind, placebo-controlled, randomised, phase 3 trial. Lancet. 2023;402(10407):1043–51.
20. Chamie K, Donin NM, Klöpfer P, et al. Adjuvant weekly girentuximab following nephrectomy for high-risk renal cell carcinoma: the ARISER randomized clinical trial. JAMA Oncol. 2017;3(7):913–20.

21. Flanigan RC, Salmon SE, Blumenstein BA, et al. Nephrectomy followed by interferon alfa-2b compared with interferon alfa-2b alone for metastatic renal-cell cancer. N Engl J Med. 2001;345(23):1655–9.
22. Mickisch GH, Garin A, Poppel H, et al. Radical nephrectomy plus interferon-alfa-based immunotherapy compared with interferon alfa alone in metastatic renal-cell carcinoma: a randomised trial. Lancet. 2001;358(9286):966–70.
23. Flanigan RC, Mickisch G, Sylvester R, et al. Cytoreductive nephrectomy in patients with metastatic renal cancer: a combined analysis. J Urol. 2004;171(3):1071–6.
24. Méjean A, Ravaud A, Thezenas S, et al. Sunitinib alone or after nephrectomy in metastatic renal-cell carcinoma. N Engl J Med. 2018;379(5):417–27.
25. Méjean A, Ravaud A, Thezenas S, et al. Sunitinib alone or after nephrectomy for patients with metastatic renal cell carcinoma: is there still a role for cytoreductive nephrectomy? Eur Urol. 2021;80(4):417–24.
26. Bex A, Mulders P, Jewett M, et al. Comparison of immediate vs. deferred cytoreductive nephrectomy in patients with synchronous metastatic renal cell carcinoma receiving sunitinib: the SURTIME randomized clinical trial. JAMA Oncol. 2019;5(2):164–70.
27. Motzer RJ, Bacik J, Murphy BA, et al. Interferon-alfa as a comparative treatment for clinical trials of new therapies against advanced renal cell carcinoma. J Clin Oncol. 2002;20(1):289–96.
28. Heng DYC, Xie W, Regan MM, et al. Prognostic factors for overall survival in patients with metastatic renal cell carcinoma treated with vascular endothelial growth factor-targeted agents: results from a large, multicenter study. J Clin Oncol. 2009;27(34):5794–9.
29. Kavolius JP, Mastorakos DP, Pavlovich C, Russo P, Burt ME, Brady MS. Resection of metastatic renal cell carcinoma. J Clin Oncol. 1998;16(6):2261–6.
30. Vogelbaum MA, Brown PD, Messersmith H, et al. Treatment for brain metastases: ASCO-SNO-ASTRO guideline. J Clin Oncol. 2022;40(5):492–516.
31. Fokas E, Henzel M, Hamm K, et al. Radiotherapy for brain metastases from renal cell cancer: should whole-brain radiotherapy be added to stereotactic radiosurgery? Analysis of 88 patients. Strahlenther Onkol. 2010;186(4):210–7.
32. Hasanov E, Yeboa DN, Tucker MD, et al. An interdisciplinary consensus on the management of brain metastases in patients with renal cell carcinoma. CA Cancer J Clin. 2022;72(5):454–89.
33. Linehan WM. Molecular targeting of VHL gene pathway in clear cell kidney cancer. J Urol. 2003;170(2 Pt 1):593–4.
34. Zhou L, Liu XD, Sun M, Zhang X, German P, Bai S, et al. Targeting MET and AXL overcomes resistance to sunitinib ther- apy in renal cell carcinoma. Oncogene. 2016;35(21):2687–97.
35. Rodriguez-Vida A, Hutson TE, Bellmunt J, Strijbos MH. New treatment options for metastatic renal cell carcinoma. ESMO Open. 2017;2(2):e000185.
36. Buti S, Bersanelli M, Sikokis A, et al. Chemotherapy in metastatic renal cell carcinoma today? A systematic review. Anticancer Drugs. 2013;24(6):535–54.
37. Braren V, Taylor JN, Pace W. Regression of metastatic renal carinoma following nephrectomy. Urology. 1974;3(6):777–8.
38. Rosenberg SA, Lotze MT, Muul LM, et al. Observations on the systemic administration of autologous lymphokine-activated killer cells and recombinant interleukin-2 to patients with metastatic cancer. N Engl J Med. 1985;313(23):1485–92.
39. McDermott DF, Regan MM, Clark JI, et al. Randomized phase III trial of highdose interleukin-2 versus subcutaneous interleukin-2 and interferon in patients with metastatic renal cell carcinoma. J Clin Oncol. 2005;23(1):133–41.
40. Yang JC, Sherry RM, Steinberg SM, et al. Randomized study of high-dose and low-dose interleukin-2 in patients with metastatic renal cancer. J Clin Oncol. 2003;21(16):3127–32.
41. Fyfe G, Fisher RI, Rosenberg SA, et al. Results of treatment of 255 patients with metastatic renal cell carcinoma who received high-dose recombinant interleukin-2 therapy. J Clin Oncol. 1995;13(3):688–96.
42. Pyrhönen S, Salminen E, Ruutu M, et al. Prospective randomized trial of interferon alfa-2a plus vinblastine versus vinblastine alone in patients with advanced renal cell cancer. J Clin Oncol. 1999;17(9):2859–67.

43. Motzer RJ, Hutson TE, Tomczak P, et al. Sunitinib versus interferon alfa in metastatic renal-cell carcinoma. N Engl J Med. 2007;356(2):115–24.
44. Motzer RJ, Hutson TE, Cella D, et al. Pazopanib versus sunitinib in metastatic renal-cell carcinoma. N Engl J Med. 2013;369(8):722–31.
45. Sternberg CN, Motzer RJ, Hutson TE, et al. COMPARZ post hoc analysis: characterizing pazopanib responders with advanced renal cell carcinoma. Clin Genitourin Cancer. 2019;17(6):425–435.e4.
46. Escudier B, Eisen T, Stadler WM, et al. Sorafenib in advanced clear-cell renal-cell carcinoma. N Engl J Med. 2007;356(2):125–34.
47. Escudier B, Eisen T, Stadler WM, et al. Sorafenib for treatment of renal cell carcinoma: final efficacy and safety results of the phase III treatment approaches in renal cancer global evaluation trial. J Clin Oncol. 2009;27(20):3312–8.
48. Rini BI, Escudier B, Tomczak P, et al. Comparative effectiveness of axitinib versus sorafenib in advanced renal cell carcinoma (AXIS): a randomised phase 3 trial. Lancet. 2011;378(9807):1931–9.
49. Motzer RJ, Escudier B, Tomczak P, et al. Axitinib versus sorafenib as second-line treatment for advanced renal cell carcinoma: overall survival analysis and updated results from a randomised phase 3 trial. Lancet Oncol. 2013;14(6):552–62.
50. Choueiri TK, Escudier B, Powles T, et al. Cabozantinib versus everolimus in advanced renal-cell carcinoma. N Engl J Med. 2015;373(19):1814–23.
51. Choueiri TK, Escudier B, Powles T, et al. Cabozantinib versus everolimus in advanced renal cell carcinoma (METEOR): final results from a randomised, open-label, phase 3 trial. Lancet Oncol. 2016;17(7):917–27.
52. Motzer RJ, Escudier B, Powles T, et al. Long-term follow-up of overall survival for cabozantinib versus everolimus in advanced renal cell carcinoma. Br J Cancer. 2018;118(9):1176–8.
53. Motzer RJ, Hutson TE, Glen H, et al. Lenvatinib, everolimus, and the combination in patients with metastatic renal cell carcinoma: a randomised, phase 2, open-label, multicentre trial. Lancet Oncol. 2015;16(15):1473–82.
54. Motzer RJ, Alekseev B, Rha SY, et al. Lenvatinib plus pembrolizumab or everolimus for advanced renal cell carcinoma. N Engl J Med. 2021;384(14):1289–300.
55. Choueiri TK, Eto M, Motzer R, et al. Lenvatinib plus pembrolizumab versus sunitinib as first-line treatment of patients with advanced renal cell carcinoma (CLEAR): extended follow-up from the phase 3, randomised, open-label study. Lancet Oncol. 2023;24(3):228–38.
56. Motzer RJ, Escudier B, Oudard S, et al. Efficacy of everolimus in advanced renal cell carcinoma: a double-blind, randomised, placebo-controlled phase III trial. Lancet. 2008;372(9637):449–56.
57. Motzer RJ, Escudier B, Oudard S, et al. Phase 3 trial of everolimus for metastatic renal cell carcinoma: final results and analysis of prognostic factors. Cancer. 2010;116(18):4256–65.
58. Motzer RJ, Hutson TE, Ren M, et al. Independent assessment of lenvatinib plus everolimus in patients with metastatic renal cell carcinoma. Lancet Oncol. 2016;17(1):e4–5.
59. Motzer RJ, Escudier B, McDermott DF, et al. Nivolumab versus everolimus in advanced renal-cell carcinoma. N Engl J Med. 2015;373(19):1803–13.
60. Motzer RJ, Escudier B, George S, et al. Nivolumab versus everolimus in patients with advanced renal cell carcinoma: updated results with long-term follow-up of the randomized, open-label, phase 3 CheckMate 025 trial. Cancer. 2020;126(18):4156–67.
61. Hammers HJ, Plimack ER, Infante JR, et al. Safety and efficacy of Nivolumab in combination with Ipilimumab in metastatic renal cell carcinoma: the CheckMate 016 study. J Clin Oncol. 2017;35(34):3851–8.
62. Lee C, Shah AY, Rasco D, et al. Lenvatinib plus pembrolizumab in patients with either treatment-naive or previously treated metastatic renal cell carcinoma (Study 111/KEYNOTE-146): a phase 1b/2 study. Lancet Oncol. 2021;22(7):946–58.

63. Incorvaia L, Bronte G, Bazan V, Badalamenti G, Rizzo S, Pantuso G, Natoli C, Russo A. Beyond evidence-based data: scientific rationale and tumor behavior to drive sequential and personalized therapeutic strategies for the treatment of metastatic renal cell carcinoma. Oncotarget. 2016;7(16):21259–71. https://doi.org/10.18632/oncotarget.7267. PMID: 26872372; PMCID: PMC5008283.

Management of Renal Pelvis, Ureter, and Urethral Cancer

12

Tripti Saxena

12.1 Renal Pelvis and Ureteral Cancer

12.1.1 Introduction

About 4000 cases per year are diagnosed with renal pelvis and ureteral cancer (also known as upper tract urothelial cancers or UTUCs), which account for 5–10% of all renal malignancies in the USA and 700 cases per year in India [1, 2]. Males are affected twice as often as females, and the median age of diagnosis is 75 years [3, 4].

12.1.1.1 Risk Factors

Several environmental [5] and hereditary factors are associated with the development of UTUCs, i.e., smoking, arsenic exposure, alcohol consumption, phenacetin use, plant extract having aristolochic acid, Lynch syndrome [6, 7] and Balkan endemic nephropathy [8].

12.1.1.2 Histology

Renal pelvis and ureteral cancers are clonally related to bladder carcinomas and 15–20% present with synchronous bladder cancer [9, 10]. Most of the renal pelvis and ureteral tumors (>90%) are of urothelial origin and are multifocal. Approximately 8% of tumors are squamous cell carcinoma, which is sessile, deeply invasive, and carries a poor prognosisLo [11]. Other histological types, i.e., adenocarcinoma, small cell carcinoma, or sarcomatoid variant, are rare [12].

12.1.1.3 Clinical Presentation

A total of 70–80% of patients with UTUCs present with gross or microscopic hematuria [8, 13, 14]. Flank pain because of obstruction of the ureter either by a tumor

T. Saxena (✉)
Department of Radiation Oncology, Max Superspecialty Hospital, Patparganj, Delhi, India

R. Madan, S. Goyal (eds.), *Essentials of Radiotherapy in Uro-Genital Malignancies*, https://doi.org/10.1007/978-981-95-5945-9_12

growth or clot may occur in 20–40% of patients. Patients with systemic complaints such as anorexia, nausea, weight loss, fever, fatigue, or cough should be evaluated for metastatic disease.

12.1.1.4 Diagnosis

The diagnosis is usually incidental and the entire urinary tract should be evaluated carefully as multiple synchronous tumors may be present [9, 15].

12.1.1.5 Radiological

- *Multi-detector Computed Tomographic Urography (MDCTU)* is an excellent tool with the highest diagnostic accuracy with a sensitivity of 67–100% and a specificity of 93–99% [16, 17]. The limitation of MDCTU is it does not detect epithelial flat lesions without mass effect or urothelial thickening.
- *Magnetic Resonance Urography (MRU):* Gadolinium-enhanced magnetic resonance urography is a promising alternative to assess upper urinary tract lesions. It can be used for the surveillance of high-risk populations or in patients with hydronephrosis when MDCTU or excretory urography is contraindicated [18]. Patients with a ureteral stent or nephrostomy tube should not be evaluated by MRU alone.
- Typical findings on radiological imaging are mass in the upper urinary tract. CT/MRI abdomen may detect tumor extension, any adjacent organ involvement, or distant metastasis.
- If the patient is allergic to contrast or can't tolerate contrast, retrograde ureteropyelography with non-contrast CT or USG is to be done.
- CT chest should be done as a part of metastatic workup.
- Bone scan should be considered if symptomatic and high suspicion of metastasis.

Ureteropyeloscopy with cystoscopy Ureteropyeloscopy with cystoscopy allows direct visualization of the entire urinary tract and biopsy to confirm the diagnosis [19, 20]. It's an integral part of diagnosis and can rule out synchronous multiple primaries [21].

Brush Biopsy Retrograde brushing of the upper urinary tract was first described in 1973 [22]. This technique is more sensitive to high-grade lesions [23]. Although ureteroscopy and biopsy have replaced brush biopsy, they may be useful in evaluating patients with positive urinary cytology with no visible lesion on radiological or ureteroscopic assessment.

Staging and Classification TNM 2017 classification is widely used to stage UTUCs (Table 12.1) [24].

Risk Stratification The major prognostic factor in patients with UTUCs is initial stage and grade. EAU2023 update has given recommendations for risk stratification [8].

Table 12.1 TNM 2017 classification for upper UTUCs

T: Primary tumor			
TX	Primary tumor cannot be assessed		
T0	No evidence of primary tumor		
Ta	Noninvasive papillary carcinoma		
Tis	Carcinoma in situ		
T1	Tumor invades the subepithelial connective tissue		
T2	Tumor invades the muscularis		
T3	Renal pelvis: Tumor invades beyond the muscularis into peripelvic fat or renal parenchyma		
	Ureter: Tumor invades beyond the muscularis into periureteric fat		
T4	Tumor invades adjacent organs or through the kidney into perinephric fat		
N: Regional lymph nodes			
NX	Regional lymph nodes cannot be assessed		
N0	No regional lymph node metastasis		
N1	Metastasis in a single lymph node 2 cm or less in greatest dimension		
N2	Metastasis in a single lymph node more than 2 cm, or multiple lymph nodes		
M: Distant metastasis			
M0	No distant metastasis		
M1	Distant metastasis		
Stage grouping			
Stage 0a	Ta	N0	M0
Stage 0is	Tis	N0	M0
Stage I	T1	N0	M0
Stage II	T2	N0	M0
Stage III	T3	N0	M0
Stage IV	T4	N0	M0
	Any T	N1 or N2	M0
	Any T	Any N	M1
Histopathologic grade			
WHO/ISUP recommended grading for urothelial histologies			
LG	Low grade		
HG	High grade		
Histology: Squamous cell carcinoma and adenocarcinoma			
GX	Grade cannot be assessed		
G1	Well differentiated		
G2	Moderately differentiated		
G3	Poorly differentiated		
G4	Undifferentiated		

Low-risk upper tract urothelial carcinomas (UTUCs) necessitate the presence of unifocal disease, a tumor size less than 2 cm, negative for high-grade cytology, low-grade findings on ureteroscopic biopsy, and the absence of any invasive aspect on computed tomography (CT). Several characteristics are associated with *high-risk upper tract urothelial carcinomas (UTUCs)*. These factors include multifocal disease, tumor size larger than 2 cm, high-grade cytology, high-grade ureteroscopic biopsy, evidence of local invasion on computed tomography (CT), presence of hydronephrosis, history of previous radical cystectomy for high-grade bladder cancer, and specific histological subtype.

12.2 Treatment Recommendations

Surgery Surgery is the standard of care for the management of renal pelvis and ureter cancer. In the early stage (T1/T2N0), the surgical outcome is excellent in terms of local control and overall survival [25, 26]. The kind of surgery depends on the location of the tumor in the ureter (upper/mid/distal) and the grade of the tumor. The bladder cancer NCCN guidelines (version 3.3023) recommend nephroureterectomy with a cuff of bladder or endoscopic resection ± postsurgical intrapelvic chemotherapy or BCG for low-grade tumors and nephroureterectomy with a cuff of bladder and regional lymphadenectomy for high-grade tumors/locally advanced tumors [27]. In selected patients, neoadjuvant chemotherapy can be considered.

Chemotherapy Chemotherapy regimens are similar to what is used for urinary bladder cancer.

- *Neoadjuvant or adjuvant regimen:* Dose-dense methotrexate, vinblastine, doxorubicin, and cisplatin (ddMVAC) for 3 or 4 cycles and gemcitabine and cisplatin for 4 cycles
- *As a radiosensitizer:* Cisplatin, 5-FU, taxanes, capecitabine or low-dose gemcitabine

Radiation Therapy With limited data and no prospective randomized controlled trials, the exact role of nonsurgical interventions is unclear. Neoadjuvant or adjuvant radiation therapy is usually not recommended for upper urinary tract cancers.

- *Early-Stage Medically Unresectable disease:* Highly conformal hypofractionated or stereotactic body radiation therapy can be considered in early-stage, medically unresectable diseases. Stereotactic body radiation therapy was offered to three elderly patients who were medically unresectable, but surgically amenable to a dose of 50–60 Gy in 5 fractions. One of the three developed bladder cancers and the other two had good local control. All three died of unrelated diseases [28]. In another case report, SBRT was delivered to a dose of 50 Gy I 4 fractions to an elderly patient with 31-month follow-up. There were no acute/chronic side effects and no evidence of recurrence [29].
- *Adjuvant radiotherapy after surgery for pT3–pT4 disease:* The role of adjuvant radiation therapy who had a complete resection of an upper urinary tract cancer is unknown. Patients with high-grade tumors or deep invasion have a significantly high local recurrence rate after nephroureterectomy. A retrospective study showed that adjuvant radiation therapy markedly reduces the local recurrence in

T3/T4NN0-1 M0 disease after undergoing successful curative resection. However, it has shown no impact on distant failures which occurred in approximately 50% of patients and such patients will need effective systemic therapy [30]. In a retrospective study, prophylactic radiation therapy was offered as adjuvant treatment in 67 patients vs. intravesical chemotherapy in 66 patients, with upper urinary tract malignancy. The author observed a significant difference in survival rates and bladder tumor relapse rates and concluded that radiation therapy may improve overall survival for patients with T3/4 stage cancer and delay bladder tumor recurrences [31]. Several studies confirm higher local recurrences and distant metastasis in T3/4 cancers [32, 33].

12.3 Principles of External Beam Radiotherapy Treatment Planning

Reviewing the at-risk volumes with the surgeon who performed the resection is helpful to gain insight into the regions and nodal basins at the highest risk of relapse.

Simulation Pelvic immobilization and CT-based simulation with IV contrast are helpful for defining the target volumes. Use of IV contrast may be contraindicated due to single-kidney or poor kidney function.

12.3.1 Contouring

GTV Primary Any gross disease on imaging and involved lymph nodes.

CTV

- For gross disease: 5 mm radial expansion, 2 cm proximal and distal margin expansion
- Renal fossa, the entire length of the ureter, the whole bladder, and draining lymph nodes (paraaortic and para-caval lymph nodes) [31].

PTV expansions should be based on institutional setup considerations and the level of accuracy required with the treatment approach (i.e., conventional vs. SBRT) (Fig. 12.1).

Doses (Fig. 12.2)

- *Subclinical and microscopic disease:* 45–50.4 Gy in 1.8–2 Gy per fraction
- *Extensive disease (R1/R2 resection, node-positive disease):* additional boost dose of 5–10 Gy to high-risk volumes

- *Unresectable or gross residual disease:* further higher doses, up to 60–64 Gy may be necessary

Planning 3D-CRT plan with various lateral and oblique field arrangements is necessary to reduce toxicity to organs at risk. IMRT with image guidance and motion management can be considered to avoid underdosing to target volumes.

Organ-at-Risk (OAR) Dose Constraints OARs include liver, spleen, stomach, duodenum, bowel, spinal cord, and bilateral kidney. For conventional fractionation, dose constraints as per QUANTEC [34] and for SBRT as per AAPM TG101 [35] are to be followed.

12.3.2 Follow-Up [8, 27]

After a radical nephroureterectomy Low risk involves cystoscopy at the third month, followed by subsequent cystoscopy and cytology every third month for 2 years, and every 6 months thereafter up to 5 years. High risk involves cystoscopy, urinary cytology, CT urography, and chest CT every 6 months for 2 years, and then yearly.

After kidney-sparing management Low risk involves cystoscopy and CT urography at 3 and 6 months, followed by ureteroscopy at 3 months. High risk involves cystoscopy, urinary cytology, CT urography, and chest CT at 3 and 6 months.

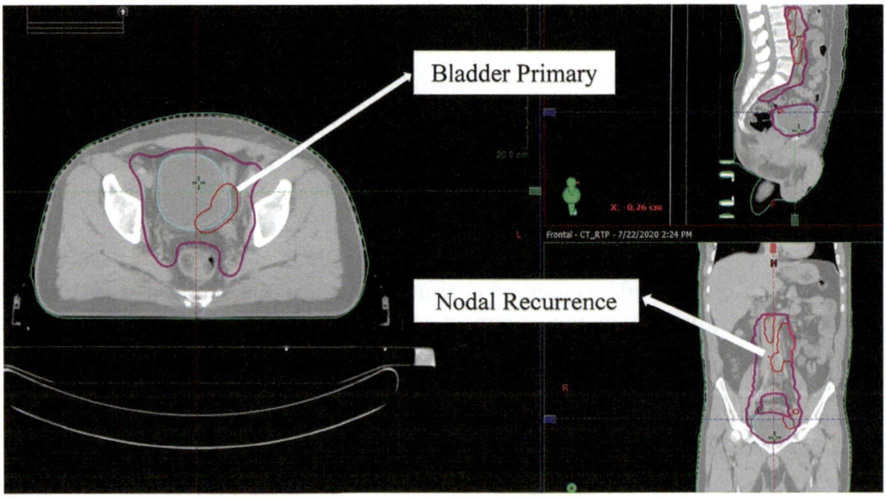

Fig. 12.1 Diagnosed case of carcinoma ureter with nodal recurrence and metachronous bladder primary, bladder primary and nodal recurrence (Red), bladder (Cyan), at-risk volume—CTV (magenta)

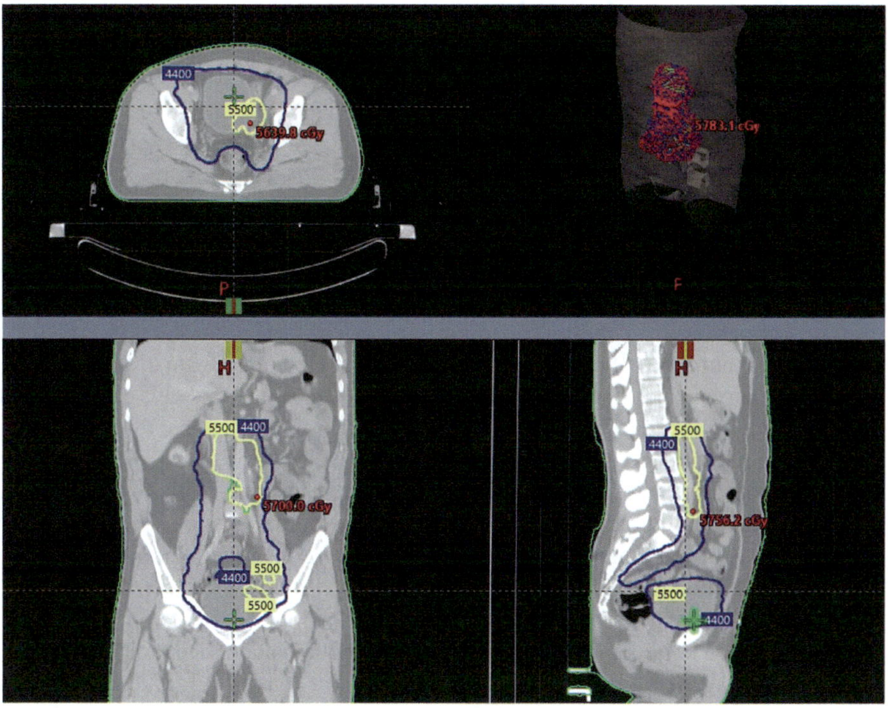

Fig. 12.2 VMAT plan with isodose lines, PTV bladder and nodal basins (Blue-45 Gy), PTV gross bladder primary and nodal basin (Yellow-55Gy)

12.4 Urethral Cancer

Introduction Primary urethral cancer is an extremely rare form, accounting for less than 1% of all genitourinary cancers worldwide and is more frequent among African-Americans [36–38]. Males are more affected than females.

Risk Factors The following factors have been linked to the development of urethral cancer.

- In men, persistent inflammation and stricture [39] (as a result of sexually transmitted illnesses such as condylomata linked with HPV16), lichen sclerosus, urethral trauma [40], external beam irradiation, radioactive seed implantation are also possible causes [41].
- Urethral diverticuli in females, most likely due to secondary chronic inflammation [42] and recurrent urinary tract infections.
- Human papilloma virus 16 (HPV16): in both sexes [43].
- Urethral cancers are frequently multifocal and appear concurrently with other GU tract malignancies.

12.5 Anatomy and Histology

Male Urethra The male urethra is 21 cm long and extends from the bladder neck to the urethral meatus. It is divided into three parts [44]:

- *Prostatic Urethra:* lined with transitional epithelium
- *Bulbomembranous Urethra:* lined with transitional epithelium, most common site of involvement
- *Penile Urethra:* lined with pseudostratified columnar epithelium up to meatus and stratified squamous epithelium at meatus

The predominant types of cases observed are those originating from urothelial cells, accounting for around 55–65% of cases, followed by squamous cell carcinoma at 16–22% and adenocarcinoma at 10–16% [45]. Urethral tumors have the potential to exhibit direct extension to neighboring organs, such as the penis. Malignancies located in the proximal urethra exhibit lymphatic drainage into the external iliac, internal iliac, and obturator lymph nodes. Conversely, malignancies situated in the distal urethra demonstrate lymphatic drainage into either the superficial or deep inguinal lymph nodes [46].

Female Urethra The female urethra extends from the bladder neck to the introitus, having an average length of 3–4 cm. It has two distinct parts [44]. The anterior segment of the urethra is composed of the distal one-third and is characterized by a lining of stratified squamous epithelium (Fig. 12.3). On the other hand, the posterior segment encompasses the proximal two-thirds of the urethra and is lined with transitional epithelium. Throughout the female urethra, submucosal glands are present, which are characterized by a columnar epithelium.

About 60% of the cases are squamous cell carcinomas, with urothelial carcinomas (15–20%) and adenocarcinomas (5–7%) following in order of prevalence [44]. Proximal urethral cancers drain into external iliac, internal iliac, and obturator lymph nodes, while distal urethral cancers drain into superficial or deep inguinal lymph nodes [46].

12.6 Clinical Presentation

- *Male Urethral Cancer:* The majority of the cases (45–57%) are detected in the advanced stage due to nonspecific symptoms. Symptoms may overlap with benign strictures. Hence any patient presenting with recurrent urethral stricture merits biopsy from the stricture. Patients may exhibit hematuria, dysuria, urethral discharge, urine retention, additional urethral mass, and difficulties voiding in locally advanced stages [47].
- *Female Urethral Cancer:* The majority of the cases present with hematuria or irritative voiding symptoms. Few may present with persistent or recurrent pelvic symptoms.

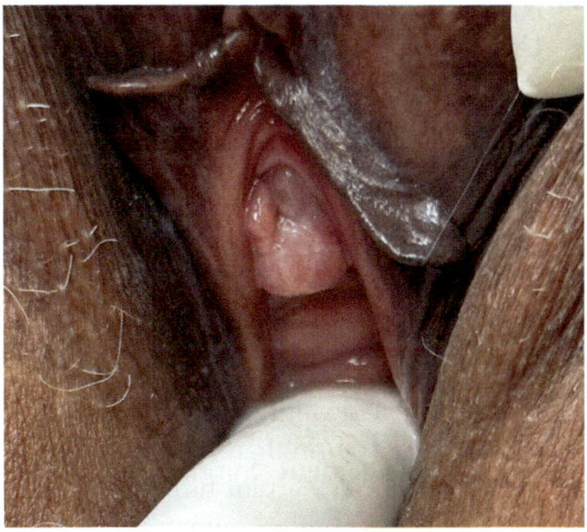

Fig. 12.3 Female urethral cancer

12.6.1 Diagnosis

- *Physical examination:* Careful inspection and palpation of genital organs should be done in both sexes. In females, the bimanual examination, and in males, digital rectal examination should also be done. The bilateral inguinal lymph nodes should be examined and location, size, and mobility should be documented [47].
- *Urinary Cytology:* Urinary cytology should be done in suspected cases of primary urethral cancer [48]. The sensitivity of urinary cytology ranges from 55% to 59% in primary urethral cancer. The detection rates vary depending on the histological entity.
- *Diagnostic Cystourethroscopy and Biopsy:* Diagnostic cystourethroscopy and biopsy allow to evaluate the exact location, extent, and histology. This should be done to evaluate the entire urethra and urinary bladder to rule out synchronous bladder primary.
- *Radiological Imaging:* MRI is helpful to determine the locoregional spread of disease and to assess the response to neoadjuvant chemotherapy [49]. CT imaging chest/abdomen/pelvis helps to evaluate disease at distant sites. PET CT has no proven role.

Staging and Classification The TNM 2017 classification is commonly employed for the staging of urethral malignancies (Table 12.2) [24].

Prognosis The predictors of decreased survival in patients with urethral cancer are [47]:

- Age > 65 years
- Proximal urethral involvement
- Higher T stage and high grade

- N2 nodes or metastatic disease
- Underlying histology
- Presence of synchronous bladder malignancy
- The extent of surgery and treatment modality adopted
- Non-urethral vs urethral recurrence

Treatment Recommendation There are no prospective randomized trials or guidelines to recommend the management of primary urethral cancer. Treatment approaches are based on small case reports or recommendations from other urinary tract cancers.

Surgical Management Surgical approaches depend upon location, extent of disease, and sex.

Male urethral cancer In the past, partial penectomy was the predominant option. But nowadays penis-preserving surgery is the preferred approach with good local control.

- *Non-invasive prostatic urethral carcinoma:* endoscopic transurethral resection along with adjuvant Bacillus Calmètte-Guerin therapy [50, 51].
- *Invading stroma of the prostate:* neoadjuvant chemotherapy followed by radical cystoprostatectomy, urinary diversion and lymphadenectomy.
- *Low-grade tumors or high-grade non-invasive tumors:* endoscopic resection or segmental resection [52].
- *Larger tumors or more invasive disease:* segmental resection with primary anastomosis or distal urethrectomy with the creation of hypospadias for lesions near to meatus.
- *Tumors involving corpus spongiosum (T2) but not corpus cavernosum:* subtotal uretherectomy and perineal urethrostomy [53]. Role of neoadjuvant or adjuvant chemotherapy is limited at this stage. However, if T3/4 or node-positive disease is revealed postoperatively, adjuvant chemotherapy should be considered.
- *Locally advanced disease (T3/4):* The treatment approach involved the administration of neoadjuvant chemotherapy guided by histological analysis, followed by a comprehensive surgical procedure encompassing penectomy, cystoprostatectomy, perineal reconstruction, and anterior pelvic exenteration. Tumors that are in close proximity to the pubic ramus should be treated by performing en bloc inferior pubectomy, while tumors that involve the inguinal lymph nodes should be managed with inguinal lymph node dissection.

Table 12.2 TNM 2017 classification for primary urethral carcinomas

Male penile urethra and female urethra			
T: Primary tumor			
TX	Primary tumor cannot be assessed		
T0	No evidence of primary tumor		
Ta	Non-invasive papillary carcinoma		
Tis	Carcinoma in situ		
T1	Tumor invades the subepithelial connective tissue		
T2	Tumor invades any of the following: Corpus spongiosum, periurethral muscle		
T3	Tumor invades any of the following: Corpus cavernosum, anterior vagina		
T4	Tumor invades other adjacent organs (e.g., invasion of the bladder wall)		
Prostatic urethra			
T: Primary tumor			
TX	Primary tumor cannot be assessed		
T0	No evidence of primary tumor		
Ta	Non-invasive papillary carcinoma		
Tis	Carcinoma in situ involving the prostatic urethra or periurethral or prostatic ducts without stromal invasion		
T1	Tumor invades urethral subepithelial connective tissue immediately underlying the urothelium		
T2	Tumor invades the prostatic stroma surrounding ducts either by direct extension from the urothelial surface or by invasion from prostatic ducts		
T3	Tumor invades the periprostatic fat		
T4	Tumor invades other adjacent organs (e.g., extraprostatic invasion of the bladder wall, rectal wall)		
N: Regional lymph nodes			
NX	Regional lymph nodes cannot be assessed		
N0	No regional lymph node metastasis		
N1	Single regional lymph node metastasis in the inguinal region or true pelvis [perivesical, obturator, internal (hypogastric) and external iliac], or presacral lymph node		
N2	Multiple regional lymph node metastasis in the inguinal region or true pelvis [perivesical, obturator, internal (hypogastric), and external iliac], or presacral lymph node		
M: Distant metastasis			
M0	No distant metastasis		
M1	Distant metastasis		
Stage grouping			
Stage 0a	Ta	N0	M0
Stage 0is	Tis	N0	M0
Stage I	T1	N0	M0
Stage II	T2	N0	M0
Stage III	T1	N1	M0
	T2	N1	M0
	T3	N0	M0
	T3	N1	M0

(continued)

Table 12.2 (continued)

Male penile urethra and female urethra			
Stage IV	T4	N0	M0
	T4	N1	M0
	Any T	N2	M0
	Any T	Any N	M0
Histopathologic grade [47]			
WHO/ISUP recommended grading for urothelial histologies			
PUNLMP	Papillary urothelial neoplasm of low malignant potential		
Low grade	Well differentiated		
High grade	Poorly differentiated		
For squamous cell carcinoma and adenocarcinoma			
GX	Grade cannot be assessed		
G1	Well differentiated		
G2	Moderately differentiated		
G3	Poorly differentiated		

12.7 Female Urethral Cancer

- *Low-grade tumors:* Endoscopic resection or segmental resection is essential for low-grade or small high-grade non-invasive cancers. In cases of invasive disease, it may be necessary to perform a urethrectomy with bladder neck closure, along with either a suprapubic cystotomy, incontinent diversion (ileovesicostomy), or a continent catheterizable stoma.
- *Advanced locoregional disease:* Neoadjuvant chemotherapy followed by surgical resection to include anterior pelvic exenteration, including anterior vaginectomy. Tumors abutting the pubic ramus should be addressed with en bloc inferior pubectomy and those having inguinal lymph nodes should undergo inguinal lymph node dissection [27].

Chemotherapy For locally advanced and metastatic disease, patients should be offered chemotherapy regimens similar to metastatic bladder cancer using gemcitabine + cisplatin or high dose methotrexate, vinblastine, doxorubicin, and cisplatin (MVAC) + growth factors (G-CSF) [47, 54].

12.8 Radiation Therapy

External Beam Radiation Therapy (EBRT) There are no prospective randomized trials comparing definitive radiation to urethral cancer surgery. Several case series have examined women's outcomes after definitive radiation with or without chemotherapy. The variability of tumor stages, histology, radiation treatments, and research eras makes these studies challenging to evaluate [55, 56]. Several limited patient series, especially in non-surgical patients, demonstrate that definitive chemoradiation therapy alone can achieve durable local control and overall survival in locally advanced urethral malignancies (≥T3, node-positive) [57–59]. One small case series suggests that mitomycin C and 5-fluorouracil-based final chemoradiation therapy for squamous cell carcinoma may work [60]. A recent US population database analysis of 2614 people with non-metastatic urethral tumors found that adding radiation to surgery improved survival and that final treatment had similar survival [61].

12.9 Principles of External Beam Radiotherapy Treatment Planning

Simulation Pelvic immobilization and CT-based simulation with IV contrast are helpful for defining the target volumes. Use of IV contrast may be contraindicated due to single-kidney or poor kidney function.

12.9.1 Delineation

Male Urethral Cancer

Penile Urethra

- *GTV:* gross urethral disease as determined by clinical and radiological examination and gross involved lymph nodes (suspicious inguinal/pelvic lymph nodes)
- *CTV:*
  - *T1–2 lesions:* GTV (urethral primary and gross lymph nodes) + 5 mm radial expansion, 2 cm proximal and distal margin expansion
  - *T2-T4 lesions:*
    - *CTV Primary:* GTV urethral primary +5 mm radial expansion; entire penile urethra up to bulb
    - *CTV Lymph Nodes:* GTV gross nodes +5 mm radial expansion + bilateral inguinal and pelvic lymph nodes up to common iliac region [62]
- *PTV:* expansions should be based on institutional setup considerations and the level of accuracy required with the treatment approach

Prostatic Urethra

- *GTV:* gross urethral disease and involved lymph nodes.
- *CTV:* entire prostate +2 cm into bladder neck, and 2 cm distal to lesion seen on imaging with in-transit lymphatics to the respective draining lymph nodes.

- *PTV:* expansions should be based on institutional setup considerations and the level of accuracy required with the treatment approach.

Female Urethral Cancer

- *GTV Primary:* gross urethral disease and involved lymph nodes.
- *CTV:* contour the entire urethra with in-transit lymphatics to the respective draining lymph nodes.
- *PTV:* expansions should be based on institutional setup considerations and the level of accuracy required with the treatment approach.

Doses

Definitive Radiation Therapy:
- *Stage ≤ T2:* 66–70 Gy @ 1.8–2 Gy per fraction [27]
- *Stage cT3-T4 or N+:*
  - At-risk pelvis and lymph nodal basin: 45–50.4 Gy @ 1.8–2 Gy per fraction
  - Gross primary +5 mm radial margin and 2 cm proximal and distal margin: 66–70 Gy @ 1.8–2 Gy per fraction
  - Gross lymph nodes +5 mm margin: 54–66 Gy @ 1.8–2 Gy per fraction
- Concurrent chemotherapy should be considered and regimens used are similar to what has been used for bladder cancer. Radiation dose reduction might be needed to minimize the toxicity.

Adjuvant Radiation Therapy:
- *R0 Resection:* 45–50.4 Gy @ 1.8 Gy per fraction to tumor bed and nodal basin
- *R1 Resection or extracapsular extension:* 54–60 Gy @ 1.8–2 Gy per fraction to tumor bed with positive margin and pelvic nodal irradiation. Consider for concurrent chemotherapy.
- *R2 Resection:* 60–70 Gy @ 1.8–2 Gy per fraction for gross disease with concurrent chemotherapy

Planning 3D-CRT plan with various field arrangements is necessary to reduce toxicity to organs at risk. IMRT with image guidance can be considered to avoid underdosing to target volumes.

Dose Constraints [34]

- PTVs should be covered at least 95% of the volume to 95% of the dose.
- *Rectum:* V60 Gy < 50%, V65 Gy < 25%, V70 Gy < 20%, and V75 Gy <15%.
- *Bladder:* V75 Gy <15%, V70 Gy <35%, V65 Gy <15%.

- *Femoral Head:* Dmax <50 Gy.
- *Small Bowel:* V45 Gy < 195 cc.

12.9.2 Normal Tissue Toxicity

Acute Pain, dysuria, hematuria, urinary urgency, diarrhea, fatigue, mucositis/dermatitis.

Chronic

- Urethral stenosis, necrosis, fistula formation, cystitis, and hemorrhage
- Glans necrosis and meatal stenosis in men
- Reproductive considerations
- Erectile dysfunction/sexual dysfunction in men
- Chronic proctitis
- Lymphedema

Brachytherapy There are no prospective randomized trials for urethral brachytherapy. Small meatal and distal urethral tumors are curable with brachytherapy. A case series of 10 patients, who were treated by high dose rate interstitial brachytherapy (HDR-IBT) either alone or as a boost post external beam radiation therapy (EBRT), suggests the following [63]:

- *Tumors < 3 cm, node-negative:* HDR-IBT alone.
- *Tumors > 3 cm, node-positive disease:* EBRT followed by HDR-IBT, but patients may be preferred for HDR-IBT first as the tumor is well demarcated and post EBRT, due to acute inflammation, this may be challenging.
- *Brachytherapy Implant Procedure:*
  - The procedure should be done under spinal anesthesia.
  - Foley's catheterization and clinical examination to assess tumor dimensions.
  - The gross tumor with 5 mm margin should be implanted.
  - Transvaginal ultrasonography should be used to guide needle insertion.
  - Two- to three-plane free-hand implant should be performed with free hand/template based.
  - Intra-planar or inter-planar distance should ideally be kept between 0.8 and 1.2 cm.
- *Brachytherapy Planning and Dosimetry:*
  - Planning CT scan with slice thickness 2.5 mm.
  - Contour urethra from bladder neck to meatus around Foley's catheter.
  - CTV and various organs at risk should be contoured.
  - No PTV margin should be given around CTV.
  - The plan should be generated for the prescription dose to the CTV. If needed, both graphic and geometrical optimization should be done.

   - Pre-planning parameter for CTV: V100% = 90% and D90% = 115–135%.
   - For OARs: D1cc to rectum ≤100% and Dmax to the unaffected urethra ≤150%.
   - *HDR-IBT Doses:*
     - *Definitive Therapy:* 42 Gy in 14 fractions over 7 days
     - *As a boost after EBRT:* 18–21 Gy in 6–7 fractions
     - Twice daily fractionation schedule
- *Brachytherapy Treatment Delivery:*
   - Minimum 6 hours interval between two fractions.
   - Brachytherapy catheters should be removed immediately after completion of treatment.
   - Foley catheter should be removed after 5–7 days of brachytherapy catheter removal.

Follow-Up

- *Tumors up to T1:* clinical examination every 3–6 months and local radiological imaging every 1–2 years.
- *Tumors > T2 and/or node-positive disease:* clinical examination, radiological imaging (MRI/CT) for local disease and chest, abdomen, and pelvis.

References

1. Cancer Statistics, 2022 8 CA: A Cancer Journal for Clinicians Materials and Methods Data Sources. Available from: https://acsjournals.onlinelibrary.wiley.com/doi/10.3322/caac.21708.
2. Sathishkumar K, Chaturvedi M, Das P, Stephen S, Mathur P. Cancer incidence estimates for 2022 & projection for 2025: Result from National Cancer Registry Programme, India. Indian J Med Res. 2022;156:598.
3. Neuzillet Y, Seisen T, Traxer O, Allory Y, Audenet F, Leon P, et al. French AFU cancer committee guidelines - update 2022-2024: upper urinary tract urothelial cancer (UTUC). Prog Urol [Internet]. 2022 [cited 2023 Sep 11];32(15):1164–94. Available from: http://www.ncbi.nlm.nih.gov/pubmed/36400481.
4. Shariat SF, Favaretto RL, Gupta A, Fritsche HM, Matsumoto K, Kassouf W, et al. Gender differences in radical nephroureterectomy for upper tract urothelial carcinoma. World J Urol. 2011;29(4):481–6.
5. Colin P, Koenig P, Ouzzane A, Berthon N, Villers A, Biserte J, et al. Environmental factors involved in carcinogenesis of urothelial cell carcinomas of the upper urinary tract. BJU Int. 2009;104:1436–40.
6. Gylling A, Nieminen T, Abdel-Rahman WM, Nuorva K, Juhola M, Joensuu E, et al. Differential cancer predisposition in lynch syndrome: insights from molecular analysis of brain and urinary tract tumors. Downloaded from [Internet]. Vol. 2, Carcinogenesis Advance Access; 2008. Available from: http://carcin.oxfordjournals.org/.
7. Lynch HT, Ens JA, Lynch JF. The Lynch syndrome II and urological malignancies. J Urol. 1990;143(1):24–8.
8. Rouprêt M, Seisen T, Birtle AJ, Capoun O, Compérat EM, Dominguez-Escrig JL, et al. European association of urology guidelines on upper urinary tract urothelial carcinoma: 2023 update. Eur Urol. Elsevier B.V. 2023;84:49–64.

9. van Doeveren T, van de Werken HJG, van Riet J, Aben KKH, van Leeuwen PJ, Zwarthoff EC, et al. Synchronous and metachronous urothelial carcinoma of the upper urinary tract and the bladder: are they clonally related? A systematic review. Urol Oncol. Elsevier Inc. 2020;38:590–8.
10. Margulis V, Shariat SF, Matin SF, Kamat AM, Zigeuner R, Kikuchi E, et al. Outcomes of radical nephroureterectomy: a series from the upper tract urothelial carcinoma collaboration. Available from: https://acsjournals.onlinelibrary.wiley.com/doi/10.1002/cncr.24135.
11. Holmäng S, Lele SM, Johansson SL. Squamous cell carcinoma of the renal pelvis and ureter: incidence, symptoms, treatment and outcome. J Urol. 2007;178(1):51–6.
12. Ouzzane A, Ghoneim TP, Udo K, Verhasselt-Crinquette M, Puech P, Betrouni N, et al. Small cell carcinoma of the upper urinary tract (UUT-SCC): report of a rare entity and systematic review of the literature. Cancer Treat Rev. 2011;37:366–72.
13. Inman BA, Tran VT, Fradet Y, Lacombe L. Carcinoma of the upper urinary tract predictors of survival and competing causes of mortality. Available from: https://acsjournals.onlinelibrary.wiley.com/doi/10.1002/cncr.24339.
14. Cowan NC. CT urography for hematuria. Nat Rev Urol. 2012;9:218–26.
15. Hafner C, Knuechel R, Zanardo L, Dietmaier W, Blaszyk H, Cheville J, et al. Evidence for oligoclonality and tumor spread by intraluminal seeding in multifocal urothelial carcinomas of the upper and lower urinary tract [Internet]. Available from: http://www.uni-regensburg.de/Fakultaeten/Medizin/.
16. Cowan NC, Turney BW, Taylor NJ, McCarthy CL, Crew JP. Multidetector computed tomography urography for diagnosing upper urinary tract urothelial tumour. BJU Int. 2007;99:1363–70.
17. Janisch F, Shariat SF, Baltzer P, Fajkovic H, Kimura S, Iwata T, et al. Diagnostic performance of multidetector computed tomographic (MDCTU) in upper tract urothelial carcinoma (UTUC): a systematic review and meta-analysis. World J Urol. 2020;38(5):1165–75.
18. Takahashi N, Glockner JF, Hartman RP, King BF, Leibovich BC, Stanley DW, et al. Gadolinium enhanced magnetic resonance urography for upper urinary tract malignancy. J Urol. 2010;183(4):1330–6.
19. Bagley DH, Rivas D. Upper urinary tract filling defects: flexible ureteroscopic diagnosis. J Urol. 1990;143(6):1196–200.
20. Blute ML, Segura JW, Patterson DE, Benson RC, Zincke H. Impact of endourology on diagnosis and management of upper urinary tract urothelial cancer. J Urol. 1989;141(6):1298–301.
21. Cosentino M, Palou J, Gaya JM, Breda A, Rodriguez-Faba O, Villavicencio-Mavrich H. Upper urinary tract urothelial cell carcinoma: location as a predictive factor for concomitant bladder carcinoma. World J Urol. 2013;31(1):141–5.
22. Gill WB, Lu CT, Thomsen S. Retrograde brushing: a new technique for obtaining histologic and cytologic material from ureteral, renal pelvic and renal caliceal lesions. J Urol. 1973;109(4):573–8.
23. Blute RD, Gittes RR, Gittes RF. Renal brush biopsy: survey of indications, techniques and results. J Urol. 1981;126(2):146–9.
24. Brierley JD, Gospodarowicz MK, Wittekind C. TNM classification of malignant tumours. Wiley; 2017.
25. Box GN, Lehman DS, Landman J, Clayman RV. Minimally invasive management of upper tract malignancies: renal cell and transitional cell carcinoma. Urol Clin North Am. 2008;35:365–83.
26. Lughezzani G, Sun M, Perrotte P, Shariat SF, Jeldres C, Budaus L, et al. Should bladder cuff excision remain the standard of care at nephroureterectomy in patients with urothelial carcinoma of the renal pelvis? A population-based study. Eur Urol. 2010;57(6):956–62.
27. Flaig TW, Spiess PE, Chair V, Abern M, Agarwal N, Buyyounouski MK, et al. NCCN Guidelines Version 3.2023 Bladder Cancer Rick Bangs, MBA ¥ Patient Advocate [Internet]; 2023. Available from: https://www.nccn.org/home/member-.
28. Maehata Y, Kuriyama K, Aoki S, Araya M, Marino K, Onishi H. Case report stereotactic body radiotherapy for localized ureter transitional cell carcinoma: three case reports. Case Rep Urol. 2015; https://doi.org/10.1155/2015/519897.

29. Evans JD, Hansen CC, Tollefson MK, Hallemeier CL. Stereotactic body radiation therapy for medically inoperable, clinically localized, urothelial carcinoma of the renal pelvis: a case report. Adv Radiat Oncol. 2018;3(1):57–61.
30. Cozad SC, Smalley SR, Austenfeld M, Noble M, Jennings S, Reymond R. Adjuvant radiotherapy in high stage transitional cell carcinoma of the renal pelvis and ureter. Int J Radiat Oncol Biol Phys. 1992;24
31. Chen B, Zeng ZC, Wang GM, Zhang L, Lin ZM, Sun LA, et al. Radiotherapy may improve overall survival of patients with T3/T4 transitional cell carcinoma of the renal pelvis or ureter and delay bladder tumour relapse. BMC Cancer. 2011;11
32. Hall MC, Womack S, Sagalowsky AI, Carmody T, Erickstad MD, Roehrborn CG. Prognostic factors, recurrence, and survival in transitional cell carcinoma of the upper urinary tract: a 30-year experience in 252 patients. Urology. 1998;
33. Catton CN, Warde P, Gospodarowicz MK, Panzarella T, Catton P, McLean M, et al. Transitional cell carcinoma of the renal pelvis and ureter: outcome and patterns of relapse in patients treated with postoperative radiation. Urol Oncol. 1996;2(6):171–6.
34. Bentzen SM, Constine LS, Deasy JO, Eisbruch A, Jackson A, Marks LB, et al. Quantitative analyses of Normal tissue effects in the clinic (QUANTEC): an introduction to the scientific issues. Int J Radiat Oncol Biol Phys. 2010;76(3 Suppl)
35. Benedict SH, Yenice KM, Followill D, Galvin JM, Hinson W, Kavanagh B, et al. Stereotactic body radiation therapy: the report of AAPM task group 101. Med Phys. Wiley. 2010;37:4078–101.
36. Mailankody S, Bajpai J, Budukh A, Swaminathan R, Dikshit R, Dhimal M, et al. Epidemiology of rare cancers in India and South Asian countries-remembering the forgotten [Internet]; 2023. Available from: www.thelancet.com.
37. Swartz MA, Porter MP, Lin DW, Weiss NS. Incidence of primary urethral carcinoma in the United States. Urology. 2006;68(6):1164–8.
38. Visser O, Adolfsson J, Rossi S, Verne J, Gatta G, Maffezzini M, et al. Incidence and survival of rare urogenital cancers in Europe. Eur J Cancer. 2012;48(4):456–64.
39. Mcmillan A, Pakianathan M, Mao JH, Macintyre CA. Urethral stricture and urethritis in men in Scotland. Genitourin Med [Internet]. 1994;70:403–5. Available from: http://sti.bmj.com/
40. Park S, McAninch JW. Straddle injuries to the bulbar urethra: management and outcomes in 78 patients. J Urol. 2004;171(2 I):722–5.
41. Kaplan GW, Bulkey GJ, Grayhack JT. Carcinoma of the male urethra. J Urol. 1967;98(3):365–71.
42. Rajan N, Tucci P, Mallouh C, Choudhury M. Carcinoma in female urethral diverticulum: case reports and review of management. J Urol. 1993;150(6):1911–4.
43. Wiener JS, Liu ET, Walther PJ. Oncogenic human papillomavirus type 16 is associated with squamous cell cancer of the male urethra. Cancer Res. 1992;52(18):5018–23.
44. Humphrey PA, Moch H, Cubilla AL, Ulbright TM, Reuter VE. The 2016 WHO classification of tumours of the urinary system and male genital organs—part B: prostate and bladder tumours. Eur Urol. 2016;70(1):106–19.
45. Zhang M, Adeniran AJ, Vikram R, Tamboli P, Pettaway C, Bondaruk J, et al. Carcinoma of the urethra. Hum Pathol. 2018;72:35–44.
46. Carroll PR, Dixon CM. Surgical anatomy of the male and female urethra. Urol Clin North Am. 1992;19(2):339–46.
47. Gakis G, Bruins HM, Cathomas R, Compérat EM, Cowan NC, van der Heijden AG, et al. European association of urology guidelines on primary urethral carcinoma—2020 update. Eur Urol Oncol. 2020;3(4):424–32.
48. Barkan GA, Wojcik EM, Nayar R, Savic-Prince S, Quek ML, Kurtycz DFI, et al. E-mail the Paris system for reporting urinary cytology: the quest to develop a standardized terminology. Acta Cytol [Internet]. 2016;60:185–97. Available from: www.karger.com/acy
49. Dayyani F, Hoffman K, Eifel P, Guo C, Vikram R, Pagliaro LC, et al. Management of advanced primary urethral carcinomas. BJU Int. 2014;114(1):25–31.

50. Palou Redorta J, Schatteman P, Huguet Pérez J, Segarra Tomás J, Rosales Bordes A, Algaba F, et al. Intravesical instillations with bacillus calmette-guérin for the treatment of carcinoma in situ involving prostatic ducts. Eur Urol. 2006;49(5):834–8; discussion 838.
51. Palou J, Baniel J, Klotz L, Wood D, Cookson M, Lerner S, et al. Urothelial carcinoma of the prostate. Urology. 2007;69(1 Suppl):50–61.
52. Konnak JW. Conservative management of low grade neoplasms of the male urethra: a preliminary report. J Urol. 1980;123(2):175–7.
53. Salgado CJ, Monstrey S, Hoebeke P, Lumen N, Dwyer M, Mardini S. Reconstruction of the penis after surgery. Urol Clin North Am. 2010;37(3):379–401.
54. Babjuk M, Burger M, Compérat EM, Gontero P, Mostafid AH, Palou J, et al. European association of urology guidelines on non-muscle-invasive bladder cancer (TaT1 and carcinoma in situ) - 2019 update. Eur Urol. 2019;76(5):639–57.
55. Milosevic MF, Warde PR, Banerjee D, Gospodarowicz MK, McLean M, Catton PA, et al. Urethral carcinoma in women: results of treatment with primary radiotherapy. Radiother Oncol. 2000;56(1):29–35.
56. Bagshaw HP, Williams NL, Huang YJ, Tward JD, Gaffney DK. Palladium interstitial implant in combination with external beam radiotherapy and chemotherapy for the definitive treatment of a female urethral carcinoma. Gynecol Oncol Rep. 2015;13:40–3.
57. Wang EH, Yu JB. Chemoradiation therapy for organ preservation in localized male urethral carcinoma. Oncology (Williston Park). 2016;30(6):520–3.
58. Kent M, Zinman L, Girshovich L, Sands J, Vanni A. Combined chemoradiation as primary treatment for invasive male urethral cancer. J Urol. 2015;193(2):532–7.
59. Cohen MS, Triaca V, Billmeyer B, Hanley RS, Girshovich L, Shuster T, et al. Coordinated chemoradiation therapy with genital preservation for the treatment of primary invasive carcinoma of the male urethra. J Urol. 2008;179(2):536–41. discussion 541
60. Oberfield RA, Zinman LN, Leibenhaut M, Girshovich L, Silverman ML. Management of invasive squamous cell carcinoma of the bulbomembranous male urethra with co-ordinated chemo-radiotherapy and genital preservation. Br J Urol. 1996;78(4):573–8.
61. Son CH, Liauw SL, Hasan Y, Solanki AA. Optimizing the role of surgery and radiation therapy in urethral cancer based on histology and disease extent. Int J Radiat Oncol Biol Phys. 2018;102(2):304–13.
62. De Hertogh O, Le Bihan G, Zilli T, Palumbo S, Jolicoeur M, Crehange G, et al. Consensus delineation guidelines for pelvic lymph node radiation therapy of prostate cancer: on behalf of the francophone Group of Urological Radiation Therapy (GFRU). Int J Radiat Oncol Biol Phys. 2023;
63. Sharma DN, Gandhi AK, Bhatla N, Kumar S, Rath GK. High-dose-rate interstitial brachytherapy for female peri-urethral cancer. J Contemp Brachytherapy. 2016;8(1):41–7.

Management of Seminoma

13

Jaspreet Kaur and Anu Agrawal

Abbreviations

3DCRT/IMRT	3D conformal Radiation Therapy/Intensity Modulated Radiation therapy
CT	Computed Tomography
CTV	Clinical Target Volume
FNAC	Fine Needle Aspiration Cytology
GTV	Gross Tumor Volume
MRI	Magnetic resonance Imaging
PET	Positron Emission Tomography
PTV	Planning Target Volume
RPLND	Retroperitoneal lymph node dissection
UICC	International Union against Cancer

13.1 Introduction

Testicular cancer is one of the most common malignancies among young adults, comprising around 1% of the general male population. Worldwide, 72,040 new cases and 9,068 deaths of testicular cancer were reported in Globocan 2022 [1]. More than 95% of testicular cancers are germ cell tumors [2]. Germ cell tumors (GCT) are divided into seminoma and non-seminoma. The incidence of GCTs has

J. Kaur (✉) · A. Agrawal
Department of Radiation Oncology, Vardhman Mahavir Medical College and Safdarjung Hospital, New Delhi, India

R. Madan, S. Goyal (eds.), *Essentials of Radiotherapy in Uro-Genital Malignancies*, https://doi.org/10.1007/978-981-95-5945-9_13

doubled in the past 30 years, with presentation of disease at an early age and in young population in the United States, followed by European countries. The peak age of occurrence for seminoma is 35–39 years [3]. Based on the histologic type and extent of the disease, it is managed with surgery, radiation therapy, and chemotherapy with the adoption of imaging and multidisciplinary care.

13.2 Anatomy

Testes originate from the genital ridge corresponding to L2 vertebrae. It descends into the scrotum through the inguinal canal along with its blood supply and lymphatics. The first site of metastases for seminoma is locoregional lymphatics, the first echelon being retroperitoneal lymph nodes, followed by mediastinal lymph nodes and then supraclavicular lymph nodes. The retroperitoneal lymph nodes are anterior to D11 to L4 vertebral bodies. However, skip metastases can occur, and retroperitoneal lymph nodes can directly drain to supraclavicular lymph nodes through the thoracic duct in the absence of mediastinal lymph nodes. Hematogenous spread is rare in seminoma. The most common site of distant metastases is the lung, followed by bone, liver, and brain.

13.3 Histopathology

On gross examination, it is well demarcated and has foci of necrosis or hemorrhages. On microscopic examination, the cells have typically round, hyperchromatic, or vesicular nuclei with prominent nucleoli. There are lymphocytic infiltrates, macrophages, plasma cells, and multinucleated giant cells. On immunohistochemistry (IHC), placental leukocyte alkaline phosphatase (PLAP), D2–40 (podoplanin), and OCT3/4 are positive in seminomas [4]. Variants of seminoma are:

(a) Classical seminoma (Fig. 13.1a and b)
(b) Anaplastic seminoma
(c) Spermatocytic seminoma
(d) Atypical or mixed seminoma

When three or more mitoses are seen per high-power field, anaplastic seminoma is diagnosed. Spermatocytic seminoma is distinct in its histologic characteristics, i.e., three different cell sizes, spherical nuclei, sparse or no lymphocytic infiltrate with lack of cytoplasmic glycogen [5]. Spermatocytic seminomas are very rare, comprising only 0.6% of all germ cell tumors. However, in contrast to other types, these are generally less aggressive and occur at an older age (50–54 years) [2]. In atypical type, there is no lymphocytic infiltrate, and cells have less cytoplasm compared to the classical seminoma type. It appears to have similar prognosis as of the classical type [6].

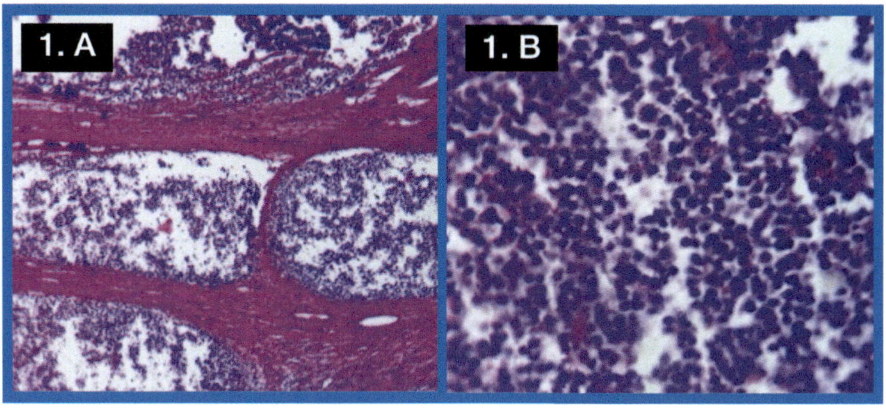

Fig. 13.1 Classical seminoma with foci of haemorrhages, Oct 3/4 positive, PLAP positive and CD 117 focal positive. (1. **a**: 40× zoom and 1. **b**: 100× zoom)

13.4 Clinical Presentation

Testicular tumor usually presents with painless scrotal swelling. Patients who have retroperitoneal lymph nodal involvement present with back pain or abdominal swelling. Metastatic disease can be diagnosed with biopsy or elevated level of serum tumor markers without any testicular swelling. Rarely, extra testicular presentation—mediastinal, retroperitoneal, or pineal might be there with no evidence of primary tumor.

13.5 Diagnostic Workup

13.5.1 Patient Evaluation

Complete history and physical examination along with evaluation of the lymph node sites should be done.

Testicular cancer usually presents as a solid mass in testis. Occasionally, inguinal lymph nodes may be enlarged. For any suspicious and clinically palpable lymph node, ultrasound-guided FNAC from the lymph node is recommended. History of previous inguinal and scrotal surgery, cryptorchidism, orchidopexy, and retractile testes should be obtained. Ultrasonography and a diagnostic and therapeutic orchiectomy should be done when there is no evidence of metastasis.

13.5.2 Staging Investigations

Includes chest X-ray, CT scan of abdomen and pelvis. CT scan of the chest is to be considered for stage II seminoma and above. A bone scan may be performed in

Table 13.1 International Germ Cell Cancer Collaborative Group Consensus Classification of Metastatic Germ Cell Cancer (IGCCCG)

Seminoma
Good prognosis group with all of the following:
Any primary site
No non-pulmonary visceral metastases
Normal AFP
Any HCG
Any LDH
Intermediate prognosis group with all of the following:
Any primary site
Non-pulmonary visceral metastases
Normal AFP
Any HCG
Any LDH
Poor prognosis group with all of the following:
There is no poor prognosis group in seminoma

stage II and III seminoma patients with bulky retroperitoneal disease. Baseline renal and pulmonary function tests should be performed in patients requiring chemotherapy.

13.5.3 Tumor Markers

Serum tumor markers Alpha Feto Protein (AFP), beta-Human Chorionic Gonadotropin (HCG), and Serum Lactate Dehydrogenase (LDH) should be done pre-treatment, as it has significant prognostic value. Also, it has utmost importance in staging, diagnosis, and surveillance of seminomas as well as non-seminomatous testicular cancers.

These tumor markers are for risk assessment according to UICC/IGCCCG stage and prognostic index (Table 13.1). The good prognosis group with no non-pulmonary visceral metastases (NPVMs) for seminoma has a 5-year overall survival of 86%, and the intermediate prognosis group with NPVMs has 72% [7].

LDH is elevated in patients with advanced seminomas, AFP and beta-HCG are often elevated in non-seminomas. The metabolic half-life of AFP is approximately 5 days, and beta-HCG is 18–24 hours. Markers are obtained before orchiectomy and repeated 7 days after the surgery.

13.6 Management

The management of seminoma is based on the staging system by the American Joint Cancer Committee on Cancer 8th edition/International Union against Cancer (AJCC/UICC), 2017 TNM classification [8].

The initial management involves high inguinal radical orchiectomy. Post-orchiectomy management is based on the histologic type and disease extent. Sperm banking should be considered before radiation therapy/systemic therapy because of the potential toxic effects on fertility.

Stage I seminoma Most patients are cured by orchiectomy alone. Post orchiectomy, adjuvant retroperitoneal radiation therapy and/or adjuvant platinum-based single-agent chemotherapy were the most widely used treatments historically.

Surveillance Approximately 20% of the patients will relapse if no adjuvant therapy is given. Either adjuvant single-agent chemotherapy with carboplatin or adjuvant radiation therapy is associated with >98% disease-specific survival and disease-free survival in selected cases. Hence, surveillance is the recommended standard management approach [9]. One of the largest population-based surveillance studies of 1,954 patients from Denmark showed that the median time to relapse was 13.7 months with 73.4% of patients developing relapse during the first 2 years, 22.2% between 3 and 5 years, and 4.3% after year 5. 15 year disease-specific survival and overall survival were 99.3% and 91.6%, respectively [10]. Most of the recurrences after surveillance occur in the retroperitoneal lymph nodes. Salvage therapy after surveillance, with either radiotherapy or chemotherapy, is highly effective with cause specific survival rates reaching 95% to 100%.

Recommended option for stage I seminoma is surveillance after orchiectomy. It is recommended to take history and do physical examination (H & P) every 3–6 months in first year, every 6 months in second year, and every 6–12 months for third year and then annually. Serum tumor markers and ultrasound abdomen are recommended for equivocal examination findings. CT abdomen and pelvis is recommended at 3, 6, and 12 months at first year, 6 monthly in second year, 6–12 monthly in third year, and every 12–24 monthly in fourth and fifth year. Chest X ray as clinically indicated, and CT chest if symptomatic [11].

Radiation therapy The relapse rate ranges from 15% to 20% of patients on surveillance, with most disease relapses detected in the infra-diaphragmatic lymph nodes. In a systemic review of 19 trials for tumor recurrence, the only important factor determining the probability of relapse is tumor size [12]. Management of relapse includes retroperitoneal radiation therapy and cisplatin-based chemotherapy. When there is local recurrence, repeat biopsy is recommended to rule out non-seminomatous or another malignant tumor. The most common sites of relapse following radiation therapy are the mediastinum, lungs, left supraclavicular fossa, and inguinal nodes. For supradiaphragmatic relapse, chemotherapy results in a virtually 100% cure rate. Isolated inguinal relapse may be treated with radiation alone. Other features associated with a higher risk of relapse may include tumor invasion of the tunica albuginea, epididymis, spermatic cord and lymphovascular invasion [13, 14].

Chemotherapy Seminoma is highly chemosensitive, even in advanced disease settings; however, the use of adjuvant carboplatin (AUC 7) after orchiectomy was initiated in stage I seminoma by Oliver et al. [15]. The United Kingdom Medical

Research Council, in a phase III noninferior study, compared a single course of carboplatin in 1477 patients with adjuvant radiation therapy. There was no difference in 5-years relapse-free survival. It concluded that adjuvant carboplatin was non inferior to adjuvant radiation therapy for stage I seminoma [16]. Regardless, in an adjuvant setting, chemotherapy may no longer be considered a preferred treatment option in stage one seminoma [9].

RPLND: The use of RPLND in seminoma is routinely not advocated unless patient is unwilling to comply with surveillance or is unable or unwilling to be treated with adjuvant radiation therapy or chemotherapy.

13.6.1 Stages II and III Seminoma

The most important prognostic factor in stage II seminoma is the presence of retroperitoneal lymph nodes. The management is based on disease substage, i.e., Stage IIA, B, and C and overall tumor bulk. In stage IIB and IIC, patients should be treated with adjuvant chemotherapy because of the disease bulk and higher risk of distant relapse even after adjuvant radiation therapy (RT). However, the patient can be considered for RPLND, where the patient has contraindications to both chemotherapy and RT or has residual disease after treatment completion. The most common sites of relapse are mediastinal or supraclavicular nodes, lung, and bone following RT in patients [17–20]. Patients with stage III seminoma are less than 5% and are usually managed with cisplatin-based regimens. According to the IGCCCG system, for the patients in the good prognostic group, three cycles of bleomycin, etoposide, and cisplatin or four cycles of etoposide and cisplatin is considered as the standard of care. For patients in the intermediate prognosis group, 4 cycles of BEP is standard [21, 22].

For stage IIA and non-bulky IIB seminoma after adjuvant therapy, recommended surveillance is H & P every 3 months in the first year, every 6 months in second year, and every 6 months in the 3rd–fifth years. CT or MRI of the abdomen and pelvis at 3 months, then at ninth or 12th month, then annually in the second and third years, then as clinically indicated. Chest X-ray every 6 months for 2 years and CT chest if symptomatic. Serum tumor markers are optional, and an abdominal ultrasound is recommended for equivocal examination findings.

For bulky stage IIB, IIC, and III seminoma, the recommended follow-up is H & P every 2 months in first year, every 3 months in the second year, every 6 months in third and fourth years, and then annually. CT or MRI abdomen and pelvis every 4 months in first year, 6 months in second year, then annually in third and fourth year, then as clinically indicated. Chest X-ray every 2 months for 1 year, every 3 months in second year, then annually, and CT chest if symptomatic. Serum tumor markers are optional, and an abdominal ultrasound is recommended for equivocal examination findings [11].

13.6.2 Radiation Dose and Technique

2D technique The intended target volume for stages I and II seminoma includes ipsilateral pelvic nodes and para-aortic lymph nodes with anteroposterior parallel opposed fields and 10 MV–18 MV photons. This classic technique is known as "hockey stick" in the United Kingdom and "dogleg" field in Europe.

- Stage I seminoma:
  A. *Para-aortic lymph node irradiation* (Fig. 13.2):
  Upper border—D10–11 interface
  Inferior border—L5-S1 interface
  Laterals—to cover the spinous process
  B. *Para-aortic and pelvic lymph node irradiation* (Fig. 13.3):
  Upper border—D10–11 interface
  Inferior border—L5-S1 interface, diagonally to the lateral/superior acetabulum then vertically to the level of mid obturator.

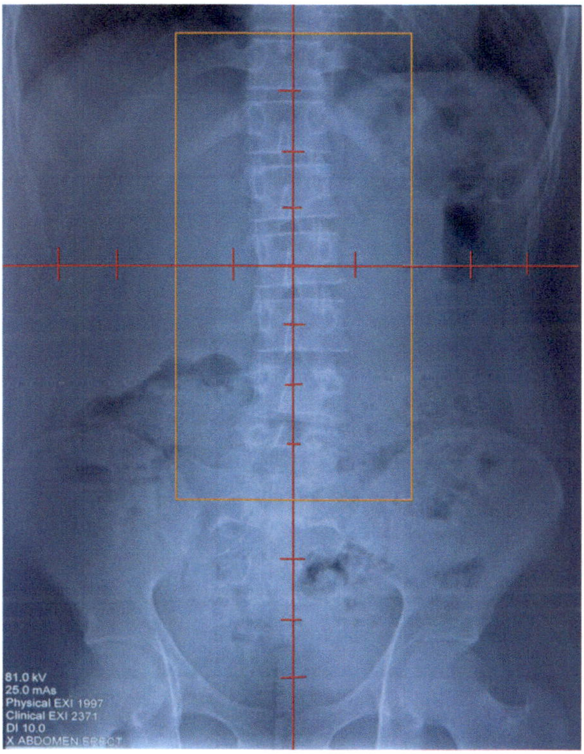

Fig. 13.2 Para-aortic lymph node field

Radiation Dose and Fractionation [23, 24]:

20 Gy in 10 fractions at 2 Gy per fraction over 2 weeks—5 days a week.

Stage II seminoma: The target volume includes the para-aortic, ipsilateral common iliac, and external iliac lymph node chain and macroscopically enlarged lymph node (Figs. 13.4 and 13.5) [25]

Superior border—D10–11 interface

Inferior border—cranial border of ipsilateral acetabulum

Lateral borders for:

(a) Para-aortic field—lateral vertebral processes
(b) Pelvic field—line from cranial border of acetabulum to the lateral process of the fourth lumbar vertebrae.

Radiation Dose and Fractionation: 20 Gy at 2 Gy per fractions followed by boost to macroscopic lymph node to a total dose of 30 Gy in stage IIA and 36 Gy in stage IIB at 2 Gy per fractions.

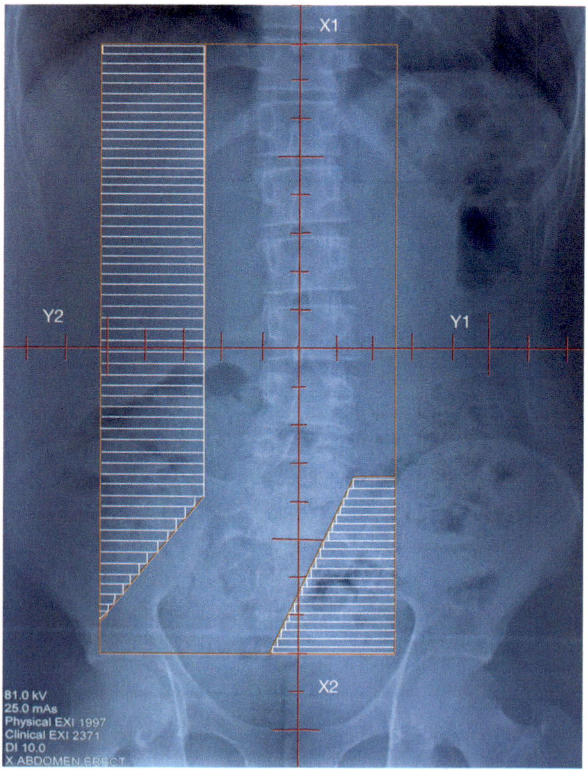

Fig. 13.3 Para-aortic and pelvic lymph node field (modified dog leg field)

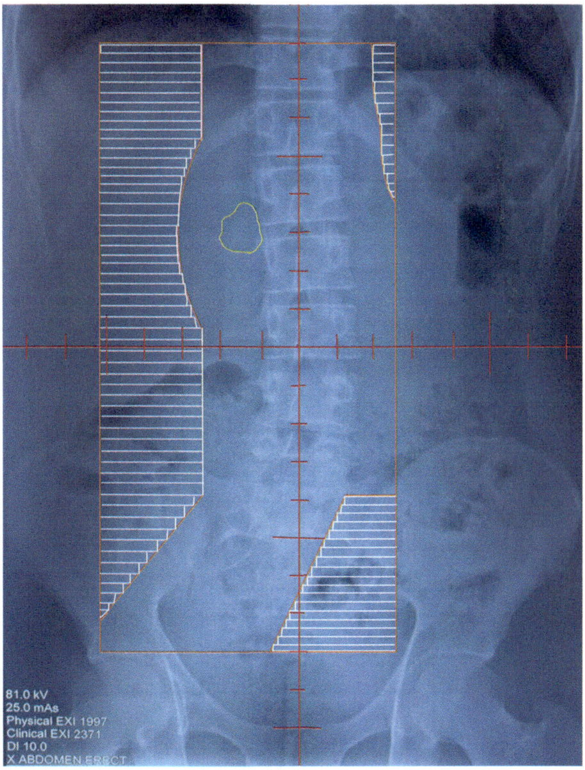

Fig. 13.4 Dog leg field—para-aortic and pelvic lymph node field encompassing gross node indicated by yellow arrow

13.6.3 3D CRT/IMRT Contouring Guidelines

The patient is made to lie down in the supine position and immobilized using a thermoplastic mask with arms above the head. IV contrast is used to help delineate gross nodal disease. Planning CT with a 2–5 mm slice thickness is taken. A PET scan can also be fused with a CT simulation scan. Target volumes for the para-aortic strip field are depicted in Table 13.3 and for para-aortic, pelvic, and gross nodal disease in Table 13.4.

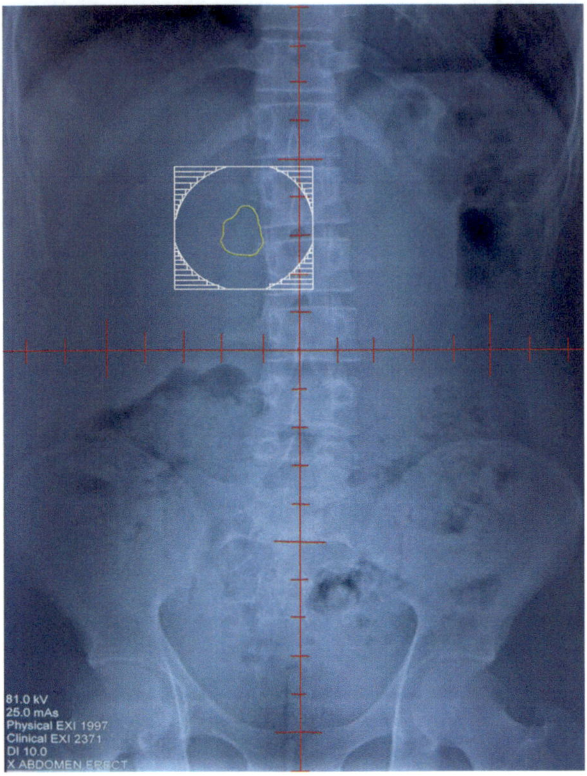

Fig. 13.5 Boost to para-aortic gross lymph node

Table 13.3 Suggested target volumes for paraaortic strip fields [26]

Target volume	Contouring based on CT imaging and vascular anatomy
CTV	Contour inferior vena cava (IVC) and aorta from 2 cm below top of kidney superiorly to bifurcation of iliac vessels inferiorly Expand IVC contour by 1–1.5 cm and aorta by 1.5–2 cm Combine both the volumes and edit it off bone and muscle
PTV	Expand CTV by 5–7 mm

Table 13.4 Suggested target volumes for para-aortic, pelvic field and gross nodal disease [26]

Target volumes	Contouring based on CT imaging and vascular anatomy
CTV 1	CTV vessels— (a) IVC/aorta contours and expansions as in Table 13.3 (b) Contour common iliac, external iliac to the upper rim of acetabulum and proximal internal iliac vessels (c) Give expansion of 1–1.5 cm CTV nodes—Contour gross node and give expansion of 1–1.5 cm Combine CTV vessels and CTV node to form CTV 1
PTV 1	Expand CTV 1 by 5–7 mm
PTV boost	Expand CTV nodes by 5–7 mm

References

1. Bray F, Laversanne M, Sung H, Ferlay J, Siegel RL, Soerjomataram I, et al. Global cancer statistics 2022: GLOBOCAN estimates of incidence and mortality worldwide for 36 cancers in 185 countries. CA Cancer J Clin. 2024;74(3):229–63.
2. Park JS, Kim J, Elghiaty A, Ham WS. Recent global trends in testicular cancer incidence and mortality. Medicine (Baltimore). 2018;97(37):e12390.
3. Giona S. The epidemiology of testicular cancer. In: Urologic cancers. Exon Publ; 2022. p. 107–16.
4. Ulbright TM. Germ cell neoplasms of the testis. Am J Surg Pathol. 1993;17(11):1075–91.
5. Aggarwal N, Parwani AV. Spermatocytic seminoma. Arch Pathol Lab Med. 2009;133(12):1985–8.
6. Tickoo SK, Hutchinson B, Bacik J, Mazumdar M, Motzer RJ, Bajorin DF, et al. Testicular seminoma: a clinicopathologic and immunohistochemical study of 105 cases with special reference to seminomas with atypical features. Int J Surg Pathol. 2002;10(1):23–32.
7. International germ cell consensus classification: a prognostic factor-based staging system for metastatic germ cell cancers. International Germ Cell Cancer Collaborative Group. J Clin Oncol. 1997;15(2):594–603.
8. Amin MB, Greene FL, Edge SB, Compton CC, Gershenwald JE, Brookland RK, et al. The eighth edition AJCC cancer staging manual: continuing to build a bridge from a population-based to a more "personalized" approach to cancer staging. CA Cancer J Clin. 2017;67(2):93–9.
9. Van De Wetering RAW, Sleijfer S, Feldman DR, Funt SA, Bosl GJ, De Wit R. Controversies in the management of clinical stage I seminoma: carboplatin a decade in—time to start backing out. J Clin Oncol. 2018;36(9):837–40.
10. Mortensen MS, Lauritsen J, Gundgaard MG, Agerbæk M, Holm NV, Christensen IJ, et al. A Nationwide cohort study of stage I seminoma patients followed on a surveillance program. Eur Urol. 2014;66(6):1172–8.
11. testicular.pdf [Internet]. [cited 2024 Jul 8]. Available from: https://www.nccn.org/professionals/physician_gls/pdf/testicular.pdf.
12. Zengerling F, Kunath F, Jensen K, Ruf C, Schmidt S, Spek A. Prognostic factors for tumor recurrence in patients with clinical stage I seminoma undergoing surveillance—a systematic review. Urol Oncol Semin Orig Investig. 2018;36(10):448–58.
13. Bayens YC, Helle PA, Van Putten WLJ, Mali SPM. Orchidectomy followed by radiotherapy in 176 stage I and II testicular seminoma patients: benefits of a 10-year follow-up study. Radiother Oncol. 1992;25(2):97–102.
14. Warde P, Gospodarowicz MK, Panzarella T, Catton CN, Sturgeon JF, Moore M, et al. Stage I testicular seminoma: results of adjuvant irradiation and surveillance. J Clin Oncol. 1995;13(9):2255–62.
15. Oliver RTD, Edmonds PM, Ong JYH, Ostrowski MJ, Jackson AW, Baille-Johnson H, et al. Pilot studies of 2 and 1 course carboplatin as adjuvant for stage I seminoma: should it be tested in a randomized trial against radiotherapy? Int J Radiat Oncol Biol Phys. 1994;29(1):3–8.
16. Oliver RTD, Mead GM, Rustin GJS, Joffe JK, Aass N, Coleman R, et al. Randomized trial of carboplatin versus radiotherapy for stage I seminoma: mature results on relapse and contralateral testis cancer rates in MRC TE19/EORTC 30982 study (ISRCTN27163214). J Clin Oncol. 2011;29(8):957–62.
17. Chung PWM, Gospodarowicz MK, Panzarella T, Jewett MAS, Sturgeon JFG, Tew-George B, et al. Stage II testicular seminoma: patterns of recurrence and outcome of treatment. Eur Urol. 2004;45(6):754–60.
18. Vallis KA, Howard GCW, Duncan W, Cornbleet MA, Kerr GR. Radiotherapy for stages I and II testicular seminoma: results and morbidity in 238 patients. Br J Radiol. 1995;68(808):400–5.
19. Zagars GK, Pollack A. Radiotherapy for stage II testicular seminoma. Int J Radiat Oncol. 2001;51(3):643–9.

20. Oldenburg J, Horwich A. Appendix 9: testicular seminoma and non-seminoma: eUpdate published online 29 June 2017 (www.esmo.org/Guidelines/Genitourinary-Cancers). Ann Oncol. 2017;28:iv165–6.
21. Beyer J, Albers P, Altena R, Aparicio J, Bokemeyer C, Busch J, et al. Maintaining success, reducing treatment burden, focusing on survivorship: highlights from the third European consensus conference on diagnosis and treatment of germ-cell cancer. Ann Oncol. 2013;24(4):878–88.
22. Hamilton RJ, Canil C, Shrem NS, Kuhathaas K, Jiang MD, Chung P, et al. Canadian Urological Association consensus guideline: management of testicular germ cell cancer. Can Urol Assoc J. 2022;16(6):155–73.
23. Mead GM, Fossa SD, Oliver RTD, Joffe JK, Huddart RA, Roberts JT, et al. Randomized trials in 2466 patients with stage I seminoma: patterns of relapse and follow-up. JNCI J Natl Cancer Inst. 2011;103(3):241–9.
24. Leung E, Warde P, Jewett M, Panzarella T, O'Malley M, Sweet J, et al. Treatment burden in stage I seminoma: a comparison of surveillance and adjuvant radiation therapy. BJU Int. 2013;112(8):1088–95.
25. Classen J, Schmidberger H, Meisner C, Souchon R, Sautter-Bihl ML, Sauer R, et al. Radiotherapy for stages IIA/B testicular seminoma: final report of a prospective multicenter clinical trial. J Clin Oncol. 2003;21(6):1101–6.
26. Wilder RB, Buyyounouski MK, Efstathiou JA, Beard CJ. Radiotherapy treatment planning for testicular seminoma. Int J Radiat Oncol. 2012;83(4):e445–52.

Non-seminomatous Germ Cell Tumors

14

Divya Khosla, Samreen Zaheer, Treshita Dey,
and Rakesh Kapoor

14.1 Introduction

Testicular tumors most commonly affect males between the ages of 15 and 35 years and are classified into two main types, germ cell tumors and non-germ cell tumors. Approximately 95% of all testicular cancers are germ cell tumors [1].

The germ cell tumors (GCTs) are further subdivided into two main subtypes: seminomatous GCT and the non-seminomatous GCT (NSGCT).

According to the 2022 WHO classification [2, 3] of "tumor of the urinary system and male genital system," the non-seminomatous germ cell tumors include following types:

Embryonal carcinoma
Yolk sac tumor, postpubertal type
Choriocarcinoma
Placental site trophoblastic tumor
Epithelioid trophoblastic tumor
Teratoma, postpubertal type
Teratoma with somatic-type malignancy

While pure histology of a single subtype can occur in NSGCT, it is more common to find mixed subtypes on histology. In this chapter, we will review the management and outcomes of NSGCTs.

D. Khosla (✉) · T. Dey · R. Kapoor
Department of Radiotherapy and Oncology, Postgraduate Institute of Medical Education and Research, Chandigarh, India

S. Zaheer
Department of Radiotherapy, Jawaharlal Nehru Medical College Hospital, Aligarh, India

R. Madan, S. Goyal (eds.), *Essentials of Radiotherapy in Uro-Genital Malignancies*, https://doi.org/10.1007/978-981-95-5945-9_14

14.2 Clinical Features and Diagnostic Workup

Most of the patients present with unilateral testicular mass, which is usually painless. Other less common symptoms include lower abdominal discomfort or feeling of heaviness. Clinical examination for any evidence of supraclavicular lymph nodes or gynecomastia also needs to be done [4]. Gynecomastia, seen in approximately 5% of males with testicular germ cell tumors, is an endocrine-related symptom of these cancers [5].

Clinical examination plays a crucial role in the evaluation of testicular tumors and should include a thorough bimanual palpation, starting with the normal testis for comparison. This method allows the examiner to assess the size, consistency, and mobility of the testes and helps in identifying any abnormalities. The testis should be palpated gently with the thumb and first two fingers to ensure a thorough examination. Any firm, hard, or fixed areas within the testis should raise suspicion for malignancy and warrant further investigation. Early detection through a careful and systematic clinical examination is vital for timely diagnosis and intervention in testicular cancer. The examination should also involve palpating the abdomen to check for signs of nodal disease or visceral involvement. Routine examination of the supraclavicular lymph nodes can help detect adenopathy, which may be present in males with advanced disease. Additionally, a chest examination should be conducted to assess for gynecomastia, which can be an indicator of endocrine changes associated with testicular cancer.

The investigations needed for diagnostic workup and staging of NSGCT include scrotal ultrasound, chest X-ray, serum tumor markers, and contrast-enhanced tomography (CECT) of abdomen and pelvis. Complete hemogram, renal function tests (RFT), and liver function tests are needed to assess the baseline status of the patient. Ultrasound is the first radiological investigation to be done when a patient presents with a testicular lump. It helps to exclude other causes of testicular pain and lump such as epididymitis, epididymo-orchitis, or cystic testicular masses. It is an important imaging investigation to see the status of contralateral testis. The sensitivity of USG ranges from 92% to 98% while the specificity is 95% to 99.8% [6]. Color Doppler USG with high-frequency USG probe is used to characterize the lesion and rule out the benign causes. A solid testicular mass on USG is highly suggestive of the need for radical orchiectomy and histological diagnosis.

CECT abdomen and pelvis is the investigation of choice to look for the retroperitoneal lymph node involvement and rule out distant metastasis to intra-abdominal sites. In case of equivocal findings, image-guided biopsy may be needed [7, 8]. CECT chest is recommended in case of suspicion of metastatic disease.

Serum tumor markers, such as human chorionic gonadotropin (hCG), lactate dehydrogenase (LDH), and alpha-fetoprotein (AFP), are crucial for both diagnostic and prognostic assessment. Serum tumor markers should be assessed before any intervention, including orchiectomy. Both pre- and post-orchiectomy levels should be measured. The American Joint Committee on Cancer (AJCC) staging system for testicular tumors includes tumor marker levels as a distinct “S” category, which is considered when determining the stage. Tumor markers are also used to monitor treatment response and detect relapse during follow-up. AFP levels are increased in 50–70% of individuals with NSGCTs. Pure choriocarcinoma and pure seminoma do not secrete AFP. β-hCG is frequently produced by syncytiotrophoblasts, especially in cases of choriocarcinoma, and is found to be elevated in about 15% of seminomas. Yolk sac tumors, embryonal carcinomas, and some teratomas are also associated with AFP secretion [9]. Elevated AFP level in a patient diagnosed solely with seminoma suggests the presence of undetected NSGCT elements. LDH, a non-specific tumor marker, is elevated in 20–60% of NSGCT cases and is generally considered an indicator of disease burden. Alpha-fetoprotein (AFP) is secreted by yolk sac tumors, embryonal carcinomas, and some teratomas [9]. Both AFP and β-hCG can also be elevated in a variety of other cancers, including lung, liver, gastrointestinal, bone, and liver tumors. Noncoding microRNAs, particularly the miR-371-373 cluster, are emerging as potential tumor marker for both seminomas and NSGCTs [10].

Radical inguinal orchiectomy serves the purpose of tissue diagnosis and is also needed for local tumor control. NCCN recommends against the routine use of positron emission tomography (PET) for NSGCT.

14.3 Staging

The staging of testicular cancer is based on the eighth edition of the tumor, node, metastasis (TNM) classification system by the American Joint Committee on Cancer (AJCC) and the Union for International Cancer Control (UICC) [11]. Testicular cancer does not have a stage IV classification in its staging system. The highest stage is stage III, which accounts for advanced disease with distant metastases, such as those involving non-regional lymph nodes or other organs. This system is used for both seminomas and non-seminomatous germ cell tumors (NSGCTs). Confirmatory biopsies are typically unnecessary for staging testicular cancer due to availability of reliable serum tumor markers and predictable patterns of metastasis. Biopsies are reserved for unusual cases, such as cases without elevated markers or disease at atypical locations.

14.4 Treatment

The cure rates for testicular tumors are among the highest for solid neoplasms. With advances in treatment, especially with the advent of platinum-based combination chemotherapy, over 95% of people diagnosed with either seminomatous or non-seminomatous germ cell tumors survive for at least 5 years [12].

Radical inguinal orchiectomy is required both for diagnostic purposes and for the treatment. The classical orchiectomy for testicular tumors consists of ligation of spermatic cord at the level of internal inguinal ring. This is the initial management and testis-sparing surgery should only be offered to compliant patients with only one testis. If testis-sparing surgery is planned, biopsy from the remaining testicular tissue should not reveal any evidence of germ cell neoplasia in situ [13]. Further, management depends on the histology and stage of disease. Patients desirous of maintaining fertility should be given the option of sperm banking [4].

14.4.1 Treatment of Stage I Disease

Orchiectomy is the standard management for stage 1 disease. About 75% of clinical stage I NSGCT cases are cured with orchiectomy alone and do not require further treatment. However, the risk of relapse after orchiectomy without any adjuvant treatment is approximately 25% [4]. Identifying patients at high risk for recurrence who would benefit most from adjuvant treatment is challenging. Although recurrence risk is about 25% with surveillance, treatment at recurrence is nearly always curative [14]. Long-term disease-specific survival exceeds 99%, regardless of whether patients undergo surveillance, chemotherapy, or retroperitoneal lymph node dissection (RPLND). Presence of lymphovascular invasion (LVSI) is associated with increased risk of relapse. In the presence of LVSI, 5-year risk of relapse is 50% while if LVSI is absent, 5-year risk of relapse decreases to 15% [15]. Another risk factor for relapse in stage 1 disease is high embryonal carcinoma component [16]. There are varied criteria to consider embryonal carcinoma as the predominant component of NSGCT. An agreed-upon definition is when embryonal component is more than any other histological component [17].

Patients who have elevated and rising levels of AFP, β-hCG, or both after orchiectomy, despite no radiographic evidence of metastatic disease, are classified as stage IS for NSGCT. Persistently elevated markers typically suggest metastatic disease. As a result, these patients should receive chemotherapy, similar to those with stage III disease.

There are three treatment options after orchiectomy—surveillance, retroperitoneal lymph node dissection, and one cycle of adjuvant bleomycin, etoposide, cisplatin (BEP) chemotherapy [18] (Table 14.1). Management of stage 1S is discussed in section on management of advanced NSGCT.

The 15-year disease-specific survival is as high as 99% for stage 1 disease, irrespective of post-orchiectomy management [19]. Risks and benefits of the treatment options need to be discussed with the patients and their caregivers.

In patients on active surveillance, relapses are seen most frequently in the first 2–3 years after being diagnosed with the disease [20]. Adequate compliance should be ensured for patients who are kept on surveillance. The patients should be well explained about other treatment options available along with their advantages and

Table 14.1 BEP chemotherapy regimen

Injection bleomycin	30 units	Day 1, day 8, and day 15
Injection etoposide	100 mg/m^2 per day	Days 1–5
Injection cisplatin	20 mg/m^2 per day	Days 1–5.

disadvantages. The surveillance is done with history, physical examination, CECT abdomen and pelvis, and chest X-ray.

In accordance with NCCN guidelines [21], history and physical examination should be done every 2 months in the first year and every 3 months in the second year. The frequency is reduced to 4–6 monthly in the third year, 6 monthly in the fourth year, and annually in the fifth year. With respect to imaging studies, NCCN surveillance guidelines vary for those without risk factors versus those with risk factors (Table 14.2).

RPLND is preferred in patients with somatic malignant transformation [22]. However, before choosing this treatment option, presence of a surgeon experienced in nerve-sparing RPLND needs to be ensured to minimize the risks of surgical complications, particularly loss of ejaculation. Patients should be made aware that chemotherapy might still be needed after RPLND depending on the pathological stage.

One cycle of BEP chemotherapy is given to stage 1 patient if risk-stratified approach is chosen or the patient is not a candidate for surveillance. Some patients may choose this treatment option to avoid the mental agony of living with risk of disease relapse in future. The risk of relapse is decreased to <5% with adjuvant chemotherapy [23].

However, the patients should be explained about the benefits and risks of this approach, including possible infertility, and the need of sperm banking.

In a systematic review of randomized trials and comparative observational studies in stage 1 testicular germ cell tumors, overall survival in NSGCT was >90% with only slight differences between the three treatment modalities [23]. The vast majority of relapsing patients achieve successful salvage with appropriately adjusted treatment based on the disease stage.

14.4.2 Treatment of Stage II Disease

Stage II disease is characterized by cancer that has spread to the regional (i.e., retroperitoneal) lymph nodes, without evidence of distant metastasis or substantial elevation in serum tumor markers (S0 or S1). For stage II A with normal tumor markers (S0), RPLND is the treatment of choice post orchidectomy. Further management depends on histology. Surveillance is recommended for pathological stage

Table 14.2 Surveillance schedule in stage 1 patients

	Risk factors present		Risk factors absent	
	CECT WAP	CXR	CECT WAP	CXR
1st year	4 monthly		4–6 monthly	At fourth and 12th month
2nd year	4–6 monthly		6 monthly	Annually
3rd year	6 monthly		Annually	
4th year	Annually		According to clinical indications	Annually
5th year	According to clinical indications			

[a]CECT WAP=Contrast Enhanced Computed Tomography of Whole Abdomen and Pelvis

I disease. However, for pathological stage II, adjuvant chemotherapy is preferred [24], apart from stage II A in which both chemotherapy and surveillance can be offered (Fig. 14.1). For pN1 and pN2 disease, two cycles of etoposide and cisplatin, (EP) while for pN3 disease, three cycles of BEP or 4 cycles of EP should be considered [21]. Teratomas are chemoresistant tumors and there is no role of adjuvant chemotherapy in these patients.

According to the NCCN guidelines, selected group of asymptomatic stage II B, S0 patients, in whom disease is limited to regional lymph nodes and is not multifocal, can be managed by RPLND [21]. RPLND is especially preferred in patients with teratoma histology as teratomas are chemoresistant tumors [25].

Stage II A with elevated tumor markers (S1), stage II B (apart from a small, selected subgroup with normal tumor markers as discussed above), and stage II C disease should be managed with chemotherapy post orchidectomy after stratifying these patients according to the International Germ Cell Cancer Collaborative Group (IGCCCG) prognostic classification. IGCCCG prognostic classification is discussed in Sect. 14.4.3 on treatment of advanced NSGCT.

After chemotherapy, many patients may still have residual disease. Surgical resection in the form of RPLND should be done for residual disease of >1 cm size after chemotherapy [22].

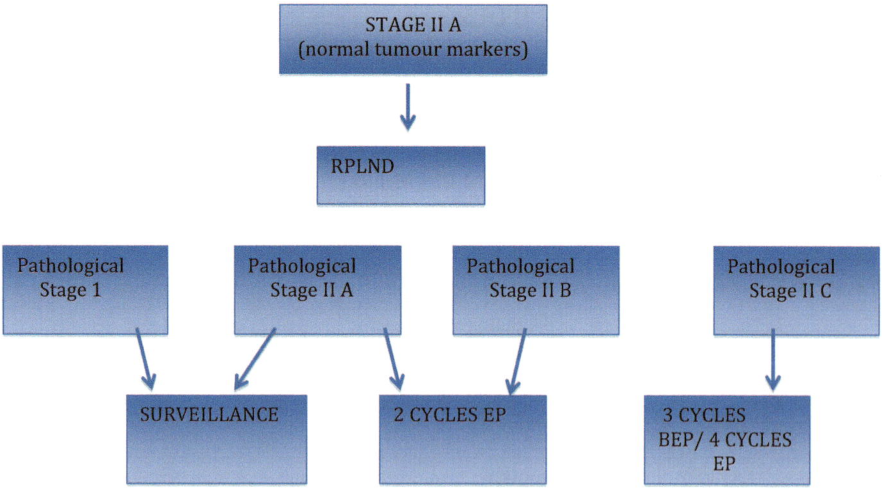

Fig. 14.1 Treatment options in stage II A disease with normal tumor markers

14.4.3 Treatment of Advanced Testicular NSGCT

In germ cell tumors, metastatic disease is the same as advanced disease, which means the disease has spread beyond the testicles. This also includes stage 1S disease.

The International Germ Cell Cancer Collaborative Group (IGCCCG) gave a prognostic grouping for metastatic germ cell tumors in 1997. According to IGCCCG, NSGCT can be divided into three risk groups (Table 14.3), with each group having significantly different progression-free survival (PFS) and overall survival (OS) [26].

However, the patients included in the IGCCC were those who were treated between 1975 and 1990. At that time the cisplatin-based chemotherapy regimen was not standardized.

The IGCCCG update consortium, published in 2021, was a collaborative study involving 9728 men with metastatic NSGCT [27]. The study included patients treated between 1990 and 2013 and was conducted across 30 institutions. Its main objectives were to assess the accuracy of the IGCCCG criteria in a contemporary patient cohort and identify new prognostic factors. PFS and OS were selected as the primary end points. There was a significant improvement in all risk groups in terms of OS; however, improvement in PFS was most pronounced in the poor prognosis group. This study concluded that the three prognostic groups as proposed by ICCCG in 1997 are still valid for standard clinical practice. Increasing age and lung metastasis were proposed as additional poor prognostic factors with 2.5 times the upper limit of normal as the new cut off for LDH values [27].

The tumor markers levels for risk stratification should be done post orchiectomy, ideally on day 1 of first cycle of chemotherapy [22]. After orchidectomy, patients with stage II and III are treated based on the risk groups defined by the ICCCG [22, 28]. Stage 1S patients, who have persistently elevated serum tumor markers after orchidectomy, are managed according to the corresponding risk group. The elevated

Table 14.3 Risk stratification of advanced NSGCT

Good prognosis (all of these)	Intermediate prognosis	Poor prognosis
Testis or retroperitoneal primary **AND**	Testis or retroperitoneal primary **AND**	Mediastinal primary **OR**
No non-pulmonary visceral metastasis **AND**	No non-pulmonary visceral metastasis **AND**	Non-pulmonary visceral metastasis **OR**
All of these AFP < 1000 ng/ml and hCG < 5000 IU/l and LDH < 1.5 × upper limit of normal	*Any of these* AFP >= 1000 ng/ml and <= 10,000 ng/ml **or** hCG >= 5000 IU/l <= 50,000 IU/l OR LDH >= 1.5 × upper limit of normal but >= upper limit of normal	*Any of these* AFP > 10,000 ng/ml OR hCG > 50,000 IU/l **or** LDH >10 × upper limit of normal

[a]*NSGCT* non-seminomatous germ cell tumor, *AFP* alpha fetoprotein, *hCG* human chorionic gonadotrophin, *LDH* lactate dehydrogenase

Table 14.4 VIP chemotherapy regimen for intermediate and poor prognosis patients

Injection etoposide	75 mg/m^2 per day	Days 1–5
Injection ifosfamide	1200 mg/m^2 per day	Days 1– 5
Injection cisplatin	20 mg/m^2 per day	Days 1–5
Injection mesna	400 mg/ m^2 per day	0 h (i.e., before), then 4 hour and 8 hour after each dose of injection Ifosfamide

markers might be indicative of subclinical metastatic disease. As discussed in Sect. 14.4.2, for stage II A and selected IIB patients whose tumor markers are in normal range, RPLND is preferred.

14.4.3.1 Good Prognostic Group

Cisplatin-based combination chemotherapy is recommended. Three cycles of bleomycin, etoposide, cisplatin (BEP) or four cycles of EP is the standard treatment for good risk group. The recommended doses are mentioned in Table 14.1.

The cycles are administered at 3 weeks interval. A randomized trial of the Genito-Urinary Group of the French Federation of Cancer Centers (GETUG T93BP) concluded that the results of four cycles of EP were similar to three cycles of BEP [29]. A randomized study of the European Organization for Research and Treatment of Cancer showed that four cycles of BEP were equivalent to three cycles of BEP. Also there was no difference in the toxicities in these groups [30].

14.4.3.2 Intermediate and Poor Prognostic Group

For this group of patients, four cycles of BEP are recommended. The alternative chemotherapy regimen is four cycles of injection etoposide, ifosfamide, and cisplatin (VIP) (Table 14.4), although the standard remains BEP regimen [28]. The alternative regimen may be used in patients who have underlying risk of pulmonary toxicity and thus are poor candidates for bleomycin. Both the chemotherapy regimens are associated with similar results, but myelosuppression is more common with VIP regimen [31].

Post chemotherapy, if residual disease measuring >1 cm is present on CECT abdomen, resection should be done [32].

14.5 Relapsed and Refractory Disease

The risk of relapse or refractory disease is higher in poor prognostic group as compared to early-stage disease with good prognostic factors [33]. The term relapsed germ cell tumor is used when the disease recurs after initial platinum-based chemotherapy, while the disease is said to be refractory if it progresses while on platinum-based therapy or recurs within 1 month of treatment completion [34]. Refractory disease also includes the subset of patients who progress after multiple lines of chemotherapy [35].

If surgery is feasible, RPLND is a treatment option, especially for relapse limited to retroperitoneum [36]. If the disease is considered inoperable, chemotherapy is the treatment of choice. The chemotherapy regimens include combination of paclitaxel, ifosfamide, cisplatin (TIP), etoposide, ifosfamide, cisplatin (VIP), or vinblastin, ifosfamide, cisplatin (VeIP) [37–39].

14.6 Summary

In conclusion, NSGCTs are highly treatable malignancies with a generally favorable prognosis, particularly when diagnosed and managed appropriately. Treatment strategies depend on the stage of disease and include orchiectomy as the primary intervention, followed by additional therapies such as chemotherapy or RPLND in advanced stages. For patients with clinical stage I disease, the majority can be cured with orchiectomy alone, while those at higher risk of recurrence may benefit from adjuvant treatment. Surveillance remains a viable option for many, with a high cure rate even in the event of recurrence. Overall, the prognosis for NSGCT patients remains excellent, with long-term disease-specific survival exceeding 99%, regardless of the treatment approach, making early detection and tailored management crucial in optimizing outcomes.

References

1. Manecksha RP, Fitzpatrick JM. Epidemiology of testicular cancer. BJU Int. 2009;104(9 Pt B):1329–33. https://doi.org/10.1111/j.1464-410X.2009.08854.x.
2. Moch H, Amin MB, Berney DM, Compérat EM, Gill AJ, Hartmann A, et al. The 2022 World Health Organization classification of tumours of the urinary system and male genital organs-part a: renal, penile, and testicular tumours. Eur Urol. 2022;82(5):458–68. https://doi.org/10.1016/j.eururo.2022.06.016. Epub 2022 Jul 16
3. Berney DM, Cree I, Rao V, Moch H, Srigley JR, Tsuzuki T, et al. An introduction to the WHO 5th edition 2022 classification of testicular tumours. Histopathology. 2022;81(4):459–66. https://doi.org/10.1111/his.14675. Epub 2022 Jul 1.
4. Albers P, Albrecht W, Algaba F, Bokemeyer C, Cohn-Cedermark G, Fizazi K, et al; European Association of Urology. Guidelines on testicular cancer: 2015 update. Eur Urol 2015;68(6):1054–68. https://doi.org/10.1016/j.eururo.2015.07.044.
5. Tseng A Jr, Horning SJ, Freiha FS, Resser KJ, Hannigan JF Jr, Torti FM. Gynecomastia in testicular cancer patients. Prognostic and therapeutic implications. Cancer. 1985;56(10):2534–8. https://doi.org/10.1002/1097-0142(19851115)56:10<2534::aid-cncr2820561036>3.0.co;2-q.
6. Zhang L, Yu H, Hemminki O, Försti A, Sundquist K, Hemminki K. Familial associations in testicular cancer with other cancers. Sci Rep. 2018;8(1):10880. https://doi.org/10.1038/s41598-018-28819-7.
7. Coursey Moreno C, Small WC, Camacho JC, Master V, Kokabi N, Lewis M, et al. Testicular tumors: what radiologists need to know--differential diagnosis, staging, and management. Radiographics. 2015;35(2):400–15. https://doi.org/10.1148/rg.352140097.
8. Hedgire SS, Pargaonkar VK, Elmi A, Harisinghani AM, Harisinghani MG. Pelvic nodal imaging. Radiol Clin North Am. 2012;50(6):1111–25. https://doi.org/10.1016/j.rcl.2012.08.002. Epub 2012 Oct 11

9. Milose JC, Filson CP, Weizer AZ, Hafez KS, Montgomery JS. Role of biochemical markers in testicular cancer: diagnosis, staging, and surveillance. Open Access J Urol. 2011;4:1–8. https://doi.org/10.2147/OAJU.S15063.
10. Regouc M, Belge G, Lorch A, Dieckmann KP, Pichler M. Non-coding microRNAs as novel potential tumor markers in testicular cancer. Cancers (Basel). 2020;12(3):749. https://doi.org/10.3390/cancers12030749.
11. Amin MB, Greene FL, Edge SB, Compton CC, Gershenwald JE, Brookland RK, et al. The Eighth Edition AJCC Cancer Staging Manual: Continuing to build a bridge from a population-based to a more "personalized" approach to cancer staging. CA Cancer J Clin. 2017;67(2):93–9. https://doi.org/10.3322/caac.21388. Epub 2017 Jan 17
12. Smith ZL, Werntz RP, Eggener SE. Testicular cancer: epidemiology, diagnosis, and management. Med Clin North Am. 2018;102(2):251–64. https://doi.org/10.1016/j.mcna.2017.10.003. Epub 2017 Dec 21
13. Dieckmann KP, Kulejewski M, Pichlmeier U, Loy V. Diagnosis of contralateral testicular intraepithelial neoplasia (TIN) in patients with testicular germ cell cancer: systematic two-site biopsies are more sensitive than a single random biopsy. Eur Urol. 2007;51(1):175–83; discussion 183–5. doi:https://doi.org/10.1016/j.eururo.2006.05.051. Epub 2006 Jun 13.
14. Kollmannsberger C, Moore C, Chi KN, Murray N, Daneshmand S, Gleave M, et al. Non-risk-adapted surveillance for patients with stage I nonseminomatous testicular germ-cell tumors: diminishing treatment-related morbidity while maintaining efficacy. Ann Oncol. 2010;21(6):1296–301. https://doi.org/10.1093/annonc/mdp473. Epub 2009 Oct 29
15. Tandstad T, Dahl O, Cohn-Cedermark G, Cavallin-Stahl E, Stierner U, Solberg A, et al. Risk-adapted treatment in clinical stage I nonseminomatous germ cell testicular cancer: the SWENOTECA management program. J Clin Oncol. 2009;27(13):2122–8. https://doi.org/10.1200/JCO.2008.18.8953. Epub 2009 Mar 23. Erratum in: J Clin Oncol. 2009;27(19):3263. Erratum in: J Clin Oncol. 2010;28(8):1438. Dosage error in article text
16. Alexandre J, Fizazi K, Mahé C, Culine S, Droz JP, Théodore C, et al. Stage I non-seminomatous germ-cell tumours of the testis: identification of a subgroup of patients with a very low risk of relapse. Eur J Cancer. 2001;37(5):576–82. https://doi.org/10.1016/s0959-8049(00)00442-1.
17. Lago-Hernandez CA, Feldman H, O'Donnell E, Mahal BA, Perez V, Howard S, et al. A refined risk stratification scheme for clinical stage 1 NSGCT based on evaluation of both embryonal predominance and lymphovascular invasion. Ann Oncol. 2015;26(7):1396–401. https://doi.org/10.1093/annonc/mdv180. Epub 2015 Apr 17
18. Motzer RJ, Agarwal N, Beard C, Bhayani S, Bolger GB, Buyyounouski MK, et al. Testicular cancer. J Natl Compr Canc Netw. 2012;10(4):502–35. https://doi.org/10.6004/jnccn.2012.0050.
19. Baird DC, Meyers GJ, Hu JS. Testicular cancer: diagnosis and treatment. Am Fam Physician. 2018;97(4):261–8.
20. Kollmannsberger C, Tandstad T, Bedard PL, Cohn-Cedermark G, Chung PW, Jewett MA, et al. Patterns of relapse in patients with clinical stage I testicular cancer managed with active surveillance. J Clin Oncol. 2015;33(1):51–7. https://doi.org/10.1200/JCO.2014.56.2116. Epub 2014 Aug 18
21. National Comprehensive Cancer Network (NCCN) [Internet]. NCCN clinical practice guidelines in oncology: Testicular cancer (version 2024). NCCN; 2024. Available from: https://wwwnccnorg/. Accessed 2024 Dec 09.
22. Patrikidou A, Cazzaniga W, Berney D, Boormans J, de Angst I, Di Nardo D, et al. European Association of urology guidelines on testicular cancer: 2023 update. Eur Urol. 2023;84(3):289–301. https://doi.org/10.1016/j.eururo.2023.04.010. Epub 2023 May 12
23. Ruf CG, Schmidt S, Kliesch S, Oing C, Pfister D, Busch J, et al. Testicular germ cell tumours' clinical stage I: comparison of surveillance with adjuvant treatment strategies regarding recurrence rates and overall survival-a systematic review. World J Urol. 2022;40(12):2889–900. https://doi.org/10.1007/s00345-022-04145-6. Epub 2022 Sep 15
24. Neuenschwander A, Lonati C, Antonelli L, Papachristofilou A, Cathomas R, Rothermundt C, et al. Treatment outcomes for men with clinical stage II nonseminomatous germ cell tumours

treated with primary retroperitoneal lymph node dissection: a systematic review. Eur Urol Focus. 2023;9(3):541–6. https://doi.org/10.1016/j.euf.2022.11.003. Epub 2022 Nov 12
25. Cary C, Kern SQ, Jacob JM, Calaway AC, Foster RS, Einhorn LH. Management of metastatic pure teratoma in chemotherapy naive patients with testicular primaries. Am J Clin Oncol. 2020;43(10):690–3. https://doi.org/10.1097/COC.0000000000000731.
26. International germ cell consensus classification: a prognostic factor-based staging system for metastatic germ cell cancers. International Germ Cell Cancer Collaborative Group. J Clin Oncol. 1997;15(2):594–603. https://doi.org/10.1200/JCO.1997.15.2.594.
27. Gillessen S, Sauvé N, Collette L, Daugaard G, de Wit R, Albany C, et al; International Germ Cell Cancer Classification Update Consortium. Predicting Outcomes in Men With Metastatic Nonseminomatous Germ Cell Tumors (NSGCT): Results From the IGCCCG Update Consortium. J Clin Oncol. 2021;39(14):1563–1574. https://doi.org/10.1200/JCO.20.03296. Epub 2021 Apr 6. Erratum in: J Clin Oncol. 2022;40(20):2283. 10.1200/JCO.22.01243.
28. Nair LM, Krishna KMJ, Kumar A, Mathews S, Joseph J, James FV. Prognostic factors and outcomes of nonseminomatous germ cell tumours of testis-experience from a tertiary cancer centre in India. Ecancermedicalscience. 2020;14:1145. https://doi.org/10.3332/ecancer.2020.1145.
29. Culine S, Kerbrat P, Kramar A, Théodore C, Chevreau C, Geoffrois L, et al; Genito-Urinary Group of the French Federation of Cancer Center (GETUG T93BP). Refining the optimal chemotherapy regimen for good-risk metastatic nonseminomatous germ-cell tumors: a randomized trial of the Genito-Urinary Group of the French Federation of Cancer Centers (GETUG T93BP). Ann Oncol. 2007;18(5):917–24. https://doi.org/10.1093/annonc/mdm062. Epub 2007 Mar 9.
30. de Wit R, Roberts JT, Wilkinson PM, de Mulder PH, Mead GM, Fosså SD, et al. Equivalence of three or four cycles of bleomycin, etoposide, and cisplatin chemotherapy and of a 3- or 5-day schedule in good-prognosis germ cell cancer: a randomized study of the European Organization for Research and Treatment of Cancer Genitourinary Tract Cancer Cooperative Group and the Medical Research Council. J Clin Oncol. 2001;19(6):1629–40. https://doi.org/10.1200/JCO.2001.19.6.1629.
31. Nichols CR, Catalano PJ, Crawford ED, Vogelzang NJ, Einhorn LH, Loehrer PJ. Randomized comparison of cisplatin and etoposide and either bleomycin or ifosfamide in treatment of advanced disseminated germ cell tumors: an Eastern Cooperative Oncology Group, Southwest Oncology Group, and Cancer and Leukemia Group B Study. J Clin Oncol. 1998;16(4):1287–93. https://doi.org/10.1200/JCO.1998.16.4.1287.
32. Sheinfeld J. The role of adjunctive postchemotherapy surgery for nonseminomatous germ-cell tumors: current concepts and controversies. Semin Urol Oncol. 2002;20(4):262–71. https://doi.org/10.1053/suro.2002.36977.
33. Daugaard G, Skoneczna I, Aass N, De Wit R, De Santis M, Dumez H, et al. A randomized phase III study comparing standard dose BEP with sequential high-dose cisplatin, etoposide, and ifosfamide (VIP) plus stem-cell support in males with poor-prognosis germ-cell cancer. An intergroup study of EORTC, GTCSG, and Grupo Germinal (EORTC 30974). Ann Oncol. 2011;22(5):1054–61. https://doi.org/10.1093/annonc/mdq575. Epub 2010 Nov 8
34. Allen JC, Kirschner A, Scarpato KR, Morgans AK. Current management of refractory germ cell tumors and future directions. Curr Oncol Rep. 2017;19(2):8. https://doi.org/10.1007/s11912-017-0572-y.
35. Einhorn LH, Stender MJ, Williams SD. Phase II trial of gemcitabine in refractory germ cell tumors. J Clin Oncol. 1999;17(2):509–11. https://doi.org/10.1200/JCO.1999.17.2.509.
36. Hamilton RJ, Nayan M, Anson-Cartwright L, Atenafu EG, Bedard PL, Hansen A, et al. Treatment of relapse of clinical stage I nonseminomatous germ cell tumors on surveillance. J Clin Oncol. 2019;37(22):1919–26. https://doi.org/10.1200/JCO.18.01250. Epub 2019 Feb 25
37. Kondagunta GV, Bacik J, Donadio A, Bajorin D, Marion S, Sheinfeld J, et al. Combination of paclitaxel, ifosfamide, and cisplatin is an effective second-line therapy for patients with relapsed testicular germ cell tumors. J Clin Oncol. 2005;23(27):6549–55. https://doi.org/10.1200/JCO.2005.19.638.

38. McCaffrey JA, Mazumdar M, Bajorin DF, Bosl GJ, Vlamis V, Motzer RJ. Ifosfamide- and cisplatin-containing chemotherapy as first-line salvage therapy in germ cell tumors: response and survival. J Clin Oncol. 1997;15(7):2559–63. https://doi.org/10.1200/JCO.1997.15.7.2559.
39. Loehrer PJ Sr, Gonin R, Nichols CR, Weathers T, Einhorn LH. Vinblastine plus ifosfamide plus cisplatin as initial salvage therapy in recurrent germ cell tumor. J Clin Oncol. 1998;16(7):2500–4. https://doi.org/10.1200/JCO.1998.16.7.2500.

Management of Penile Cancer

15

Bharti Devnani, Harjot Kaur Bajwa,
and Dharma Ram Poonia

15.1 Introduction and Risk Factors

Penile cancer is an uncommon tumour that arises from the squamous epithelium of the glans, coronal sulcus, and prepuce or foreskin. The etiology of penile cancer is multifactorial, with several risk factors contributing to its development. A study involving more than 1000 patients from different countries found that 25–33% of penile cancer cases were associated with HPV, with HPV-16 being the most common strain. Early-age circumcision has been shown to prevent the development of penile cancer. Poor hygiene, chronic inflammation, and sexually transmitted diseases are significant risk factors. [1, 2]. Phimosis, a condition where the foreskin cannot be fully retracted over the glans, increases the risk by 25–60%. Other risk factors mentioned in the literature include trauma, tobacco use, and lichen sclerosis.

Globally, the incidence of penile cancer varies significantly across socioeconomic and cultural groups. Developed countries generally report a low incidence, while higher rates are observed in South America, Southeast Asia, and parts of Africa. In India, the annual age-adjusted incidence rate is reported to be between 0.7 and 3 per 100,000 population [3]. The mortality rate of penile cancer remains high in developing countries.

B. Devnani (✉)
Department of Radiation Oncology, All India Institute of Medical Sciences, Jodhpur, India
e-mail: devnanib@aiimsjodhpur.edu.in

H. K. Bajwa
Department of Radiation Oncology, American Oncology Institute, Hyderabad, India

D. R. Poonia
Department of Surgical Oncology, All India Institute of Medical Sciences, Jodhpur, India

R. Madan, S. Goyal (eds.), *Essentials of Radiotherapy in Uro-Genital Malignancies*, https://doi.org/10.1007/978-981-95-5945-9_15

15.2 Diagnostic Evaluation

A thorough history and physical examination are essential before proceeding with the treatment of penile cancer. Patients commonly present with a nonhealing ulcer or proliferative growth on the penis, often accompanied by bleeding and foul-smelling discharge due to secondary infection. Key details to be recorded include the location, size, and gross appearance of the lesion, as well as the extent of deep invasion into corporal bodies, spongiosum, urethra, and the healthy non-involved parts of the penis. These details should ideally be depicted pictorially. Retraction of the prepuce is necessary for assessing the glans and corona glandis. In cases of tight phimosis, circumcision or a dorsal slit might be required to properly examine the lesion. A thorough clinical evaluation of the inguinal area is also crucial, noting any palpable groin nodes, their number, diameter, consistency, laterality, fixity, skin involvement, and presence of fungation. Advanced cases may present with large inguinal nodes, femoral artery invasion, and fungating masses (Fig. 15.1).

For early-stage disease, a physical examination is generally sufficient, except in obese patients, where it should be supplemented by ultrasonography (USG) or cross-sectional imaging. USG is useful for determining the depth of tumor involvement. Multiparametric MRI is increasingly used to guide organ-preserving strategies, with high-resolution T2-weighted images helping to evaluate the extent of the tumor and differentiate hypodense lesions from hyperdense corporal bodies. In advanced primary or clinically node-positive cases, a formal metastatic workup is necessary, including a CT scan of the abdomen and pelvis. PET-CT is promising for identifying pelvic nodes with positive inguinal nodes and evaluating distant metastasis.

A punch or incisional biopsy is required to establish a histological diagnosis. For small prepuce lesions, excision with wider margins is sometimes performed. The patient's HIV status should be ascertained due to the common etiology of sexually transmitted diseases. Palpable groin nodes should be subjected to FNAC. Staging of

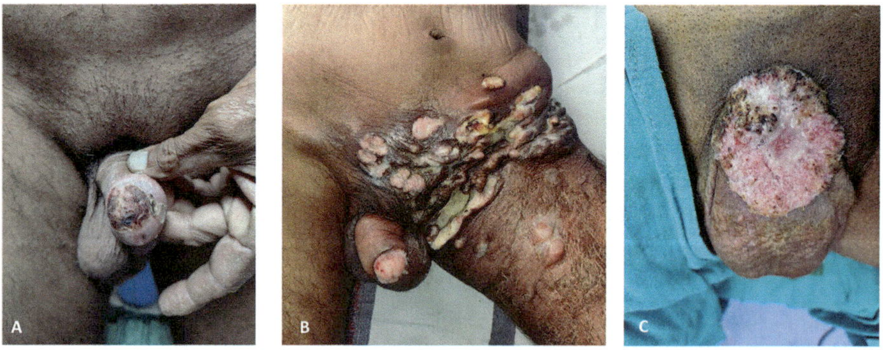

Fig. 15.1 Clinical Presentation of Ca penis; (**a**) An ulcerated lesion involving the Glans Penis; (**b**) Fungating mass involving left groin with ulcerated lesion in penis; (**c**) Penis is completed destroyed with non- healing ulcer

the groin nodes is a critical prognostic factor and must be accurately determined before initiating treatment. Dynamic sentinel lymph node biopsy (DSNB) combined with fine-needle aspiration cytology (FNAC) reduces the false-negative rate to less than 5% and is a standard staging procedure for clinically node-negative patients. Additionally, patients should be evaluated for systemic spread and constitutional symptoms like fatigue and weight loss.

15.3 Pathology

The histopathological examination (HPE) of penile cancer should include a detailed report on histology, grade, lymphovascular invasion, depth of invasion, perineural invasion, and HPV status. The 2016 WHO classification initially categorized tumours based on the presence or absence of human papillomavirus (HPV) [4]. The 2022 WHO classification further refined this by subclassifying tumours into HPV-associated and HPV-independent types [5]. The commonly used 3-tier grading system is proposed by Broder and WHO/ISUP classification, which is based on the level of keratinization, mitosis, and nuclear pleomorphism. The most common histopathological type of penile cancer is squamous cell carcinoma, accounting for 95% of cases. Basaloid variety of squamous cell carcinoma is known for early inguinal metastasis and is associated with poor prognosis. Other rare histopathological types include sarcoma, melanoma, and basal cell carcinoma. Condylomatous and basaloid carcinomas are HPV-associated tumours, while papillary, verrucous, and sarcomatoid carcinomas are HPV-independent tumours. Determining HPV status can be done through HPV DNA testing or P16 immunohistochemistry (IHC), which is crucial for prognostic purposes.

15.4 Staging

The eighth edition of the American Joint Committee on Cancer (AJCC) classifies penile cancers based on the invasion and presence of risk factors like lymphovascular invasion (LVI) or perineural invasion (PNI) [6]. T1 tumours are described as invasion of lamina propria (glans); dermis, lamina propria or dartos fascia (foreskin); or invasion of the connective tissue between epidermis and corpora regardless of the location. All sites with or without LVI or PNI and/or not high grade (i.e., grade 3 or sarcomatoid). T1 is further categorized into T1a (without LVI or PNI and is not high grade) and T1b (LVI or PNI and/or high grade). T2 tumours are defined as invasion into corpus spongiosum (either glans or ventral shaft) with or without urethral invasion, and T3 tumours are defined as invasion into corpora cavernosum (including tunica albuginea) with or without urethral invasion. Tumours invading other adjacent structures (i.e., scrotum, prostate, pubic bone) are classified as T4. The clinical nodal staging defines N0 as no palpable or visibly enlarged inguinal lymph nodes, N1 as palpable mobile unilateral inguinal lymph node, N2 as palpable mobile ≥2 unilateral inguinal nodes or bilateral inguinal lymph nodes, and N3 as palpable fixed inguinal nodal mass or pelvic lymphadenopathy unilateral or bilateral. The pathological nodal staging defines N0 as no lymph node metastasis, N1 as ≤2 unilateral inguinal metastases without ENE, N2 as ≥3 unilateral inguinal metastases or bilateral metastases, and N3 as ENE of lymph node metastases or pelvic lymph node metastases without ENE.

M0 is the absence of distant metastasis, while M1 is the presence of distant metastasis. Based on AJCC recommendations, the SCC of the penis is graded as follows:

Grade 1 is well differentiated; Grade 2 is moderately differentiated; and Grade 3 is poorly differentiated/undifferentiated. The presence of anaplastic cells categorizes the tumour as Grade 3

Based on the TNM classification, the prognostic stage groups are defined as stage I (T1a N0M0), stage IIA (T1b or T2 N0M0), stage IIB (T3 N0 M0), stage IIIA (T1-3 N1M0), stage IIIB (T1-3 N2M0) and stage IV (T4 or N3 or M1).

15.5 Stage-Wise Management of Penile Cancer

15.5.1 Treatment Approach

Penile cancer poses unique challenges beyond oncological outcomes, as the penis is integral to sexual intercourse and urination and symbolizes masculinity for men. The two most common treatment approaches for penile cancer are surgery and radiotherapy. For localized disease, surgical treatment options include circumcision, partial penectomy, or total penectomy with urethrostomy. Disfiguring radical treatments significantly impact sexual function, which in turn affects the quality of life of these patients [7]. The European Association of Urology (EAU) guidelines recommend organ-preserving approaches over radical penectomy [8]. These approaches can include organ-preserving surgery, external beam radiotherapy (EBRT), or brachytherapy. Due to limited data from randomized controlled trials comparing radiotherapy and surgery, management often depends on institutional protocols and expertise. Lymph node involvement is a poor prognostic factor in penile cancer. In patients with regional metastatic disease, overall survival ranges from 10% to 80%, depending on the nodal disease burden and type of treatment [9, 10].

15.5.2 Treatment of Superficial Non-invasive Disease (PeIN Ta)

Penile intraepithelial neoplasia (PeIN) is a rare entity and a known precursor to penile cancer. The incidence of transformation from PeIN to penile cancer ranges from 2.6% to 13% [11]. The most common locations for PeIN are the glans or prepuce. Surgery is the treatment of choice, which may involve circumcision, wide local excision, or partial glans resurfacing [11, 12]. Non-invasive alternatives include topical therapy with imiquimod or 5-fluorouracil (5-FU). These agents have variable response rates, ranging from 40% to 100% [13, 14]. Nd:YAG or CO_2 lasers are also used for tumor ablation, with response rates ranging from 52% to 100% and recurrence rates from 7% to 48% [14, 15]. Surgery has the advantage of providing adequate histopathological data and assessing invasiveness and should be the preferred treatment modality unless contraindicated.

15.5.3 Surgery as a Definitive Treatment for Invasive Penile Cancer

For invasive diseases confined to the glans (clinically T1/T2 disease), there has been a shift from radical approaches to organ-sparing surgery. It is essential to perform a complete excision of the tumor, including the surrounding erythema and an adequate margin of normal skin, to reduce local recurrence [16]. Although the exact margin for penectomy is not well defined in the literature, the EAU guidelines suggest a margin of 3–5 mm. In cases of cT3 disease with corpora cavernosa infiltration, partial amputation is performed. The primary goals of treatment are to maintain upright urination and sexual function without compromising oncological control, which the sine qua non of the treatment. Penile-sparing surgery has been reported to be associated with better erectile and sexual function, as measured by the International Index of Erectile Function-15 (IIEF-15) questionnaire, compared to penectomies. Although organ-preserving surgeries should be offered to highly motivated and compliant patients, recurrence-free survival rates vary, with 77% reported for penile-sparing surgeries and up to 93% for penectomies [10]. In patients where resection would result in an inability to void urine while standing or without wetting the scrotum, radical amputation and diversion via a perineal urethrostomy are recommended. The surgical defect can be covered using flaps in cases of locally advanced or ulcerated disease.

For large proximal shaft tumours, total penectomy with perineal urethrostomy is required. In cases of extensive proximal tumours invading adjacent structures, total emasculation (total penectomy, scrotectomy, and orchiectomy) is recommended (Fig. 15.2). In extreme cases, a hemipelvectomy or even a hemicorporectomy has been described; however, modern treatment guidelines now recommend concurrent chemotherapy and radiotherapy (RT) for unresectable disease.

Lymph node involvement is a poor prognostic factor in penile carcinoma. Penile lymphatic drainage involves the superficial and deep inguinal lymph nodes first, followed by pelvic lymph nodes. The optimal management for patients with clinically node-negative (cN0) disease has evolved from inguinal lymph node dissection to sentinel lymph node mapping or modified superficial lymphadenectomy [17–19] (Fig. 15.3).

In low-risk tumours (pTa, pTis, and pT1a G1), surgical staging can be avoided due to the low risk of metastasis and the significant morbidity associated with the procedure. Intermediate-risk tumours (pT1a G2) are associated with a 6–8%

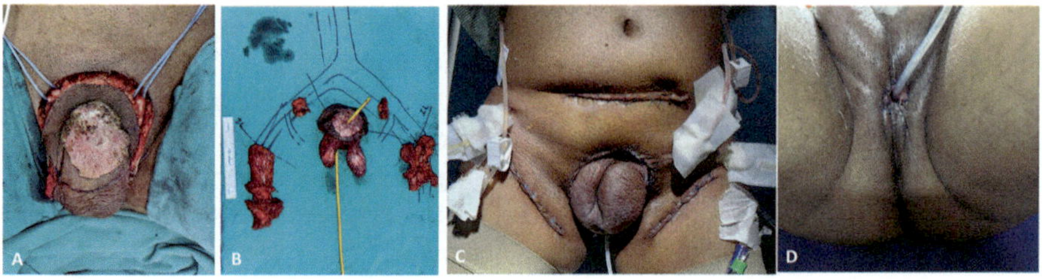

Fig. 15.2 Total Emasculation with Radical Penectomy for Ca Penis: (**a**) Intraoperative picture showing wide surgical margin and cord structure looped; (**b**) Surgical Specimen including enblock resected penile stump with bilateral testes and LNs; (**c**) Surgical bed after closure; (**d**) Perineal Urethrostomy with catheter insitu

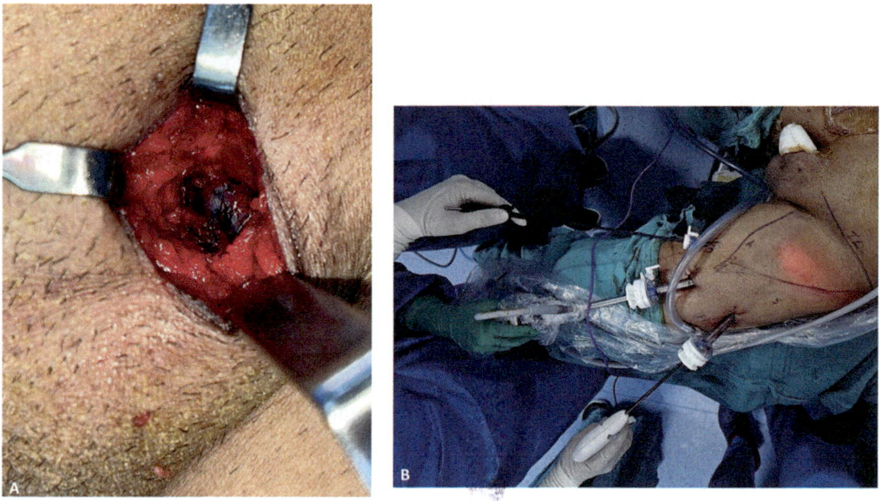

Fig. 15.3 Management of inguinal LNs: (**a**) Left inguinal LN basin-Sentinel LN Biopsy in N0 Setting; (**b**) Intraoperative image showing Video Endoscopic Inguinal Lymph node dissection (VEIL) in N0 setting

probability of micrometastatic disease. Surgical staging can be considered on a case-by-case basis, weighing the benefits against the potential morbidity for the patient. High-risk tumours (pT1b G2) have a 22–30% risk of micrometastasis, and surgical staging is recommended for all high-risk tumours.

For node-positive disease, bilateral radical inguinal lymph node dissection (ILND) is the standard of care. However, radical ILND carries significant morbidity, including wound infections, skin necrosis, lymphedema, lymphocele formation, and seroma [20, 21]. These complications may be reduced by minimally invasive approaches such as videoendoscopic ILND and robot-assisted videoendoscopic ILND, or by using fascial-sparing ILND templates. Literature reviews indicate that these minimally invasive approaches provide similar lymph node yields compared to open ILND, with faster postoperative recovery, fewer wound complications, and similar rates of lymphocele formation and readmission [22–24] (Fig. 15.4).

Prophylactic pelvic lymph node dissection is recommended for intermediate/high-risk patients. For radiologically negative patients, certain predictive factors can help identify those at risk of positive pelvic lymph nodes. The presence of three or more positive inguinal lymph nodes without perinodal spread is associated with positive pelvic lymph nodes in 33–67% of patients [25]. Additionally, the presence of perinodal spread is a significant factor associated with positive pelvic lymph nodes [25–27].

15.5.4 Radiotherapy as a Definitive Treatment for Penile Cancer

The radiotherapy technique used for penile cancer depends on the size and location of the tumor. The NCCN recommendations for organ-preserving definitive radiotherapy in penile cancer patients are as follows [25]:

For clinically T1/2N0 tumours smaller than 4 cm, the recommended approach is circumcision followed by either brachytherapy alone (interstitial implant) or external beam radiotherapy (EBRT) delivering 65–70 Gy with conventional fractionation using an appropriate bolus to the primary penile lesion with 2 cm margins. Prophylactic EBRT can be considered for the inguinal lymph nodes in patients who are inoperable or who decline surgical management.

For clinically T1/2N0 tumours larger than 4 cm, the recommended approach is circumcision followed by either EBRT with concurrent chemotherapy, delivering 45–50.4 Gy to a portion of or the whole penile shaft depending on the bulk and extent of the lesion plus pelvic/inguinal nodes, and then boosting the primary lesion with 2 cm margins to 65–70 Gy, or brachytherapy alone in select cases with careful post-treatment surveillance.

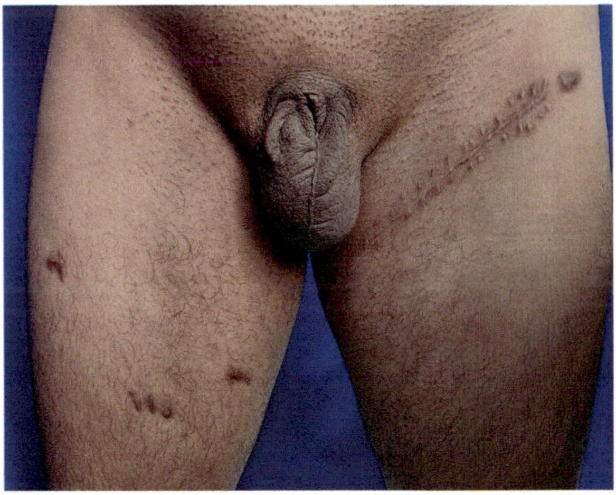

Fig. 15.4 Long-term outcomes: 6 month follow-up after partial penectomy with Left open inguinal lymph node dissection and Right video endoscopic inguinal Lymph node dissection

For clinically T3–4 or N+ (surgically unresectable) tumours, the recommended approach is circumcision followed by EBRT with concurrent chemotherapy, delivering 45–50.4 Gy to the whole penile shaft, pelvic lymph nodes, and bilateral inguinal lymph nodes, followed by a boost to the tumor with 2 cm margins and gross lymph nodes to 60–70 Gy.

15.5.5 EBRT for Definitive Management of Penile Cancers

Data describing outcomes of external beam radiotherapy (EBRT) for the definitive management of penile cancer is limited. Definitive EBRT provides penile preservation rates between 36% and 66% at 5 years and a 5-year local control rate of around 62% (Table 15.1). Radiotherapy results in organ preservation and improved quality of life with satisfactory clinical outcomes, particularly in cases of advanced disease or in patients who are not suitable candidates for surgery [11].

15.5.6 EBRT Technique

Before planning definitive external beam radiotherapy (EBRT) for penile cancer, it is recommended to perform a radical circumcision to reduce the risk of

Table 15.1 EBRT studies reporting outcomes using EBRT as the definitive treatment of penile squamous cell carcinoma

Study & number of patients	RT Dose	Median FUP Months	5 year LC %	5 year CSS %	5 year penile preservation %	Stenosis/ necrosis rate	Tumour characteristic
Sarin et al. (1997) *N* = 59 [12]	60 Gy	62	55	66	50	3% necrosis 14% stenosis	T1 – 86.4% T2 – 8.5% T3 – 1.7% T4 – 3.4%
Gotsadze et al. (2000) *N* = 155 [29]	40–60 Gy	40	65	86	65	1% necrosis 7% stenosis	T1 – 36.8% T2 – 55.5% T3 – 7.7%
Azrif et al. (2006) *N* = 41 [30]	50–52.5 Gy/16#	41	62	96	62	8% necrosis 29% stenosis	T1 – 90.2% T2 – 9.8%
Ozsahin et al. (2006) *N* = 21 [31]	52 Gy	62	49	NR	52	10% stenosis	T1 – 37% T2 – 53% T3 – 8%

FUP follow up, *LC* local control, *CSS* cancer specific survival, *NR* not reported paraphimosis, foreskin contracture, or tissue necrosis. Sperm preservation options should be discussed with the patient when necessary. Very small superficial tumours involving the glans or prepuce and not suitable for brachytherapy can be treated with a direct electron field, with a lead cut-out to shield the scrotum and testis. A 2 cm margin around the gross tumor is added to account for penumbra and microscopic disease, and a bolus must be used to ensure adequate skin coverage. The electron energy chosen should achieve coverage at a depth by the 90% isodose line, with 100% at the skin surface.

To treat the full thickness of the penis in locally advanced disease, the penis should be positioned in a way that is reproducible, provides adequate target coverage and spares the normal tissues. Generally, a tissue-equivalent block with a central cylinder is used to immobilize the penis (Fig. 15.1). Parallel opposed lateral fields are used for treatment with scrotum and testis shielded by lead sheets. Transparent Plexiglass or Lucite chambers are preferred over wax blocks as they allow for better daily treatment verification. Different-sized blocks are used to account for anatomical variation, and some patients may develop penile edema during treatment, requiring replanning with a larger block. The distal aspect of the chamber beyond the penis should be filled with tissue-equivalent material to ensure adequate dose coverage to the tip of the glans. During contouring, the Clinical Target Volume (CTV) should include the full thickness of the penis with at least a 1 cm margin added proximally and distally beyond the tumor, and the Planning Target Volume (PTV) is created by adding a 5 mm to 1 cm margin around the CTV to account for setup variations. Conventional fractionation to a total dose of 60–70 Gy is the regimen used most frequently in clinical practice, with inferior outcomes reported in penile cancer patients treated with a biologically effective dose (BED) value <60 Gy ($\alpha/\beta = 10$) [12]

There is a doubtful role of prophylactic groin EBRT in cN0 patients. The EAU guidelines recommend groin radiation only for palliation [7], whereas the NCCN guidelines suggest considering prophylactic EBRT (45 Gy in 25 fractions) to inguinal lymph nodes in patients who are inoperable or those who refuse surgery. In case of gross disease involving the nodes, if the patient is inoperable, treatment of the primary and concomitant nodal regions along with concurrent chemotherapy should be considered. Typically, the gross nodal disease needs to be boosted to 54–57 Gy for adequate regional control.

15.5.7 Brachytherapy for Definitive Management of Penile Cancers [19]

Though used infrequently due to non-availability or lack of expertise, brachytherapy is a highly effective organ-preserving approach with excellent cosmetic and functional results [10]. Interstitial brachytherapy is associated with penile preservation in 85% of men at 5 years, maintained in 70% by 10 years. Brachytherapy is suitable for clinical stage T1b or T2 tumours with a maximum diameter of less than 4 cm. The ideal location for brachytherapy is lesions over the glans penis. If the target area can be covered with an additional plane of needles, then lesions with minor extension across the coronal sulcus can also be treated with brachytherapy. Larger lesions, especially those extending into the corpora cavernosa, have a higher risk of local failure and complications with brachytherapy compared to surgery or external radiotherapy. Before considering brachytherapy for primary penile cancer, lymph node assessment via sentinel lymph node evaluation or inguinal node dissection is recommended. In the case of positive lymph nodes, a combined approach using brachytherapy for the primary tumour and surgery for the lymph nodes can be considered.

15.5.7.1 Technique

The most common technique of penile brachytherapy is interstitial, which must be performed under general anaesthesia or penile block with sedation. Low-dose-rate (LDR), pulse-dose-rate (PDR) or high-dose-rate (HDR) brachytherapy can deliver the treatment. The implant geometry is decided based on the tumour dimensions and extent. The principles of the Paris system for interstitial implantation are useful for the placement of sources. The treatment plan is generated so that the prescription isodoses encompass the visible and palpable tumour with an appropriate margin. Minimum margins of 10 mm or greater in all directions around the gross tumour are recommended, as the depth of invasion is generally underappreciated on clinical examination.

The interstitial implant is performed using customized templates. Freehand insertion of needles can also be done, provided needle stability is ensured at the time of implantation and during planning and treatment. After insertion of a Foley's catheter, the interstitial needles or catheters are inserted in parallel planes with equal spacing to create a uniform volume implant (Fig. 15.5). The needles are inserted in

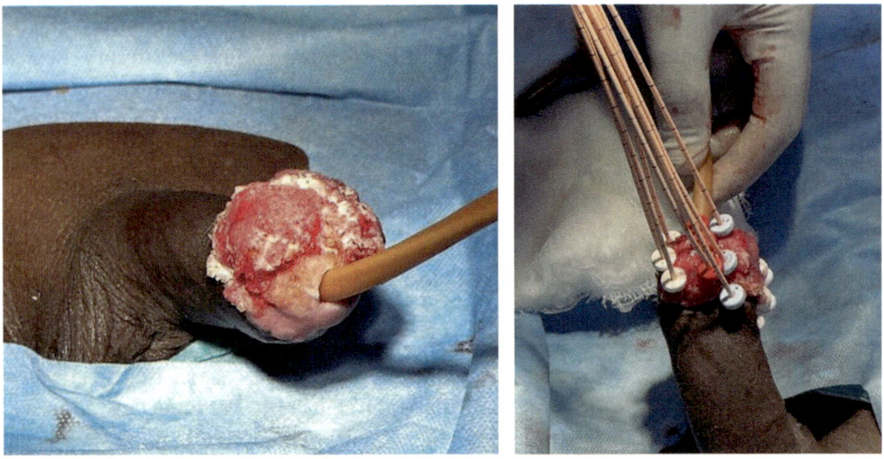

Fig. 15.5 SCC of penis cT2N0, 3.5 cm * 2.5 cm * 1.2 cm disease involving glans of the penis and minimal involvement of the corpora cavernosa, urethra free. Interstitial Brachytherapy for Penile cancer. (Brachytherapy pic courtesy—Dr Ajeet Kumar Gandhi)

a direction orthogonal to the longitudinal direction of the penis. Single-plane implants usually result in underdosing of a part of the tumour due to scalloping of isodoses at greater depths. A two- to three-plane implant ensures adequate coverage of the target in all directions. In the case of the template-based technique, the individual needles are held in a parallel array using pre-drilled Lucite or Plexiglass templates. Stabilizing devices such as Jackson–Pratt drains or fixing buttons can be used when using flexible catheters. During needle or catheter insertion, care is taken to maintain adequate spacing and avoid the urethra. A spacing of 12–18 mm is acceptable for LDR or PDR implants. For HDR brachytherapy, a spacing of 10–12 mm is used between needles or catheters to achieve uniform dosimetry. A wider separation of periurethral needles can be done to minimize the central dose to the urethra.

15.5.7.2 Dose Prescription for Brachytherapy

The patient is scanned in the supine or lateral decubitus position for CT-based planning. A CT slice thickness of less than 2 mm is recommended. Delineation of the gross tumour volume, clinical target volume, skin, and urethra is performed on CT images.

A minimum basal dose of 85% between the needle planes is used for LDR/ PDR prescriptions during brachytherapy planning. The LDR prescribed dose is generally 60 Gy at 0.5–0.6 Gy/h. The entire course of treatment is completed in about 5 days. PDR brachytherapy is based on the delivery of pulses equivalent to the hourly dose rate of an LDR implant. The dose prescription for HDR brachytherapy is generally 38.4 Gy over 6 days, with a fractionation of 3.2 Gy twice daily, 6 h apart. Doses ranging between 42 and 45 Gy over 6 days (3.5 Gy–3.75 Gy × 12) have a risk of penile necrosis. It is important to ensure dose homogeneity and restrict the high-dose regions (V_{125} less than 40% and V_{150} less than 20%). Urethra V_{115} less than or equal to 10% and the V_{90} less than 95% decreases the incidence of urethral strictures. Skin necrosis risk can be reduced by restricting the skin dose to less than 125% of the prescription dose. CT-based planning is mandatory for HDR ^{192}Ir penile brachytherapy.

15.5.7.3 Sequelae and Outcomes of Penile Brachytherapy

The most common early sequela of penile brachytherapy is moist desquamation at the treated area, which usually starts within 10–15 days. It usually takes 2 months for complete healing. Patients with diabetes or vascular disease may have delayed healing extending over 3–4 months or longer. Soft tissue ulceration and urethral meatal stenosis are the most common late sequelae of penile brachytherapy. Cosmesis is excellent, as hypo- or hyperpigmentation or telangiectasia is limited. Though limited, the implant site may develop fibrosis over time. As opposed to other treatment modalities, brachytherapy usually maintains erectile function due to negligible dose to the corpora and the shaft.

The studies reporting outcomes of penile brachytherapy are depicted in Table 15.2. The 5-year local control is around 80–88% with a penile preservation rate of 80%. Delaunay et al. analysed the outcomes of penile brachytherapy and its

Table 15.2 Brachytherapy studies in penile squamous cell carcinoma

Study & number of patients	RT dose	Median FUP Months	5 year LC %	5 year CSS %	5 year penile preservation %	Stenosis/necrosis rate	Tumour characteristics
Crook et al. (2009) *N* = 67 [20]	60 Gy (PDR/LDR)	48	87.3	83.6	88	16% necrosis 12% stenosis	T1 – 56% T2 – 33% T3 – 8%
Cordoba et al. (2016) *N* = 73 [33]	60 Gy (LDR)	51	NR	91.4	87.6	6.8% necrosis 6.6% stenosis	T1 – 75.3% T2 – 15%
Kellas - Sleczka et al. (2019) *N* = 76 [22]	28–54.8 Gy (median EQD2 for superficial HDR) 47.4–55.1 Gy (median EQD2 for interstitial HDR)	76	65	85	69.5	2.6% necrosis 1.3% stenosis	T1 – 37% T2 – 53% T3 – 8%
Martz et al. (2021) *N* = 29 [23]	36 Gy (HDR)	72.4	82	88	79.3	10.3% necrosis, 17% telangiectasia	T1-2N0-2M0

impact on sexual function in patients with penile cancer [32]. The 5-year specific survival was 87.6% (95% CI, 72.4–94.7%) and the 5-year disease-free survival was 84% (95% CI, 57.6–94.7%), respectively. The penile preservation rate was 66%. 58.8% patients remained sexually active after treatment, and 94.4% patients retained erections after brachytherapy.

15.5.7.4 Surface Mould Brachytherapy

Surface mould brachytherapy is a technique that utilizes custom moulds with catheters embedded within the applicator at equal spacing. This technique is suitable for superficial tumours (Tis/1a/1b) and should not be used for tumours invading the corpus spongiosum or beyond a depth of 5 mm. It is essential to limit the dose delivered to the skin to less than 120% when performing this technique.

15.5.8 Role of Adjuvant EBRT in Penile Cancer

15.5.8.1 Adjuvant EBRT Indications for Primary Site

There is limited data regarding the role of post-operative EBRT to the primary site. In patients with positive margins, post-op RT may improve local control. Langsenlehner et al. reported a 5-year local recurrence rate of 28.5% in patients ($n = 14$) who received post-op RT following incomplete surgical resection. The dose delivered was 45–50 Gy with up to 60 Gy boost to the surgical stump [24]. Zouhair et al. reported a local recurrence rate of 25% in patients with positive margins who received post-operative radiotherapy [25].

15.5.8.2 Adjuvant EBRT Indications for Nodal Sites

The role of adjuvant inguinal node radiotherapy in penile cancer is not clear, as data from randomized control trials is lacking. Thus, guidelines for adjuvant radiotherapy in penile cancer are extrapolated from other sites like vulvar squamous cell carcinomas. The NCCN guidelines recommend adjuvant external beam radiotherapy (EBRT) in cases of high-risk features, which include positive surgical margins, more than or equal to 2 pelvic lymph node metastases, extracapsular extension, bilateral inguinal nodal involvement, or more than or equal to 4 cm tumor deposit in the lymph nodes [11, 28]. The pelvic lymph nodes are irradiated in all patients with more than 1 inguinal lymph node metastasis. In the absence of gross disease, 45 Gy in 25 fractions is the recommended dose. Pathological factors such as positive margins, presence of extracapsular extension, or gross residual disease require delivery of higher doses to the nodal regions. The studies evaluating the role of adjuvant RT to the groin/pelvis in penile squamous cell carcinoma are mentioned in Table 15.3.

Table 15.3 Adjuvant EBRT (groin /pelvis) studies in penile carcinoma

Study & number of patients	EBRT indication	RT dose	Median FUP Months	5 year LC %	5 year CSS %	5 year OS %
Langsenlehner et al. 2008 *N* = 24 [24]	Positive surgical margin or N+	45–60 Gy	58.4	100	84.3	56.6
Ager et al. (2021) *N* = 146 [34]	p N3	45 Gy/20 fx; 54 Gy/27 fx; 50–54 Gy/25–27 fx	10.6	56	51	44
Choo et al. (2020) *N* = 23 [35]	pN+ (N3 = 43%)	45 Gy/25 fx (LN not involved); 56Gy/28 fx (involved LN)	15.8	NR (2-year: 27%)	NR (2-year: 49.3%)	NR (2-year: 25%)
Chen et al. (2004) *N* = 45 [36]	pN+	40–70 Gy/20–35 fx	37	NR (3-year: 89% [AIRT group]	NR	54.3

15.5.9 Chemotherapy

15.5.9.1 Role of Neoadjuvant Chemotherapy in Penile Cancer

Over the past few years, there has been increasing interest in the use of neoadjuvant chemotherapy followed by surgery in patients who present with bulky lymph nodes at diagnosis. This treatment strategy is based on data from a phase 2 study in which patients with N2 or N3 disease received neoadjuvant chemotherapy with the TIP regimen (paclitaxel, ifosfamide, and cisplatin) [37]. Patients who had an excellent response to NACT had improved time to tumour progression and survival. The NCCN and EAU guidelines also recommend NACT as the first line of treatment for this group of patients.

15.5.9.2 Role of Adjuvant Chemotherapy in Penile Cancer

Currently, the role of adjuvant chemotherapy in penile cancer is unclear due to a lack of high-level evidence. Data from retrospective studies suggests that adjuvant chemotherapy may be beneficial in patients with pN2/N3 disease or those with extracapsular extension [38].

15.5.9.3 Role of Chemotherapy/Immunotherapy for Recurrent or Metastatic Penile Cancer

Due to limited response rates, the benefit of chemotherapy in this setting is marginal. As far as immunotherapy is concerned, there is a need for high-level evidence to define its utility in this group of patients.

References

1. Douglawi A, Masterson TA. Penile cancer epidemiology and risk factors: a contemporary review. Curr Opin Urol. 2019;29:145–9.
2. Vieira CB, Feitoza L, Pinho J, Teixeira-Júnior A, Lages J, Calixto J, et al. Profile of patients with penile cancer in the region with the highest worldwide incidence. Sci Rep. 2020;10:2965.
3. Fu L, Tian T, Yao K, et al. Global pattern and trends in penile cancer incidence: population-based study. JMIR Public Health Surveill. 2022;8:e34874.
4. Moch H, Cubilla AL, Humphrey PA, Reuter VE, Ulbright TM. The 2016 WHO classification of tumours of the urinary system and male genital organs-part A: renal, penile, and testicular tumours. Eur Urol. 2016;70(1):93–105.
5. Moch H, Amin MB, Berney DM, Compérat EM, Gill AJ, Hartmann A, et al. The 2022 World Health Organization classification of tumours of the urinary system and male genital organs-part A: renal, penile, and testicular tumours. Eur Urol. 2022;82(5):458–68.
6. Amin MB, Edge SB, Greene FL, et al., editors. AJCC cancer staging manual. 8th ed. Springer; 2017.
7. Maddineni SB, Lau MM, Sangar VK. Identifying the needs of penile cancer sufferers: a systematic review of the quality of life, psychosexual and psychosocial literature in penile cancer. BMC Urol. 2009;9:8.
8. Brouwer OR, Albersen M, Parnham A, Protzel C, Pettaway CA, Ayres B, et al. European Association of Urology-American Society of Clinical Oncology collaborative guideline on penile cancer. Eur Urol. 2023;83(6):548–60.
9. Pagliaro LC, Crook J. Multimodality therapy in penile cancer: when and which treatments? World J Urol. 2009;27:221–5.
10. Sakalis VI, Campi R, Barreto L, Perdomo HG, Greco I, Zapala Ł, et al. What is the most effective management of the primary tumor in men with invasive penile cancer: a systematic review of the available treatment options and their outcomes. Eur Urol Open Sci. 2022;40:58–94.
11. Crook J. Contemporary role of radiotherapy in the management of primary penile tumors and metastatic disease. Urol Clin North Am. 2016;43:435–48.
12. Sarin R, Norman AR, Steel GG, Horwich A. Treatment results and prognostic factors in 101 men treated for squamous carcinoma of the penis. Int J Radiat Oncol Biol Phys. 1997;38(4):713–22.
13. Gotsadze D, Matveev B, Zak B, Mamaladze V. Is conservative organ-sparing treatment of penile carcinoma justified? Eur Urol. 2000;38:306e12.
14. Azrif M, Logue JP, Swindell R, Cowan RA, Wylie JP, Livsey JE. External-beam radiotherapy in T1-2 N0 penile carcinoma. Clin Oncol. 2006;18:320e5.
15. Ozsahin M, Jichlinski P, Weber DC, Azria D, Zimmermann M, Guillou L, et al. Treatment of penile carcinoma: to cut or not to cut? Int J Radiat Oncol Biol Phys. 2006;66(3):674–9.
16. Parra RO. Accurate staging of carcinoma of the penis in men with nonpalpable inguinal lymph nodes by modified inguinal lymphadenectomy. J Urol. 1996;155(2):560–3.
17. Horenblas S, Jansen L, Meinhardt W, Hoefnagel CA, de Jong D, Nieweg OE. Detection of occult metastasis in squamous cell carcinoma of the penis using a dynamic sentinel node procedure. J Urol. 2000;163(1):100–4.
18. Coblentz TR, Theodorescu D. Morbidity of modified prophylactic inguinal lymphadenectomy for squamous cell carcinoma of the penis. J Urol. 2002;168(4 Pt 1):1386–9.
19. Crook JM, Haie-Meder C, Demanes DJ, Mazeron JJ, Martinez AA, Rivard MJ. American Brachytherapy Society–Groupe Europëen de Curiethërapie–European Society of Therapeutic Radiation Oncology (ABS-GEC-ESTRO) consensus statement for penile brachytherapy. Brachytherapy. 2013;12(3):191–8.
20. Crook J, Ma C, Grimard L. Radiation therapy in the management of the primary penile tumor: an update. World J Urol. 2009;27(2):189–96.

21. Cordoba A, Escande A, Lopez S, Mortier L, Mirabel X, Coche-Déqueant B, et al. Low-dose brachytherapy for early stage penile cancer: a 20-year single-institution study (73 patients). Radiat Oncol. 2016;11:96.
22. Kellas-Sleczka S, Bialas B, Fijalkowski M, Chicheł A, Kabacińska R, Pietraszek A, et al. Nineteen-year single-center experience in 76 patients with penile cancer treated with high-dose-rate brachytherapy. Brachytherapy. 2019;18(4):493–502.
23. Martz N, Bodokh Y, Gautier M, Granier A, Elleuch R, Chirpaz E, et al. High-dose rate brachytherapy in localized penile cancer: 5-year clinical outcome analysis. Clin Transl Radiat Oncol. 2021;27:89–95.
24. Langsenlehner T, Mayer R, Quehenberger F, Ponholzer A, Berghold A, Schmid AP, et al. The role of radiation therapy after incomplete resection of penile cancer. Strahlenther Onkol. 2008;184:359–63.
25. Zouhair A, Coucke PA, Jeanneret W, Nicoucar K, Ozsahin M, Mirimanoff RO, et al. Radiation therapy alone or combined surgery and radiation therapy in squamous-cell carcinoma of the penis? Eur J Cancer. 2001;37:198–203.
26. Djajadiningrat RS, van Werkhoven E, Horenblas S. Prophylactic pelvic lymph node dissection in patients with penile cancer. J Urol. 2015;193:1976–80.
27. Lughezzani G, Catanzaro M, Torelli T, Biasoni D, Stagni S, Buffi NM, et al. The relationship between characteristics of inguinal lymph nodes and pelvic lymph node involvement in penile squamous cell carcinoma: a single institution experience. J Urol. 2014;191:977–82.
28. National Comprehensive Cancer Network (NCCN). Penile Cancer. NCCN Clinical Practice Guidelines in Oncology (NCCN Guidelines), Version 1.2023. Available from: https://www.nccn.org/professionals/physician_gls/pdf/penile.pdf.
29. Gotsadze D, Matveev B, Zak B, Mamaladze V. Is conservative organ-sparing treatment of penile carcinoma justified? Eur Urol. 2000;38:306–12.
30. Azrif M, Logue JP, Swindell R, Cowan RA, Wylie JP, Livsey JE. External-beam radiotherapy in T1-2 N0 penile carcinoma. Clin Oncol. 2006;18:320–5.
31. Ozsahin M, Jichlinski P, Weber DC, Rouzaud M, Rijken H, Philip T, et al. Treatment of penile carcinoma: to cut or not to cut? Int J Radiat Oncol Biol Phys. 2006;66:674–9.
32. Delaunay B, Soh PN, Delannes M, Allory Y, Bachaud JM, Gabriele P, et al. Brachytherapy for penile cancer: efficacy and impact on sexual function. Brachytherapy. 2014;13(4):380–7.
33. Cordoba A, Escande A, Lopez S, Pouessel D, Hennequin C, Le Fur E, et al. Low-dose brachytherapy for early stage penile cancer: a 20-year single-institution study (73 patients). Radiat Oncol. 2016;11:96.
34. Ager M, Njoku K, Serra M, Robinson A, Pickering L, Afshar M, et al. Long-term multicentre experience of adjuvant radiotherapy for pN3 squamous cell carcinoma of the penis. BJU Int. 2021;128:451–9.
35. Choo R, Nehra A, Zattoni F, Pagliaro LC, Karnes RJ. Is there any benefit in adding postoperative adjuvant concurrent radiotherapy and chemotherapy for penile cancer with regional lymph node metastasis? Minerva Urol Nefrol. 2020;72:474–81.
36. Chen MF, Chen WC, Wu CT, Chuang CK, Ng KF, Chang JT. Contemporary management of penile cancer including surgery and adjuvant radiotherapy: an experience in Taiwan. World J Urol. 2004;22:60–6.
37. Dickstein RJ, Munsell MF, Pagliaro LC, Pettaway CA. Prognostic factors influencing survival from regionally advanced squamous cell carcinoma of the penis after preoperative chemotherapy. BJU Int. 2016;117(1):118–25.
38. Sharma P, Djajadiningrat R, Zargar-Shoshtari K, Catanzaro M, Zhu Y, Nicolai N, et al. Adjuvant chemotherapy is associated with improved overall survival in pelvic node-positive penile cancer after lymph node dissection: a multi-institutional study. Urol Oncol. 2015;33(11):496.e17–23.

Brachytherapy in Urogenital Malignancies

16

Kunhi Parambath Haresh, Suyash Pandey, and Anjali V. Ramdulari

16.1 Introduction

Brachytherapy, a specialized kind of radiation therapy, involves introducing radioactive sources directly into or around the tumor, allowing high doses of radiation to target the malignancy while minimizing exposure to adjacent healthy tissues. Brachytherapy, developed and refined over decades, has proven beneficial in treating cancers of various sites like genitourinary, gynecological, head and neck, and breast. The capacity to administer localized high doses of radiation enables brachytherapy to have higher treatment efficacy with fewer side effects than external beam radiation [1]. As a result, brachytherapy has evolved as a critical component in the multimodal approach to treating malignancies, tailored to individual patient needs and tumor characteristics. In this chapter, we will briefly review the role of brachytherapy in urogenital malignancies, its application, and the procedures employed.

16.2 Brachytherapy Can Be Classified Based on Dose Rate and Delivery Method (Table 16.1)

16.2.1 Benefits of Brachytherapy

The advantages of brachytherapy over external beam radiation therapy (EBRT) are [2]:

K. P. Haresh (✉) · S. Pandey · A. V. Ramdulari
Department of Radiation Oncology, All India Institute of Medical Sciences, New Delhi, India

R. Madan, S. Goyal (eds.), *Essentials of Radiotherapy in Uro-Genital Malignancies*, https://doi.org/10.1007/978-981-95-5945-9_16

Table 16.1 Classification of brachytherapy

Based on dose rate	Based on the delivery method
Low-dose rate (LDR) Medium-dose rate (MDR) High-dose rate (HDR)	Intracavitary Interstitial Intraluminal Surface brachytherapy

- Higher Radiation Dosage: Compared to EBRT, brachytherapy can deliver a higher radiation dosage to the tumor while exposing less healthy tissues. This can increase therapy efficacy. The capacity to give a larger radiation dose using brachytherapy has the potential to enhance tumor control rates, particularly for radiation-sensitive malignancies.
- Targeted Treatment: Brachytherapy allows for the precise positioning of radiation sources inside or next to the tumor, providing radiation exactly where it is needed. This focused strategy helps to protect healthy tissues and organs from unwanted radiation exposure.
- Brachytherapy often requires fewer treatment sessions and has a shorter overall treatment duration than EBRT, which often entails daily treatments over several weeks. This can be more convenient for patients, potentially leading to a faster recovery.
- Conformal Dose Distribution: Brachytherapy is the most conformal form of radiation, tailoring the radiation dose to the tumor's size and shape. As there is no or very little risk of movement (the tumor moves with the needles) there is no need for PTV margins.
- Reduced Side Effects: Because brachytherapy is targeted and can spare healthy tissues, patients may experience fewer side effects than EBRT, which passes through healthy tissues to the tumor.

16.3 Brachytherapy for Prostate Cancer

It is a well-known fact that higher the radiation dose, better the disease control in prostate cancer [3]. Prostate adenocarcinoma has a low a/b ratio and is highly sensitive to high doses per fraction. Brachytherapy is the most effective way to deliver hypo-fractionated dose escalation within standard tissue tolerance for OARs. Depending upon the risk group of prostate cancer that the patient belongs to, brachytherapy can be used either as the sole modality of radiation (monotherapy) or as a boost along with external beam radiation as given in Table 16.2. In either scenario, brachytherapy can be performed using permanent LDR seed implants or HDR afterloading.

Clinical evidence suggests that LDR and HDR brachytherapy have equivalent outcomes for localized prostate cancer using current dose regimens. However, the increased dose escalation possible with HDR brachytherapy regimens could increase biologically effective irradiation doses, resulting in better results. Based on large number of published studies, HDRBT is now considered to be an effective

Table 16.2 Settings for use of brachytherapy in Ca prostate [4]

Monotherapy	Boost: combination with EBRT
Low-risk disease (Gleason score 6, and PSA <10 ng/ml, and clinical tumor classification T1, T2a), or Favorable intermediate-risk disease (Gleason score 7, or PSA 10–20 ng/ml or clinical tumor classification of T2b, T2c) with primary Gleason score 3 + 4, <50% positive biopsy cores, and only a single intermediate-risk feature	HDRBT can be given both before and after EBRT as a brachytherapy boost in unfavorable intermediate-risk and high-risk Ca prostate

Table 16.3 Recommendations for HDR-BT in Ca prostate [6]

Suitable patients	Unsuitable patients
Stages T1b–T3b	TURP within 3–6 months
Any Gleason score	Maximum urinary flow rate (Qmax) <10 ml/s
Any PSA level	IPSS >20
	Rectal fistula
	Pubic arch interference
	Lithotomy position or anesthesia not possible

means of increasing the dose of radiation in the radical treatment of prostate cancer [5].

The following are the general criteria for patient selection for HDR BT. Any organ-confined prostate cancer can be taken up for brachytherapy irrespective of PSA and Gleason if they do not have any of the unsuitable criteria listed in Table 16.3.

16.3.1 Equipment Requirement

Equipment required for performing BT in Ca prostate is similar to any transperineal transrectal ultrasound-guided procedure and includes the following:

- An operating room suitable for sterile procedures and access to anesthetic support. Alternatively, a brachytherapy suite with adequate shielding to perform the HDR treatment is more advantageous.
- Trans-rectal ultrasound system (TRUS) as shown in Fig. 16.1. Stepper system either floor-mounted or couch-mounted one on which the TRUS probe can be mounted is an additional welcome resource if available.
- Interstitial implant catheters of a suitable design compatible with the TRUS-based template. The American Brachytherapy Society (ABS) recommends using template-based BT for patients as it improves overall accuracy and simplifies

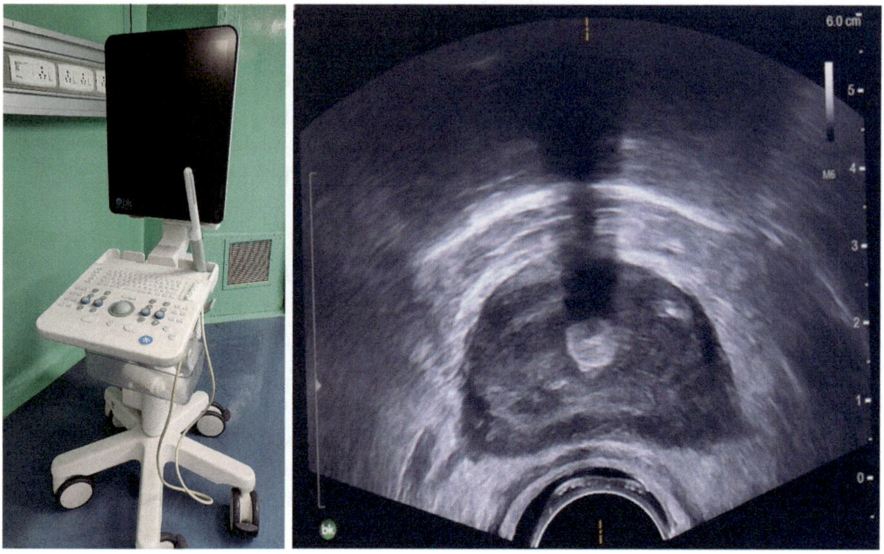

Fig. 16.1 TRUS-equipped USG for guided needle insertion

procedures. Various templates with different specifications are used routinely around the world. Some common examples are the contour prostate template, CT/MR contour prostate template, and the Martinez template set.
- Access to appropriate imaging post-implant with either TRUS, CT, or MR.
- A treatment planning system that can accurately reconstruct the implantation and is capable of three-dimensional dosimetry, along with software that enables post implant.
- Ensure the availability of appropriately sized three-way Foley catheter before the procedure.
- HDR afterloader.

16.3.2 Procedure

16.3.2.1 Pre-brachytherapy Assessment and Clearance

The following are required before the procedure taking steps to reduce procedure-associated complications.

- Pre-anesthetic clearance (spinal/epidural).
- Stop blood thinners well before the procedure (usually 1 week).
- Bowel preparation with PEGLEC, the day before the procedure.
- Part preparation.
- Ensure all required equipment are available and functional.

- Antibiotics may be started just before the procedure.
- The authors regularly do a prior TRUS evaluation and we recommend it to be performed if logistics permit.

16.3.2.2 Brachytherapy Procedure

- The anesthesia is given either in a spinal or epidural form.
- The patient is placed in a high lithotomy position (Fig. 16.2). Parts are cleaned and draped to create a sterile surgical field.
- A three-way Foley catheter is inserted, clamped, and pushed high up in the bladder to minimize the chances of balloon rupture by the needle tip during the procedure. The scrotum is also strapped high and away.
- The TRUS unit is assembled, and a preliminary scan is performed before needle insertion.
- Needles are inserted under TRUS guidance. The needle placement aims to achieve a good dose distribution (Fig. 16.3). The following general principles are adhered to get a good implant:

  1. Anterior needles are inserted first to avoid the artifact effect in USG acquisition.
  2. Implantation is done by targeting the reference plane, that is, the plane with maximum size of the prostate.
  3. 14–18 needles are inserted at least 7–10 mm to target good coverage in the reference plane.
  4. Peripheral loading: two-thirds of the needles are placed in the periphery of the gland.
  5. To reduce urethral toxicity, the needles should be at least 5 mm away from the urethra.
  6. The posterior needles should be 5 mm inside the capsule to optimize rectal dose.
  7. The tip of the needles needs to be well inside the bladder to get an adequate dose to the base of the prostate.

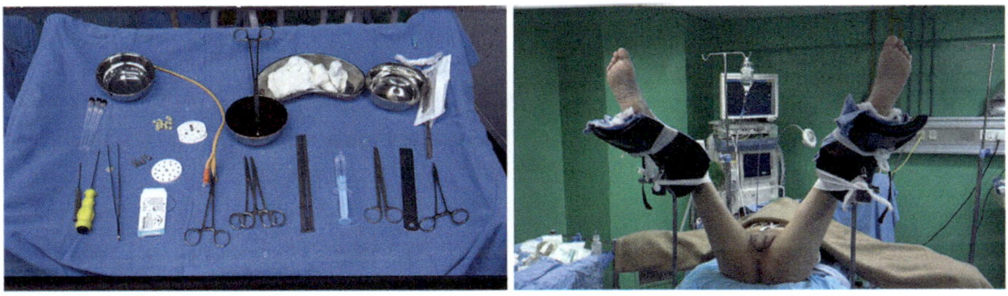

Fig. 16.2 (**a**) Requirements for prostate brachytherapy; (**b**) high lithotomy for prostate brachytherapy

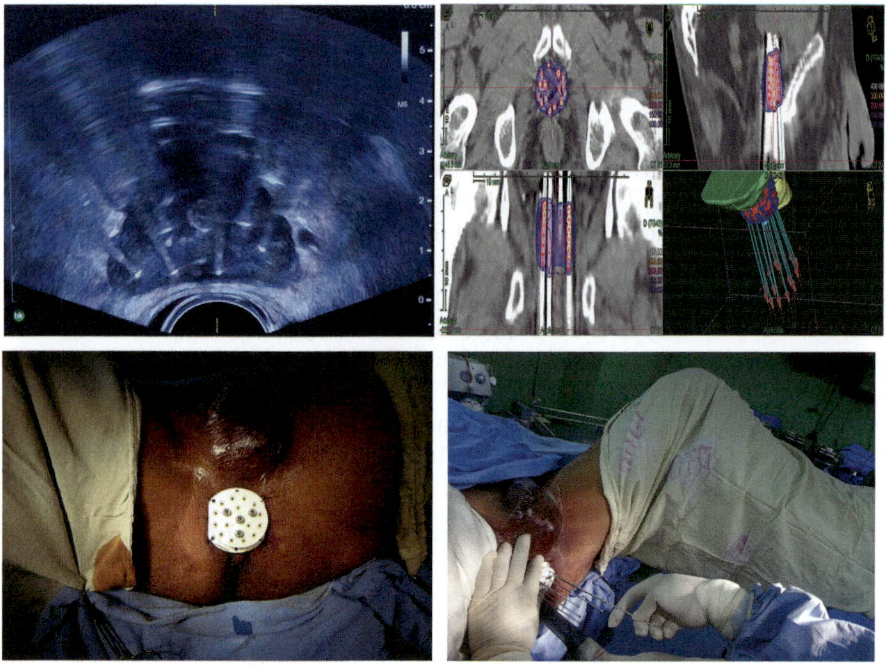

Fig. 16.3 Images depicting template fixation and needle insertion under USG guidance and CT-based planning

16.3.2.3 Post Brachytherapy

- This includes acquiring post-implantation images, which can be CT/MRI or TRUS, and transferring them to the treatment planning system. A diagnostic image sequence can be used to delineate target volumes.
- The needles are reconstructed on the TPS, and target volumes and OARs are contoured.
- Plan development as in next section.
- After plan evaluation and QA, the fraction is delivered, and the patient is shifted back to the recovery room where the implantation is removed.
- The suture fixation of the template is removed, and then the needles are removed one by one as swiftly as possible. Foley is unclamped and pulled down, and bladder irrigation is started using the three-way Foley catheter.
- Firm perineal pressure with fist is applied for 5 min with a sterile dressing pad to ensure hemostasis and avoid hematoma formation.
- The patient is observed overnight with required medicational support, and the bladder irrigation continues until hematuria subsides. Patient is discharged once the patient passes urine freely after the Foley is removed.

16.3.3 Brachytherapy Planning

16.3.3.1 Target Volumes

CTV includes the entire prostate and extraprostatic extensions identified on the diagnostic imaging and expanding it by 3 mm to include the subclinical disease if present. The expansion is reduced anteriorly and posteriorly to reduce the dose of OARs [7].

16.3.3.2 Organ at Risks

Rectum: Contouring the outer wall alone is considered adequate as per recommendations. Generally, we contour an additional 1 cm above and below the level of PTV.

Urethra: It is delineated with the help of the urethral catheter and is visible on the imaging. The contour must extend from the bladder base to 5 mm below the prostatic apex.

Bladder: the outer wall of the bladder is contoured. We usually draw it for 1 cm above the level of PTV.

Other OARs, such as the penile bulb, neurovascular bundle, and bladder neck, can also be contoured for dosimetric evaluation.

The authors prefer to use 11.5 Gy per fraction by three different implants performed every 21 days for HDR monotherapy.

The recommended doses are given in Tables 16.4 and 16.5. The authors prefer to use two implants of 9.5–10.5 Gy per fraction performed every 21 days for HDR boost.

16.3.3.3 Plan Evaluation Criteria

The following parameters are usually used for plan evaluation (Table 16.6).

The authors are regularly using and are comfortable with the following constraints: PTV—D90 > 100%, V100 > 90% V150 < 35%; Bladder—D10 < 75%, D0.1 cc <80%; Rectum D10 < 75%, D0.1 cc < 80%; Urethra—D10 < 115%, D0.1 cc < 120% (adhering to the contouring already described above).

ICRU recommendation for reporting HDR-BT in Ca prostate is given in Table 16.7.

16.3.3.4 State-of-the-Art Real-Time USG-Guided Systems

Highly efficient solutions for brachytherapy of the prostate are available commercially like Oncentra Prostate™ (previously called SWIFT) and Vitesse™ [9]. This

Table 16.4 GEC/ESTRO recommendations for dose recommendation for HDR monotherapy in Ca prostate [6]

HDR monotherapy dose recommendations:
34.5 Gy in 3 fractions (11.5 Gy/#)
27.0 Gy in 2 fractions (13.5 Gy/#)
19.0 Gy in 1 fraction
Two- and three-fraction regimens are recommended over a single-fraction regimen [8].
21 days gap between each fraction.

Table 16.5 GEC/ESTRO recommendations for dose recommendation for combined EBRT and HDR boost in Ca prostate [3]

Various EBRT dose recommendations in cases of brachytherapy boost:
45 Gy in 25 fractions over five weeks
46 Gy in 23 fractions over four and a half weeks
35.7 Gy in 13 fractions over two and a half week
37.5 Gy in 15 fractions over three weeks
HDR boost recommendations:
15 Gy in 3 fractions
11–22 Gy in 2 fractions
12–15 Gy in 1 fraction

Table 16.6 GEC/ESTRO recommendation for plan evaluation [7]

Target constraints	OARs constraint
Coverage of CTV is evaluated	Rectum: D2 cc ⩽ 75 Gy EQD2
D90 = >100% D100 = >95%	Urethra: D0.1 cc = ⩽120 Gy EQD2 D10 ⩽ 120 Gy EQD2 D30 ⩽ 105 Gy EQD2

system is an all-in-one solution for brachytherapy of prostate cancer [10]. The stepper (either floor mounted or couch mounted) with the TRUS probe inserted in the rectum is positioned. Three-way Foley of adequate size is inserted. The brachytherapy template is attached to the stepper assembly. Prostate is anchored to the template by placing two prostate anchors through the template holes. First, an initial three-dimensional ultrasound image of the prostate is obtained in the treatment position. CTV and OARs are contoured and virtual needle placement is done in the TPS and the preplan is made. Once the acceptable plan is ready, the actual implant procedure is started. The needles are inserted in the pre-decided holes of the template as per the preplan. The 3D ultrasound of the prostate is again obtained with the needles in place. Once the needles are reconstructed, a plan is made once again. The needles are connected to the HDR machine in the same room. All the personnel move to the console area and anesthetics monitor the patient with slave monitoring with audio video set up from the console area. Once the radiation delivery is complete, the personnel goes inside the room and the needles are removed in the same position and hemostasis is achieved. This is ultrasound-guided insertion and ultrasound- based planning. The advantage of this technique is that it is least traumatic and very accurate. There is no issue of needle displacement.

16.3.3.5 LDR Brachytherapy

This is performed by the insertion of radioactive seeds into the prostate under ultrasound guidance. Even though this is routinely performed in the West, in the treatment of prostate cancers, it is very little used in our country. This is mainly due to the unavailability of the seeds, lack of infrastructure for the application, and lack of expertise. Table 16.8 details the particulars of the seeds that are commonly used for the procedure.

Table 16.7 ICRU recommendation for reporting HDR-BT in Ca prostate [7]

External beam dose
Implant technique; number of catheters
Total reference air kerma (TRAK); total source exposure
Pattern of dwell times for each applicator
CTV: D90, V100, V150, V200
PTV (if defined): D90, V100, V150, V200
Organs at risk: Rectum: D2 cc, D0.1 cc Urethra: D0.1 cc, D10, D30

Table 16.8 Commonly used LDR seeds in brachytherapy of prostate cancer

LDR seed	Half-life (days)	Dose for monotherapy (Gy)	Dose for boost (Gy)
Iodine 125	59.4	145	110–115
Palladium 103	17	125	90–100
Cesium 131	9.7	115	85

16.3.4 Expected Toxicities

The most common toxicities recorded after brachytherapy are genitourinary and gastrointestinal symptoms [11]. These toxicities are comparatively more when a combined treatment [12] regimen is used. The toxicity profile is highly reduced compared to EBRT.

16.3.4.1 Acute Complications

Acute urinary symptoms following brachytherapy include increased frequency, urgency, and discomfort while urination. Some patients having brachytherapy for prostate cancer may develop acute gastrointestinal symptoms like diarrhea, bloating, or abdominal discomfort. Some individuals may have acute rectal irritation, such as rectal urgency, bleeding, or pain.

16.3.4.2 Late Complications

Erectile dysfunction is a late consequence of brachytherapy in prostate cancer treatment. Late urinary incontinence, or the inability to control urine flow, can emerge as a consequence of brachytherapy. This is more likely in patients who have received higher radiation doses or in conjunction with other treatments. Gastrointestinal problems, such as persistent diarrhea, rectal bleeding, or rectal discomfort, might develop months or years following brachytherapy treatment. Brachytherapy may cause some patients to suffer late bladder issues, such as increased frequency, urgency, or discomfort during urinating. Late urethral stricture is still another complication.

16.3.5 Outcomes of the Treatment

Brachytherapy in the treatment of prostate cancer has shown promising results, either used as monotherapy or in combination with EBRT. When used as monotherapy, it demonstrated excellent results. A major study demonstrated that the 5-year findings showed 96% overall survival, 100% cause-specific survival, 100% local control, 0% distant metastases, and 94% biochemical control (Phoenix definition nadir +2) [12]. The chronic GU toxicity rates were minimal (grades 1–3), with no grade 4 toxicity, with local control rates of 70–87% at 5 years and 70% at 10 years, and cancer-specific survival rates of 72–92% at 10 years.

In combination with EBRT, HDR-BT boost has been shown to improve survival, decrease the risk of distant metastases, and decrease the need for long-term ADT [13]. Multiple randomized controlled trials have shown better results by adding brachytherapy to EBRT [14–16].

16.4 Brachytherapy in Penile Cancer

The incidence of penile cancer varies significantly across different regions and populations. It is relatively rare in the United States and Europe, with an incidence of about 1 per 100,000 men per year. However, it is more common in parts of Asia, Africa, and South America, where it might be as high as 1–2 per 100,000 men per year.

Radical surgery (total or subtotal penectomy) is the most common treatment approach in penile cancer, with reasonable local control rates and survival outcomes. However, the negative impact of surgical resection on sexual function can have a major detrimental psychological impact, leading to a significant deterioration in patients' quality of life. Brachytherapy's role in treating penile cancer is to provide a therapeutic option that preserves the cosmetic and functional integrity of the penis while efficiently targeting the tumor [17].

16.4.1 Indications

BT is used primarily in T1 and T2 penile squamous cell carcinoma (and selected T3 lesions), ideally smaller than 4 cm with no or minimal extension onto the penile shaft [18].

16.4.2 Procedure

- The patient undergoes all required investigations to determine the disease's local extent and rule out distant metastases.
- The procedure is done under either general or spinal anesthesia.

- GTV is determined by clinical examination and using available imaging modalities, and 3–5 mm of margin is added to determine the CTV.
- The implant can be placed either by using a template or by freehand. The authors prefer freehand implants. When a template is required, the interstitial brachytherapy breast template is used to stabilize the penis during the procedure. The template comprises two square plates of plastic covered by a series of 1 cm holes. The bridge keeps the two templates in parallel at all times. A foam collar is placed around the penis to ensure the stable positioning of the organ during treatment.
- A Foley catheter is used to assist the urinary tract during the procedure.
- Hollow steel needles are placed to ensure that CTV coverage is guaranteed according to the Paris system rules.
- Needles are placed at least 10 mm apart in two to three different planes depending upon the extent of the disease.
- In the freehand technique, we first use the metallic trocar and needle and thread the flexible plastic brachytherapy catheters through the trocar and secure them with plastic buttons (Fig. 16.4).

16.4.3 Dose Prescription and Evaluation

The recommended doses are given in Table 16.9. The target and OAR constraints are given in Table 16.10.

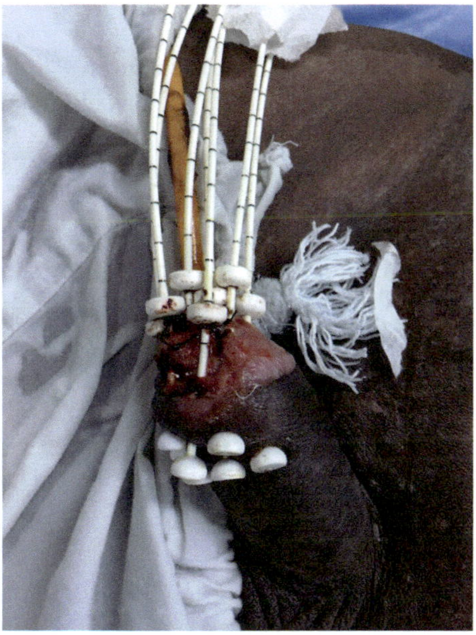

Fig. 16.4 Penile freehand brachytherapy

Table 16.9 ABS-GEC-ESTRO recommendation for dose prescription (HDR-BT) [19]

Dose	Fractionation
18 Gy (POST OP)	3 Gy × 6# over 3 days (delivered BD)
38.4 Gy	3.2 Gy × 12# over 6 days (delivered BD)
42 Gy	3.5 Gy × 12# over 6 days (delivered BD)
45 Gy	3.75 Gy × 12# over 6 days (delivered BD)

Table 16.10 ABS-GEC-ESTRO recommendation for target and OARs constraints [19]

Target constraints	OARs constraint
CTV	Urethra
V100% > =95%	V90 < 95%
V125% < 40%	V115 < 10%
V150% < 20%	Skin
V200% diameter > 10 mm (to be avoided)	V125 < 1%

The authors use 3 Gy per fraction twice a day for 14–17 fractions taking the total dose to 42–51 Gy by HDR.

16.4.4 Expected Toxicities

The most common toxicities recorded after BT in penile cancer are urethral stenosis and skin necrosis [20].

16.4.4.1 Acute Complications

Most of the acute complications observed are acute radiation dermatitis in 90% of the patients treated with brachytherapy. It is usually self-resolving with supportive management and resolves by 8 weeks post-treatment.

16.4.4.2 Late Complications

According to various literature reviews, urethral stenosis is observed in 8–45% of patients. It can be prevented by optimizing the dose received by the urethra. It is managed by dilatation or endoscopically.

Skin necrosis was observed in 0–26% of the patients in different case series. The most vital point in preventing necrosis was to keep the dose to the skin less than 120% of the prescribed dose and prevent overlap of the 200% isodose curve.

Other toxicities observed were hyperpigmentation and fibrosis at the site of catheterization.

16.4.5 Outcomes of the Treatment

Brachytherapy in the treatment of penile cancer has shown promising results [21], with local control rates of 70–87% at 5 years and 70% at 10 years, as well as cancer-specific survival rates of 72–92% at 10 years [18]. Common complications include necrosis, stenosis, meatal stenosis, and soft tissue ulceration. Penile preservation rates range from 70% to 88% at 5–10 years.

16.5 Urethral Cancer

Treatment of urethral cancer is complex due to its rarity and the diverse treatment options employed. Surgery remains the primary therapeutic option. The fundamental advantage of radiation for urethral cancer is that it preserves organ function while aiming for local disease management. This is especially useful for people in the early stages of the disease or who want non-surgical treatments.

16.5.1 Indications

Brachytherapy is quite helpful for restricted or localized illness, particularly in the anterior urethra, whether used alone or in combination with conservative surgery or EBRT. The approach can be:

- *Intraluminal* (for superficial lesions up to 5 mm deep)
- *Interstitial* (by perineal template or freehand)

16.5.2 Procedure

16.5.2.1 Intraluminal

Intraluminal is performed with a catheter (closed at one end) or the Foley's catheter and after loaded with a radioactive source. The patient is catheterized with a three-way Foley catheter (no. 22). A 34-cm-long nylon catheter is inserted through the drain channel of the Foley and securely attached at the distal end. The urine drainage bag is linked to the side tube. The patient undergoes MRI-based planning. MRI helps to delineate the gross tumor volume (GTV) accurately. The clinical target volume contains the GTV, a 10 mm margin on each extremity of the lesion, and a 5 mm margin on the infiltrating section [22].

16.5.3 Dose Prescription

ESTRO recommends 65 Gy for brachytherapy alone with LDR and 20–25 Gy for boost. The recommended dose of HDR is 4–5 sessions of 10 Gy each in 3–4 weeks [23].

16.5.4 Expected Toxicities

16.5.4.1 Acute Complications

Most commonly observed toxicities are pain and inflammation at the implantation site. Less than 5% of the patients experience worsening of urinary symptoms.

16.5.4.2 Late Complications

Late complications were observed in the form of secondary strictures, urethral fistula, or erectile dysfunction.

16.5.5 Outcomes After Brachytherapy

Brachytherapy has been described as an ideal method for organ preservation for urethral cancer. Most of the superficial lesions had excellent responses to treatment. They had an overall survival rate of about 83% compared to invasive tumors, which had a poor response to treatment with an overall response of about 23%. The treatment is well tolerated with minimal toxicities [23].

16.6 Carcinoma Urinary Bladder

The role of brachytherapy in the carcinoma of the urinary bladder has increased in recent era, particularly as part of bladder-sparing regimens or for patients who cannot undergo more invasive surgical treatments such as cystectomy. Here is an overview of the role and benefits of brachytherapy in treating bladder cancer:

16.6.1 Bladder Preservation

Brachytherapy is particularly efficient as a bladder-preserving strategy. It is frequently utilized in situations where cancer has not penetrated the muscle layer of the bladder (non-muscle-invasive bladder cancer, NMIBC) and in some selected cases of muscle-invasive bladder cancer (MIBC) where bladder preservation is a priority [24].

16.6.2 Combination with External Beam Radiation Therapy (EBRT)

After EBRT, brachytherapy can be utilized as a boost. EBRT treats a greater area, including potential microscopic illness, whereas brachytherapy increases the tumor dose, increasing radiation therapy's total efficacy.

The literature reports two schedules: a "low" EBRT dose for the bladder alone and a "high" EBRT dose for the bladder with or without pelvic nodes. Low-dosage EBRT is followed by high-dose brachytherapy and high-dosage EBRT is followed by low-dosage brachytherapy [25]. The total cumulative dose of EBRT and brachytherapy for all regimens in terms of biological equivalent dose at 2 Gy/fraction (EQD2) is roughly 70 Gy with an α/β-ratio of 10–15 Gy.

16.6.3 Treatment of Recurrent Disease

Brachytherapy is an effective treatment option for recurrent bladder tumors, especially if previous treatments such as TURBT (transurethral resection of bladder tumor) or EBRT have failed [26]. The GEC/ESTRO criteria for patient selection are given in Table 16.11.

16.6.4 Procedure

Bladder implantations are generally performed using two types of procedures:

- *The open retropubic method*—The surgical technique for brachytherapy catheter placement in bladder cancer treatment includes:
  - Making a surgical incision to gain access to the bladder.
  - Locating the tumor in the bladder.
  - Measuring tumor size to determine catheter placement.

Table 16.11 GEC/ESTRO recommendation for patient selection for brachytherapy in Ca urinary bladder [27]

Solitary tumor with maximum tumor diameter <5 cm
No concurrent carcinoma in situ elsewhere in the body
Tumor classified as cT2-T3
Tumor not located in bladder neck or prostatic urethra
No distant metastasis

- Inserting a curved hollow needle into the bladder wall.
- Inserting a flexible brachytherapy catheter via the needle.
- Ensuring that catheters exit the bladder and abdominal wall appropriately.
- Using intravenous spacers or metallic clips for guiding.
- Finishing the operation by securing the catheters.
- Taking out catheters and spacers at the end of treatment.

- *The minimally invasive endoscopic surgical approach* combines transperitoneal (robot-assisted) laparoscopy and simultaneous cystoscopy. This method uses both cystoscopy (flexible or rigid) and laparoscopy to identify the target volume. The cystoscope can detect the implantation site, the TURBT scar, or the tumor itself. During laparoscopy, the light from the cystoscope shines through the bladder wall, indicating the location to be implanted.

16.6.5 Target Volume Delineation and Plan Evaluation

The *target volume* is defined as the site of the visible TURBT scar or persistent tumor.

The *CTV* is defined as the scar or tumor with a 5 mm margin in all directions. The total detrusor thickness, including the mucosa, is part of the CTV. ICRU recommendation for reporting HDR-BT in Ca Urinary bladder is given in Table 16.12.

Table 16.12 ICRU recommendation for reporting HDR-BT in Ca urinary bladder [27]

External beam: Total dose, fraction dose
Technique of implantation: (a) Retropubic approach (b) Laparoscopic/robot-assisted technique
CTV size: Length, width, thickness
Number of catheters
Delivered dose (a) PDR: Pulse dose, number of pulses, period time (b) HDR: Fraction dose, number of fractions, time between fractions
Total reference air kerma (TRAK)
CTV dose-volume parameters (for brachytherapy): D98, D90, V100, V150
OARs dose-volume parameters (for brachytherapy) (a) Non-involved bladder (outside of CTV): V100 (b) Non-involved bladder (outside of CTV): D2 cm^3 (c) Rectum: D2 cm^3, D0.1 cm^3 (d) Sigmoid: D2 cm^3, D0.1 cm^3 (e) Small bowel: D2 cm^3, D0.1 cm^3

16.6.6 Expected Toxicities

16.6.6.1 Acute Complications

The most common acute complications seen after brachytherapy are worsening urinary symptoms in frequency, urgency, and obstruction of urine flow. Hematuria is observed in some cases and is often self-resolving. Acute gastrointestinal complications may be observed in the form of nausea, vomiting, or diarrhea.

16.6.6.2 Late Complications

Bladder fibrosis is the most commonly observed chronic toxicity after brachytherapy that leads to urinary incontinence and bladder irritation. Erectile dysfunction is a rare complication observed post brachytherapy.

16.6.7 Outcomes After Brachytherapy

The use of brachytherapy in treating carcinoma (CA) urinary bladder has improved local control with preserved bladder function. 90% of the patients maintain normal functioning bladder post-treatment. No difference in survival outcomes was observed when compared to surgical approaches, but there is a significant reduction in procedure-related morbidity and an improvement in overall quality of life. Multiple studies about brachytherapy in bladder preservation demonstrated 5-year and 10-year disease-specific survival rates of 68% and 59%, respectively [24].

16.7 Conclusion

Brachytherapy has proven great potential in treating genitourinary malignancies and has shown its benefit over various other treatments. The precision in targeting, ability for dose escalation, dose conformity, shorter duration, and potential for organ preservation make brachytherapy an attractive treatment option for genitourinary malignancies.

References

1. Chargari C, Deutsch E, Blanchard P, Gouy S, Martelli H, Guérin F, et al. Brachytherapy: an overview for clinicians. CA Cancer J Clin. 2019;69(5):386–401.
2. Marwaha G, Macklis R, Singh AD, Wilkinson A. Brachytherapy. Dev Ophthalmol. 2013;52:29–35.
3. Zaorsky NG, Davis BJ, Nguyen PL, Showalter TN, Hoskin PJ, Yoshioka Y, et al. Evolution of brachytherapy for prostate cancer. Nat Rev Urol. 2017;14(7):415–39.
4. Porter AT, Blasko JC, Grimm PD, Reddy SM, Ragde H. Brachytherapy for prostate cancer. CA Cancer J Clin. 1995;45(3):165–78.

5. Challapalli A, Jones E, Harvey C, Hellawell GO, Mangar SA. High dose rate prostate brachytherapy: an overview of the rationale, experience and emerging applications in the treatment of prostate cancer. Br J Radiol. 2012;85(Spec Iss 1):S18–27.
6. Hoskin PJ, Colombo A, Henry A, Niehoff P, Paulsen Hellebust T, Siebert FA, et al. GEC/ESTRO recommendations on high dose rate afterloading brachytherapy for localised prostate cancer: an update. Radiother Oncol J Eur Soc Ther Radiol Oncol. 2013;107(3):325–32.
7. Salembier C, Lavagnini P, Nickers P, Mangili P, Rijnders A, Polo A, et al. Tumour and target volumes in permanent prostate brachytherapy: a supplement to the ESTRO/EAU/EORTC recommendations on prostate brachytherapy. Radiother Oncol J Eur Soc Ther Radiol Oncol. 2007;83(1):3–10.
8. Behmueller M, Tselis N, Zamboglou N, Zoga E, Baltas D, Rödel C, et al. High-dose-rate brachytherapy as monotherapy for low- and intermediate-risk prostate cancer. oncological outcomes after a median 15-year follow-up. Front Oncol. 2021;11:770959.
9. Szlag M, Ślosarek K, Rembielak A, Białas B, Fijałkowski M, Bystrzycka J. Real-time brachytherapy for prostate cancer – implant analysis. Rep Pract Oncol Radiother. 2008;13(1):9–14.
10. Lavoie-Gagnon H, Martin AG, Poulin E, Archambault L, Pilote L, Foster W, et al. Advantages of TRUS-based delineation for high-dose-rate prostate brachytherapy planning. J Contemp Brachytherapy. 2022;14(1):1–6.
11. Martell K, Kollmeier MA. Complications and side effects of high-dose-rate prostate brachytherapy. Brachytherapy. 2021;20(5):966–75.
12. Mohammed N, Kestin L, Ghilezan M, Krauss D, Vicini F, Brabbins D, et al. Comparison of acute and late toxicities for three modern high-dose radiation treatment techniques for localized prostate cancer. Int J Radiat Oncol Biol Phys. 2012;82(1):204–12.
13. Miszczyk M, Magrowski Ł, Krzysztofiak T, Stando R, Majewski W, Stawiski K, et al. Brachytherapy boost improves survival and decreases risk of developing distant metastases compared to external beam radiotherapy alone in intermediate and high risk group prostate cancer patients. Radiother Oncol. 2023;183:109632.
14. Rodda S, Tyldesley S, Morris WJ, Keyes M, Halperin R, Pai H, et al. ASCENDE-RT: an analysis of treatment-related morbidity for a randomized trial comparing a low-dose-rate brachytherapy boost with a dose-escalated external beam boost for high- and intermediate-risk prostate cancer. Int J Radiat Oncol Biol Phys. 2017;98(2):286–95.
15. Sathya JR, Davis IR, Julian JA, Guo Q, Daya D, Dayes IS, et al. Randomized trial comparing iridium implant plus external-beam radiation therapy with external-beam radiation therapy alone in node-negative locally advanced cancer of the prostate. J Clin Oncol Off J Am Soc Clin Oncol. 2005;23(6):1192–9.
16. Hoskin PJ, Rojas AM, Bownes PJ, Lowe GJ, Ostler PJ, Bryant L. Randomised trial of external beam radiotherapy alone or combined with high-dose-rate brachytherapy boost for localised prostate cancer. Radiother Oncol. 2012;103(2):217–22.
17. Hasan S, Francis A, Hagenauer A, Hirsh A, Kaminsky D, Traughber B, et al. The role of brachytherapy in organ preservation for penile cancer: a meta-analysis and review of the literature. Brachytherapy. 2015;14(4):517–24.
18. Rouscoff Y, Falk AT, Durand M, Gal J, Chand ME, Gautier M, et al. High-dose rate brachytherapy in localized penile cancer: short-term clinical outcome analysis. Radiat Oncol Lond Engl. 2014;9:142.
19. Crook JM, Haie-Meder C, Demanes DJ, Mazeron JJ, Martinez AA, Rivard MJ. American Brachytherapy Society-Groupe Européen de Curiethérapie-European Society of Therapeutic Radiation Oncology (ABS-GEC-ESTRO) consensus statement for penile brachytherapy. Brachytherapy. 2013;12(3):191–8.
20. Kellas-Śleczka S, Białas B, Fijałkowski M, Wojcieszek P, Szlag M, Cholewka A, et al. Nineteen-year single-center experience in 76 patients with penile cancer treated with high-dose-rate brachytherapy. Brachytherapy. 2019;18(4):493–502.
21. Sharma DN, Joshi NP, Gandhi AK, Haresh KP, Gupta S, Julka PK, et al. High-dose-rate interstitial brachytherapy for T1-T2-stage penile carcinoma: short-term results. Brachytherapy. 2014;13(5):481–7.

22. Chakrabarti B, Ghorai S, Ray SB, Kar SK. Intraluminal urethral brachytherapy for recurrence of transitional cell carcinoma of urinary bladder in urethral stump. J Contemp Brachytherapy. 2013;5(1):42–4.
23. Lewis S, Pal M, Bakshi G, Ghadi YG, Menon S, Murthy V, et al. High-dose-rate brachytherapy – a novel treatment approach for primary clear cell adenocarcinoma of male urethra. J Contemp Brachytherapy. 2015;7(3):248–51.
24. Bos MK, Marmolejo RO, Rasch CRN, Pieters BR. Bladder preservation with brachytherapy compared to cystectomy for T1-T3 muscle-invasive bladder cancer: a systematic review. J Contemp Brachytherapy. 2014;6(2):191–9.
25. de Crevoisier R, Ammor A, Court B, Wibault P, Chirat E, Fizazi K, et al. Bladder-conserving surgery and interstitial brachytherapy for lymph node negative transitional cell carcinoma of the urinary bladder: results of a 28-year single institution experience. Radiother Oncol. 2004;72(2):147–57.
26. Zhou YM, Feng X, Zhou BC, Fan YF, Huang YL. Evaluation of therapeutic effects of 125I particles brachytherapy for recurrent bladder cancer. Oncol Lett. 2018;15(3):3453–7.
27. Pieters BR, van der Steen-Banasik E, Smits GA, Brabandere MD, Bossi A, Limbergen EV. GEC-ESTRO/ACROP recommendations for performing bladder-sparing treatment with brachytherapy for muscle-invasive bladder carcinoma. Radiother Oncol. 2017;122(3):340–6.

17 Supportive Care in Urogenital Cancer

Rajesh Mahajan, Divya Khosla, and Naine Bhadrala

17.1 Introduction

The World Health Organization (WHO) defines palliative care (PC) as an approach that enhances the well-being of patients, both adults and children, as well as their families who are confronting life-threatening illnesses. Its main objective is to prevent and alleviate suffering by quickly identifying, thoroughly assessing, and treating pain and other problems, whether they are physical, psychosocial, or spiritual [1].

The contemporary notion of palliative care (PC) originated from the hospice movement of the 1970s, spearheaded by Dame Cicely Saunders, a figure renowned for her transformative contributions to end-of-life care. In 1967, she established the world's first modern hospice in London, UK, introducing the groundbreaking concept of 'total pain'. Concurrently, Balfour Mount, a young urologist at McGill University in Canada, observed feelings of abandonment, psychological distress, and a heightened risk of suicide among cancer patients. He initiated studies on terminally ill patients at the Royal Victoria Hospital, seeking guidance from Cicely Saunders to deepen his understanding of end-of-life care. Mount introduced palliative care services in both inpatient acute-care and community settings, coining the term "palliative care" from the Latin roots "palliare" (to cloak) and "palliate" (to mitigate). Transitioning from urologic oncology, Mount dedicated himself to full-time practice in PC, eventually being appointed as the inaugural Chair in Palliative Medicine at McGill University [2]. Nonetheless, patients with genitourinary cancers still confront significant unmet needs, resulting in enduring adverse effects on their physical, functional, psychological, and socioeconomic well-being. This

R. Mahajan (✉) · N. Bhadrala
Department of Anaesthesia, Critical Care, Pain, and Palliative Medicine, Government Medical College, Jammu, India

D. Khosla
Department of Radiotherapy and Oncology, PGIMER, Chandigarh, India

R. Madan, S. Goyal (eds.), *Essentials of Radiotherapy in Uro-Genital Malignancies*, https://doi.org/10.1007/978-981-95-5945-9_17

circumstance is striking given the historical progression of PC and the close association urology maintains with its advancement [3, 4].

Genitourinary cancers encompass various types of cancers affecting the urinary system (bladder, kidneys, ureters, urethra) and the male reproductive system (prostate, testes, penis). The symptoms experienced in genitourinary cancers can vary depending on the specific type and stage of the cancer [5, 6]. Providing PC to genitourinary malignancies is one of the models of specialty-aligned palliative care (SAPC), which denotes interprofessional PC provided to a distinct patient group in close collaboration with primary or specialized healthcare professionals for diseases. Caring for patients with complex conditions requires PC clinicians to acquire more specialized medical knowledge to provide enhanced SAPC [8, 9]. The following tips mainly emphasize the foundational work that can help palliative care (PC) clinicians form new relationships and establish collaborative Specialist-Advanced Palliative Care (SAPC) programmes (Table 17.1) [10]. Another crucial aspect of this process is the significant investment in building relationships with specialists. In developing these relationships, palliative care clinicians should prioritize being easily accessible to specialists (Table 17.2) [10].

Patients in the advanced stages of terminal illness, not only restricted to genitourinary malignancy, may encounter typical urologic problems. Effectively addressing these symptoms is crucial to guarantee a high standard of care towards the end of life. Effectively addressing urologic symptoms such as pain, spasms, bladder outlet blockages, spinal cord compression, haematuria, and delirium is of utmost importance when adopting a palliative approach in advanced illness [5, 8, 11, 12].

However, patients may not readily disclose genitourinary symptoms to healthcare providers due to embarrassment, such as urinary frequency or incontinence. Further, Patients diagnosed with genitourinary malignancies, particularly bladder and prostate cancer, face an elevated risk of suicide. This risk is most pronounced

Table 17.1 Key considerations for palliative care practitioners when providing specialized palliative care

1. Invest significantly in establishing connections with experts.
2. Acquire knowledge about the fundamental causes of symptoms, usual disease progressions, and key decision junctures for patients facing severe illnesses within the specialized field.
3. When initiating a program, opt for patient groups where your influence can be maximized.
4. Set clear expectations and boundaries right from the beginning.
5. Develop initial bonds with those most inclined to collaborate and refer, allowing those who are more hesitant to be encouraged by initial achievements.
6. Integrate SAPC clinics within specialty requirements by adjusting their workflows and schedules accordingly.
7. Assume positive motives: Approach with humility, curiosity, and diplomacy to foster cooperative integration.
8. Actively identify areas of overlap and unique skill sets in primary care domains, and progressively refine roles and expectations to ensure efficient and impactful patient care.
9. View each consultation as a chance for mutual learning.
10. Broaden your primary care scope by actively involving interprofessional team members aligned with your specialized areas.

Adapted from Umbehr et al. [8] and Wu et al. [9]

Table 17.2 Enhancing accessibility for palliative care clinicians to foster relationships with specialized healthcare providers

1. Make sure to share your contact details frequently and repeatedly.
2. Aim to reply promptly.
3. Suggest holding brief meetings before tackling complex discussions. Request regular feedback on specific aspects, such as the usefulness of consultations and suggestions for improvement.
4. Create opportunities to review and discuss challenging cases, promoting mutual understanding and building rapport.
5. Engage in joint visits together to reinforce commitment, demonstrate value, and display availability.
6. Address emotionally taxing aspects of the job to connect with colleagues on an empathetic level, potentially mitigating burnout and moral distress.
7. Utilize collaborative reflection to clarify the roles related to primary care contributions.
8. Provide consistent updates about patients, particularly during transitions to comfort-oriented or hospice care, potentially aiding specialists in finding closure and relief.

Adapted from Umbehr et al. [8] and Wu et al. [9]

among males, older individuals, those of white ethnicity, those with advanced cancer stages, those living alone, and those with concurrent psychological comorbidities. Identifying patients at risk of developing these symptoms enables early investigation and management. Early detection, the implementation of risk-reduction strategies, and the timely referral to mental health experts are imperative actions in addressing this concern [13].

The primary objectives of palliative care for genitourinary malignancies encompass the following aspects [5, 7, 11]:

1. Symptom Control: Effectively addressing physical symptoms such as pain, urinary issues (such as haematuria or obstruction), sexual dysfunction, and fatigue associated with genitourinary malignancies.
2. Emotional and Psychosocial Assistance: Identifying and addressing the emotional and psychosocial hurdles encountered by both patients and their families.
3. Facilitating Communication and Shared Decision-Making: Encouraging transparent and collaborative communication among healthcare providers, patients, and their families.
4. Providing Spiritual and Cultural Guidance: Recognizing and respecting the significance of spiritual and cultural beliefs in patients' lives.
5. Supporting Caregivers: Recognizing that caregiver support significantly impacts the well-being of patients and their families.
6. Encouraging Advance Care Planning: Engaging patients in discussions about their preferences for end-of-life care, including resuscitation, life-sustaining measures, and the designation of a healthcare proxy or power of attorney.
7. Ensuring Continuity of Care: Guaranteeing consistent and coordinated support, symptom management, and emotional care as patients transition through different stages of their illness.

The overarching aim of palliative care for genitourinary malignancies is to enhance the overall quality of life for patients and their families by focusing on physical comfort, emotional well-being, effective communication, and comprehensive support throughout the course of the disease.

17.1.1 Anatomy and Neural Innervation of Lower Urinary Track

Before we proceed to discuss the specifics of administrating palliative care in cases of genitourinary malignancy, it is essential to first provide a concise overview of the anatomy and neural connections of the lower genitourinary tract. This includes a description of significant receptors in lower genitourinary tract and how frequently employed drugs in palliative care affect these receptors. (Fig. 17.1) [14, 15].

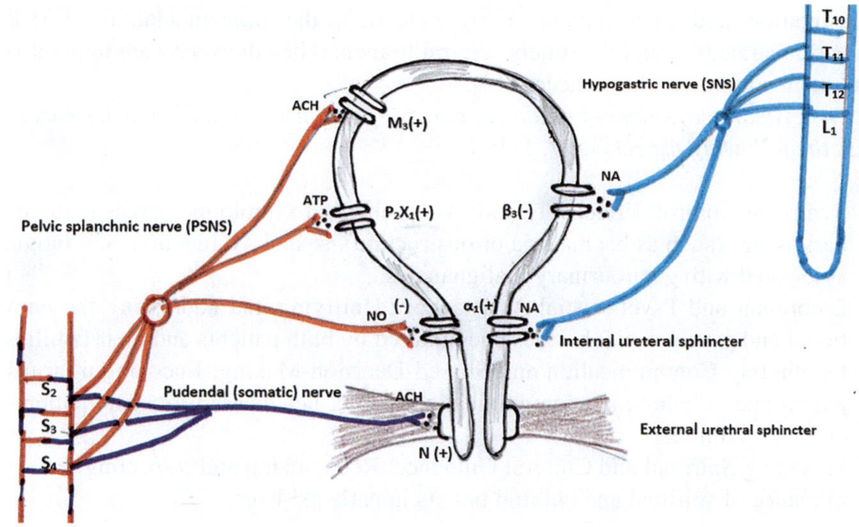

Fig. 17.1 Illustrates the innervation of the lower urinary tractThe parasympathetic nervous system (PSNS), specifically the pelvic nerve, activates the bladder detrusor muscle through the stimulation of muscarinic receptors (M3) by acetylcholine (ACH) and purinergic receptors (P2X1) by adenosine triphosphate (ATP) and relaxation of the urethral smooth muscle via nitric oxide (NO)Sympathetic nervous system (SNS), via the hypogastric nerve, stimulates the urethral smooth muscle and inhibits the bladder detrusor through α1-adrenergic and β3-adrenergic receptors, respectivelySomatic pudendal nerve triggers the striated muscle of the external urethral sphincter, facilitated by ACH activation of nicotinic (N) receptors. (NA denotes noradrenaline. Parenthesized plus and minus signs indicate neural stimulation and inhibition, respectively)

Table 17.3 Medications that affect bladder function

Antipsychotics/sedatives	Sedative effect, potentially causing confusion and relaxing the detrusor muscle, possibly leading to urinary retention
Beta-receptor antagonists	Urinary retention
Calcium channel blockers	Urinary retention, fecal impaction
Diuretics	Increase urine production (polyuria) and volume, resulting in urgency and frequency
Methylxanthines (caffeine, theophylline)	Polyuria, bladder irritation
Neuroleptics (thioridazine, chlorpromazine)	Anticholinergic effect
Opioids	Urinary retention, fecal impaction, sedation, delirium
Sedatives and hypnotics	Sedative effect, which might relax the detrusor muscle
Tricyclic antidepressants	Anticholinergic and alpha-receptor antagonist effects, resulting in postvoid dribbling, straining, and hesitancy in urine flow

Adapted from Newman and Wein [15]
UI urinary incontinence

17.1.2 Medications Acting on Urinary System

A medication assessment could prove beneficial for palliative patients who are often prescribed numerous medications, as these substances might potentially exacerbate urinary problems such as retention or incontinence (Table 17.3). Additionally, an array of medications is employed to address genitourinary symptoms, and a concise summary of these is also available (Table 17.4) [14, 15].

17.2 Symptoms Burden Associated with Genitourinary Malignancy

17.2.1 Haematuria

Haematuria is a common symptom associated with urological malignancies. It can manifest as either microscopic (not visible to the naked eye) or frank (visible) haematuria. In cases of frank haematuria, clot formation can occur, leading to bladder tamponade and urinary retention. There are several potential causes of haematuria, including tumours such as renal, ureteric, bladder, or prostate tumours; urinary tract infection; drug-induced bleeding (e.g., from aspirin, anticoagulants, or nonsteroidal anti-inflammatory drugs); systemic coagulation disorders; radiation cystitis, chemotherapy-related haemorrhagic cystitis (cyclophosphamide, doxorubicin, and ifosfamide); and urinary calculi [16–19].

To investigate haematuria, various tests and procedures may be performed, including urinalysis, microscopy, urine culture, CT urogram/IV urogram,

Table 17.4 Drugs used to treat genitourinary problems

Drugs		Indication	Dosage	Side effect
Antimuscarinic	Oxybutynin	Overactive bladder, urinary incontinence	Immediate-release tablets: 5 mg 2–3 times daily; extended-release tablets: 5–30 mg once daily.	Dry mouth, constipation, blurred vision, dizziness, drowsiness, urinary retention.
	Tolterodine		Immediate-release tablets: 1–2 mg twice daily; extended-release capsules: 2–4 mg once daily	
	Solifenacin		5–10 mg once daily	
	Darifenacin		7.5–15 mg once daily	
	Trospium		Immediate-release tablets: 20 mg twice daily	
	Fesoterodine		4–8 mg once daily	
Beta-3 Adrenergic Agonists	Mirabegron	Overactive bladder	25–50 mg once daily	Increased blood pressure, increased heart rate, urinary tract infection, headache, dizziness
Alpha-1 Adrenergic Antagonists	Tamsulosin	Benign prostatic hyperplasia (BPH).	0.4 mg once daily.	Dizziness, low blood pressure, abnormal ejaculation, headache, nasal congestion.
	Alfuzosin		Extended-release tablets: 10 mg once daily.	
	Silodosin		8 mg once daily.	

(continued)

Table 17.4 (continued)

Drugs		Indication	Dosage	Side effect
Prostaglandin Analogs	Misoprostol	Prevention of gastric ulcers caused by nonsteroidal anti-inflammatory drugs (NSAIDs)	Varies depending on the condition being treated.	Diarrhea, abdominal pain, nausea, vomiting, uterine contractions
	Alprostadil	Erectile dysfunction, patent ductus arteriosus in neonates	Varies depending on the form (injection or suppository) and condition being treated.	Pain at the injection site, dizziness, penile pain
Muscarinic Receptor Agonists	Bethanechol	Urinary retention, neurogenic bladder.	10–50 mg 3–4 times daily.	Abdominal cramps, diarrhea, excessive salivation, sweating, urinary urgency.
Desmopressin (DDAVP)		Diabetes insipidus, nocturnal enuresis	Varies depending on the condition being treated.	Headache, nausea, nasal congestion, water retention, hyponatremia
Botox		Overactive bladder, neurogenic bladder	Injected into the bladder muscle under medical supervision	Urinary tract infection, urinary retention, pain at the injection site, hematuria

ultrasound scan, and cystourethroscopy. The treatment of haematuria involves addressing any reversible causes, such as treating urinary tract infections and systemic coagulation disorders. It is also important to discontinue any medications that may be contributing to the bleeding. General measures include encouraging oral fluid intake to promote urine output and prevent clot retention. In cases of anaemia, transfusion may be considered to alleviate symptoms.

Additional treatment options for haematuria include the use of medications like ethamsylate to enhance platelet adhesion, which can help reduce bleeding. The use of tranexamic acid is controversial due to the potential formation of hard blood clots. Continuous bladder irrigation employing haemostatic agents capable of precipitating proteins can offer potential benefits. This procedure entails rinsing the bladder with a saline solution followed by the application of solutions like 1% alum, formalin (0.5–1%), silver nitrate, or epsilon aminocaproic acid for ongoing bladder irrigation. Transurethral coagulation can be performed to cauterize bleeding vessels within the bladder. In more critical conditions, embolization of the internal iliac artery may be necessary to control the bleeding.

External radiotherapy, typically delivered at a dose of 30 Gy in 10 fractions, can be beneficial. Radiation therapy can shrink tumour burden and resolve haematuria. However, radiation can itself cause haematuria, with severe haemorrhagic cystitis being a known late adverse effect occurring months to years after pelvic radiation [18]. This radiation-induced haematuria can be managed with various interventions, including catheterization, clot removal, endoscopic treatment, systemic or intravesical therapies, hyperbaric oxygen therapy, and, in extreme cases, urinary diversion with or without cystectomy. In severe cases with bladder tamponade and intense lower abdominal pain, a urinary diversion procedure like cutaneous ureterostomy may be considered when other measures fail to relieve symptoms. It's important to consult with a healthcare professional for a proper diagnosis and individualized treatment plan for haematuria.

17.2.2 Urinary Retention [20–23]

Refers to the inability to fully empty the bladder, and it can occur as either a chronic or acute condition. There are several underlying causes of urinary retention, which can be classified into different categories. Local causes include urinary tract infections, benign prostate hypertrophy, pelvic tumours, constipation, urethral stricture, haematuria with blood clots, malignant prostate enlargement, and bladder neck infiltration. Neurological causes encompass spinal cord compression, presacral plexopathy, and surgical denervation due to procedures such as radical hysterectomy or prostatectomy. Debility factors like generalized weakness, immobility, and decreased consciousness level can also contribute to urinary retention. Certain medications, such as anticholinergics, tricyclic antibiotics, phenothiazines, opioids, and α-agonists, may also induce the condition.

Acute urinary retention is considered a medical emergency, often accompanied by severe abdominal pain and a strong urge to urinate. In such cases, immediate management involves temporary urinary catheterization or, if not possible, consultation with a urologist for suprapubic catheterization or cystostomy.

Chronic urinary retention, on the other hand, presents with mild discomfort or pain, lower abdominal distention, difficulty initiating urination, weak urinary flow, and a sense of incomplete bladder emptying. It can also manifest as increased urination frequency and nocturnal enuresis, which may be misdiagnosed as incontinence. Prolonged urinary retention can lead to various complications, including kidney and bladder damage, urinary tract infections, hydronephrosis, renal failure, and stubborn constipation due to the bladder-bowel interdependency [23]. These complications can further result in agitation, confusion, and additional health issues.

Implementing simple non-pharmacological measures can be highly beneficial in managing urinary retention. These measures include establishing regular toilet habits by using a commode instead of bedpans, ensuring privacy during bathroom visits, applying suprapubic pressure, creating the sound of running water by turning on a tap, and placing a hot water bottle on the lower abdomen. It is essential to monitor fluid balance and serum electrolytes while addressing and treating the underlying causes specific to each patient's needs. Constipation can be managed with laxatives, and urinary tract infections should be promptly treated. In cases of clot retention, discontinuing anticoagulants and addressing bleeding diathesis may be necessary. It is important to review the medications and drugs the patient is taking to ensure they are not aggravating the condition. Neurological causes require careful management and treatment as needed. When it comes to catheterization, the options to consider depend on the underlying pathology and may include urethral catheterization for long-term use, suprapubic catheterization, or intermittent self-catheterization. For benign or malignant prostate enlargement, options such as transurethral resection or laser ablation of the prostate can be considered.

17.2.3 Urinary Tract Infections [24–26]

Patients in palliative care often experience urinary tract infections (UTIs), which can have a broad range of presentations, ranging from no symptoms at all to severe manifestations that can potentially result in septic shock. Common symptoms include dysuria, incontinence, urinary retention, haematuria, suprapubic or loin pain, fever, and confusion. Various risk factors contribute to UTIs, such as low urinary output (due to dehydration), bladder dysfunction (outlet obstruction, neuropathic bladder), catheterization, diabetes mellitus, immunocompromise, and vesical fistulae. The most frequently encountered pathogens causing UTIs are Escherichia coli, followed by Streptococcus faecalis, Proteus, Pseudomonas, and Klebsiella, species.

Diagnostic measures include urine testing for protein, blood, leukocytes, and nitrites, with a negative result on all tests making UTI unlikely. A midstream urine sample should be obtained for culture. In most patients, a clinical diagnosis combined with positive bedside testing is sufficient to initiate treatment.

Treatment begins with recommendation of increased fluid intake. Urinary alkalis such as potassium citrate, sodium citrate, and sodium bicarbonate can alleviate urgency symptoms for UTIs. Urine culture and antibiotic sensitivities are recommended. However, awaiting culture sensitivities reports, common antibiotic regimens like trimethoprim 200 mg twice daily for 3 days, ciprofloxacin 250–500 mg twice daily orally or intravenously, co-amoxiclav 375 mg three times daily orally or intravenously, cefalexin 250 mg four times daily orally, and cefuroxime 125–250 mg twice daily orally or intravenously can be initiated.

While the presence of an indwelling or suprapubic catheter raises the likelihood of bacterial infections, with approximately 50% of patients developing bacteriuria within 10–14 days, intervention is not required unless the patient exhibits symptoms or undergoes re-catheterization/instrumentation. For individuals experiencing recurrent urinary tract infections, using prophylactic low-dose antibiotics or antibacterial agents like hexamine Hippurate can be beneficial.

17.2.4 Bladder Spasm/Bladder Pain [27–30]

The mechanism of bladder contraction is from severe spasms of detrusor muscle causing the patient to feel the urge to urinate. Severe bladder spasms may cause urinary incontinence. There may be cramping pain with burning sensation. There are two types of bladder pain, obstructive and irritative.

Bladder pain can result from either acute or chronic obstruction. Acute obstruction often leads to intense lower abdominal pain along with restlessness, anxiety, or delirium. Treatment typically involves addressing the underlying cause or relieving symptoms through urinary catheterization. Irritative bladder pain, however, is primarily caused by inflammation triggered by various factors such as external radiation, chemotherapeutic agents like cyclophosphamide, bladder tumours, mechanical irritation from catheters, bladder calculi, or infective cystitis. Symptoms may include increased urinary frequency, dysuria, urgency, and incontinence.

Treatment focuses on removing any offending agent or treating any local disease like urinary tract infection with antibiotics. If catheterized, change the urinary catheter or reduce balloon volume. Non-pharmacological measures like adequate fluid intake and avoiding certain foods such as coffee, alcohol, spicy foods and preservatives, which can exaggerate bladder spasms. The patient should follow "bladder drill" (e.g., voiding every 1.5–2 h by the clock). Pelvic floor exercises can be helpful. TENS devices, which provide electrical stimulation through skin, may help.

Pharmacological management includes use of anticholinergic drugs to relax the bladder and prevent spasms (flavoxate, oxybutynin, tolterodine and solifenacin). Tricyclic antidepressants (amitriptyline, imipramine), and α-blockers(terazosin,doxazocin) can also be used to reduce bladder spasms. Additionally, for alleviating bladder neck irritation, alpha-blockers and phenazopyridine can be utilized. Pain may persist after dealing with the primary cause and may even require opioid and non-opioid analgesics like NSAIDs. Corticosteroids could potentially decrease inflammation related to bladder tumours, thus potentially alleviating associated pain.

Intravesically administered local anaesthetics and opioids can be helpful. Lidocaine 2% or bupivacaine 0.5% (mixed with 0.9% sodium chloride) can be introduced via a catheter in place, and the catheter should then be closed off for a duration of 20 min to 1 h. Nerve block and neurolytic procedures like neurolytic hypogastric plexus block, ganglion impar block, and phenol saddle block may be helpful after consultation with pain physician. Injection of Botox into the bladder wall at cystoscopy may provide relief for up to 3 months.

In cases of urethral irritation caused by a transurethral catheter, switching to a suprapubic catheter is a valid alternative. The choice of treatment invasiveness should align with the patient's overall condition, be tailored to their specific needs, take into account their symptom burden, and consider the potential impact of the proposed treatment.

17.2.5 Urinary Incontinence [30, 31]

It refers to the unintentional release of urine, causing distressing symptoms that impact patients physically, psychologically, socially, and sexually. This condition leads to anxiety, low self-esteem, difficulty socializing, and disrupted sleep. Caregivers are also significantly affected. There are different types of urinary incontinence (Table 17.5).

Dignity-protective continence care involves respect, empathy, trust, privacy, autonomy, and proficient communication [32, 33]. This includes providing continence pads, regularly checking pad saturation to prevent odour and excessive wetness, and ensuring privacy by closing doors or curtains during toileting. Additionally, promptly responding to calls for continence care is crucial to build trust and prevent incontinence. Timely care delivery also helps avoid incontinence-associated dermatitis. Empowering patients by involving them in their care allows them to regain a sense of control and reduces their self-perceived burden.

In cases of severe and unmanageable urinary incontinence, a condom-type collecting container or indwelling urinary catheter may be necessary. However, it is important to respect the patient's preference to urinate independently. If other options are not feasible, suprapubic catheterization can be considered. More invasive surgical procedures like urinary diversion stomas or augmentation cystoplasty are rarely performed in palliative care settings.

A medication review could be advantageous for palliative patients who are frequently prescribed multiple medications, as these drugs may potentially worsen urinary issues such as retention or incontinence (Table 17.1).

17.2.6 Genitourinary Fistulas [34, 35]

Genitourinary fistulas are abnormal connections between the genital tract and various organs like the bladder, ureter, urethra, rectum, or colon. They often occur in advanced cancer patients due to factors like radiotherapy or tumour growth. These fistulas can lead to severe symptoms, including uncontrolled discharge of urine or feaces, pelvic pain, and emotional distress. Managing them requires a multidisciplinary approach, including radiotherapy, catheterization, and, in some cases, surgery. Skin protection, absorbent products, and odour management are also essential aspects of care.

Specific types of genitourinary fistulas include vesico-vaginal, uretero-vaginal, urethra-vaginal, recto-vaginal, colo-vaginal, entero-vaginal, vesico-enteric, vesico-colonic, and recto-urethral fistulas. Each presents its own challenges and considerations in terms of diagnosis and management.

Rectovaginal fistulas involve an abnormal connection between the rectum and vagina, resulting in stool and gas leakage into the vagina. Diagnosis involves careful examination and diagnostic tests. Treatment options may include surgery or faecal diversion through a colostomy or ileostomy.

Table 17.5 Overview of urinary incontinence types

Type of UI	Description	Worsened by these agents	Treatment
Functional	Untimely urination because of physical disability, external obstacles, or problems in thinking or communicating that prevent a person from reaching a toilet	Drugs that increase fluid retention, nocturnal diuresis, sedation, or cognitive impairment (alcohol, anticholinergics, antidepressants, antihistamines, antipsychotics, NSAIDs, opioids, sedatives/hypnotics, skeletal muscle relaxants, thiazolidinediones	Eliminate causes
Overflow	Urinary retention or overdistended bladder owing to anatomical, neurogenic, and/or drug factors	Drugs that cause bladder relaxation (or decrease bladder contractions), sedation, and urinary retention (anticholinergics, antidepressants, antihistamines, antipsychotics, calcium channel blockers, dopamine agonists, opioids, skeletal muscle relaxants	Reviewing medications Alfa-adrenergic blockers (terazosin, tamsulosin) Urethral dilatation (anatomical cause) Permanent catheterization, suprapubic catheterization, or indwelling catheters may be necessary
Stress	Increased intra-abdominal pressure from physical activities (e.g., coughing, exercise, jumping, lifting. laughing)	Drugs that decrease bladder sphincter tone or contribute to coughing (ACE inhibitors (bradykinin cough), alpha-adrenergic antagonists	Lifestyle modifications like reducing caffeine intake, quitting smoking, weight loss, pelvic floor exercises Vaginal estrogen creams Suppressing cough with certain cough depressants can also be beneficial.

(continued)

Table 17.5 (continued)

Type of UI	Description	Worsened by these agents	Treatment
Urge/OAB	Involuntary leakage accompanied by or immediately preceded by urgency	Drugs that increase urine flow and bladder contractions (alcohol, caffeine, diuretics (carbonic anhydrase inhibitors, loop diuretics, thiazides), lithium)	Underlying causes like urinary tract infections should be treated. Behavioural therapy, including adjusting water intake, treating constipation, bladder training, and muscle training Anticholinergic agents (e.g., oxybutynin and tolterodine) B3 adrenergic agonists can be considered
Mixed	Typically, a combination of stress and urge\ incontinence		Dependent on symptoms that predominate

NSAID Nonsteroidal anti-inflammatory drug, *OAB* overactive Bladder, *UI* Urinary incontinence

Vesico-enteric fistulas often occur in palliative care settings due to colonic malignancy. Symptoms include gas or froth in urine, foul odour, recurrent urinary tract infections, and the presence of faecal matter in urine. Diagnosis involves various tests, and treatment may require surgical removal of affected bowel and bladder segments or bypass procedures like colostomy or ileostomy.

Vesicovaginal fistulas involve continuous urine leakage into the vagina and require differentiation from total urethral incontinence. Diagnosis is aided by various diagnostic tools, and surgical excision is the most effective treatment. In some cases, urinary diversion or nephrostomy may be considered.

Overall, the management of genitourinary fistulas in palliative care is complex and requires a tailored approach to each patient's specific condition and needs.

17.2.7 Upper Urinary Tract Obstruction [36–40]

Upper urinary tract obstruction occurs when one or both ureters or kidneys are blocked, potentially leading to kidney function impairment or failure. Causes include external factors like tumours, fibrosis, or strictures, and internal factors like tumours or stones. Bilateral or unilateral obstruction with compromised kidney function can rapidly lead to renal failure, with symptoms like drowsiness, dehydration, and reduced urine output.

Patients with ureteric obstruction may have no symptoms or experience lower back to groin pain. Sepsis and kidney dysfunction signs include nausea, vomiting, haematuria, and reduced consciousness. Diagnosis is made through ultrasound, CT, or MRI.

Management depends on cause, history, and prognosis. Electrolyte balance may require urgent treatment, fluid balance monitoring, and antibiotics for infections. Pain management should be tailored to the patient's renal function. Nonsteroidal anti-inflammatory drugs (NSAIDs) can be used to relieve pain and reduce the renal response to acute urinary obstruction, although caution is needed in impaired kidney function. Opioid analgesics may also be administered to alleviate the pain. In cases where there is tumour-related swelling, dexamethasone in doses of 8–16 mg may be beneficial. However, anticholinergic medications like hyoscine butyl bromide do not have a role in managing acute ureteric colic. Alpha-blockers relax prostatic smooth muscle and reduce outflow resistance and may be helpful specifically for individuals with distal ureteric calculi. Newer medications, such as tamsulosin and silodosin, specifically target the alpha-1a receptor, offering a better side effect profile. Definitive management can be considered for reversible obstructions, such as shockwave lithotripsy or endoscopic surgery for kidney stone disease.

The decision to perform urological intervention should consider the patient's and family's wishes and take into account the prognosis. Intervention may be beneficial for patients with rapid renal failure progression and a few months of life expectancy, while palliative care without intervention is suggested for patients with short life expectancy.

Ureteric stenting is a reasonable approach for newly diagnosed patients with potential tumour regression through radiotherapy, chemotherapy, or surgery. When stent placement is not feasible, interventional radiologists or urologists may insert percutaneous nephrostomy tubes. While interventions such as nephrostomy or ureteral stenting can enhance symptoms and quality of life, resulting in improved performance status, they do not extend survival durations. More invasive procedures like urinary diversion and reconstructive surgery for ureteral strictures or ureteropelvic junction obstruction are rarely utilized in palliative care, unless the patient's underlying condition treatment indicates a significant life expectancy.

17.2.8 Lower Urinary Tract Obstruction

Lower urinary tract obstruction involving the bladder, prostate, and urethra can lead to urinary retention. Proper emptying of the lower urinary tract depends on bladder contraction and the absence of obstruction. Abnormalities in these aspects can result from neurological conditions like traumatic brain injury, stroke, or pelvic nerve injuries.

Mechanical urinary obstruction can be caused by conditions such as benign prostatic hyperplasia (BPH), urethral strictures, or pelvic malignancies. Severe constipation can also contribute to obstruction. To evaluate lower urinary tract obstruction and retention, a comprehensive history and physical examination are crucial. Symptoms include slow urinary flow, incomplete emptying, urgency, and more. Medication history and examination findings like palpable bladder or tenderness help diagnose retention. Imaging studies like ultrasound, CT, or MRI are used to confirm the diagnosis. Cystoscopy and urodynamic evaluation provide further insights.

Treatment depends on the severity. Observation, catheter placement, pharmacological therapy (alpha-blockers, 5-alpha-reductase inhibitors), and clean intermittent catheterization (CIC) are options. Surgical procedures like transurethral resection of the prostate (TURP) may be necessary in certain cases [41–43].

17.2.9 Changes in Urine Appearance and Colour

Alterations in the colour and appearance of urine can arise from a range of factors, including underlying medical conditions and treatments, in individuals with genitourinary cancer. These changes may lead to unwarranted anxiety and should be managed effectively (Table 17.6) [29, 44].

17.2.10 Dysuria [10, 43]

Dysuria, or painful urination, can be a distressing symptom for patients with serious or terminal illnesses. Dysuria in palliative care patients can stem from various causes, including urinary tract infections (UTIs), bladder irritation, urinary retention, or underlying medical conditions. To effectively manage dysuria in this context, several considerations come into play.

First and foremost is the need for a thorough assessment to pinpoint the underlying cause. Healthcare providers should delve into the patient's medical history, conduct physical examinations, and possibly order relevant tests, such as urine cultures,

Table 17.6 Common changes in urine appearance/discoloured urine

Changes in colour	Common causes
Red/pink	Hematuria, rifampicin, phenazopyridine, senna laxatives, beetroot, dantron, doxorubicin, hematuria, nefopam
Orange/yellow	Nitrofurantoin, sulfasalazine, phenazopyridine liver or bile duct obstruction or other disease, dehydration
Blue/green	Amitriptyline, indomethacin, propofol, methylene blue, pseudomonas aeruginosa
Dark brown	Liver or kidney disease, urinary tract infection, metronidazole, nitrofurantoin, senna laxatives, methocarbamol
Foamy	Proteinuria
Strong odor	Certain foods (e.g., asparagus)
Sediment or floating material	Protein crystallization, urolithiasis, tissue shedding, or blood clots

Adapted from Sinclair et al. [30]

to determine the precise cause of dysuria. Once identified, addressing the underlying cause becomes crucial. For instance, if a UTI is the culprit, initiating appropriate antibiotic treatment based on culture and sensitivity results is vital. Tailored interventions should be applied for other identified causes.

Pain management remains a cornerstone of palliative care, and if dysuria is causing discomfort, the implementation of adequate pain relief measures is paramount. This may involve the use of analgesic medications to alleviate the associated pain. Ensuring the patient's hydration is another important aspect, as it can help prevent UTIs and maintain overall urinary tract health. However, it's essential to strike a balance and avoid overhydration, which could lead to discomfort due to increased urine production.

Maintaining good perineal hygiene is essential to prevent irritation and potential infection, necessitating caregivers to keep the patient's genital area clean and dry. Additional comfort measures such as applying a warm, moist cloth to the genital area or taking a warm bath can help ease discomfort related to dysuria. In cases of urinary retention, appropriate bladder management techniques should be considered, including catheterization or other interventions prescribed by healthcare professionals.

Dysuria is associated with significant emotional distress, and offering emotional support and fostering open communication is crucial to alleviate anxiety and address concerns related to this symptom. Regular follow-up appointments are imperative to monitor the patient's condition, assess the effectiveness of interventions, and adjust the treatment plan as needed, based on the patient's preferences, medical history, and overall care goals.

17.3 Sexual Concerns and Intimacy [45–47]

Individuals diagnosed with genitourinary malignancies, such as prostate, bladder, testicular, and kidney cancers, often face significant concerns about their sexual health. The cancer itself and its treatments, including surgery, radiation therapy, chemotherapy, and hormonal therapy, can have various impacts on sexual function and overall well-being. These effects may include issues like erectile dysfunction, decreased libido, orgasmic dysfunction, pain during intercourse, and changes in fertility.

Maintaining sexual health is essential for overall well-being, and healthcare providers should not make assumptions about what patients want or need from their sexual relationships. Instead, they should actively explore how illness affects patients' self-perception, relationships, and sexuality. Patients may be hesitant to discuss these issues, so it is important for clinicians to initiate conversations about them without judgement.

Additionally, healthcare providers should not assume that older patients or those who are single and not in long-term relationships do not desire intimacy or sexual relationships. When patients seek assistance with their sexual concerns, a comprehensive medical history should be gathered, considering the influence of medications like hormone therapy on libido and sexual function. Obtaining a sexual history is most effective when using open-ended, nonjudgmental questions. The goal is to make discussions about sexuality feel natural, address potential barriers, and provide support, assurance, or appropriate treatment. Various tools have been studied for obtaining sexual history. The Permission, Limited Information, Specific Suggestions, and Intensive Therapy (PLISSIT) model is an example of a four-step approach to sexual history and intervention. Additionally, other symptoms, such as dyspnoea, pain, fatigue, and wound issues, should be addressed in the context of sexual intimacy.

The emotional and psychological implications of a cancer diagnosis on sexual health should not be underestimated. Patients may benefit from counselling or support groups that focus on the emotional aspects of sexual health and help them cope with the changes they are experiencing.

17.4 Cancer-Related Fatigue

Cancer-related fatigue (CRF) is a prevalent issue among cancer patients, arising from factors associated with both the disease itself and its treatments. Unfortunately, many patients opt not to disclose this symptom to their healthcare providers, often perceiving it as something they cannot avoid, inconsequential, or untreatable. Management of CRF includes routine screening, systematic assessment, and multidisciplinary interventions for prevention and treatment. CRF screening should be incorporated into routine patient assessments, alongside vital sign measurements. Once these symptoms are acknowledged, a systematic process for identifying modifiable causes (such as anaemia, hormone imbalances, and the direct or indirect effects of cancer and its treatments) can help dispel the notion of inevitability and the belief that fatigue cannot be addressed. Initiating discussions about CRF right from the beginning of cancer treatment can also facilitate the implementation of non-pharmacological preventive measures, such as exercise before, during, and after cancer treatments [48].

17.5 Caregiver Burden [49–51]

Caregivers supporting patients with genitourinary malignancies face several significant challenges and issues, including emotional distress, coping with uncertainty, physical care tasks, treatment-related responsibilities, communication and advocacy, balancing personal life, emotional challenges, spiritual requirements, intimacy concerns, financial strain, and neglecting self-care. To address these challenges, a multidisciplinary approach is needed, involving healthcare providers who recognize and support caregivers, offer information and referrals to supportive services, and encourage caregivers to seek help and prioritize self-care.

17.6 Advance Planning in Genitourinary Malignancies [11, 52]

It involves proactive discussions and decision-making processes to prepare patients and their families for future healthcare decisions [11, 52, 53]. Effective advance care planning can be achieved within an integrated urology-palliative care clinic, with many patients with terminal illnesses preferring a less aggressive approach to end-of-life care. Key components include:

1. Advance Directives: Legal documents like living wills and durable power of attorney for healthcare enable patients to specify their medical treatment preferences.
2. Goals of Care Discussions: Healthcare providers engage in conversations to understand the goals and values of patients and their families, guiding treatment decisions to align with patient preferences.
3. Treatment Preferences: Patients discuss their treatment preferences, considering risks, benefits, and outcomes, and these are documented in their medical records.
4. Communication and Shared Decision-Making: Continuous communication ensures that patients and families make informed decisions regarding the disease, treatments, and potential outcomes.
5. Prognostic Discussions: Healthcare providers inform patients and families about disease progression, complications, and expected survival, assisting in decision-making.
6. Palliative Care and Hospice Referrals: Discussions include referrals to palliative care and hospice services, providing symptom management, quality of life enhancement, and end-of-life support.
7. Supportive Care and Survivorship Planning: Addressing long-term effects and survivorship needs, including surveillance, follow-up care, and strategies for well-being post-treatment.

Advance planning in genitourinary malignancies upholds patient values, fosters patient-centred decision-making, and ensures continuity of care throughout the disease trajectory.

17.7 End-of-Life Care [11, 53]

End-of-life care (EOLC) pertains to the provision of support for individuals in various circumstances:

(a) Those in the final stages of life, typically expected to pass away within a few hours or days due to advanced, progressive, incurable conditions.
(b) Individuals experiencing frailty alongside coexisting conditions, with an anticipated life expectancy of no more than 12 months.

(c) People with pre-existing conditions who face the risk of sudden acute crises leading to death.
(d) Individuals dealing with life-threatening acute conditions resulting from sudden catastrophic events. A 'good death' is characterized by the absence of pain, the presence of support from loved ones, and the ability to choose one's preferred setting for end-of-life care. Crucial elements of this care encompass:

1. Acknowledgement of the patient's terminal phase.
2. Symptom Management: Addressing pain and other distressing symptoms, including anticipatory prescribing for pain, respiratory issues, agitation, nausea, vomiting, and difficulty breathing.
3. Regular review of clinical interventions to ensure they align with the patient's best interests.
4. Effective Communication and Shared Decision-Making: Facilitating open discussions about prognosis, treatment choices, and advance care planning, involving both patients and their families.
5. Assessment of hydration and nutrition needs, including considerations for initiation or discontinuation.
6. Ongoing reassessment of the patient's condition.
7. Support for caregivers, including education, respite care, and emotional assistance to sustain their well-being.
8. Provision of emotional and psychosocial support, offering counselling and resources to address emotional challenges.
9. Ensuring dignified and respectful care following death.
10. Offering bereavement support to family members after the patient's passing, including counselling and connection with support groups.

In essence, end-of-life care for genitourinary malignancies aims to respect patients' preferences, alleviate suffering, and foster a compassionate environment for patients and their families.

17.8 Bereavement Support [54, 55]

Comprehensive PC should encompass exceptional bereavement assistance, which can commence well before the death of the patient. Initiating discussions about the impending event and outlining the available support mechanisms can significantly alleviate stress for the caregiver. Following the patient's demise, it is essential to extend support to the family members. This support may encompass various aspects, including the provision of information, financial aid, social support, psychological assistance, counselling, and connecting them with support groups. The interventions may need to involve individual, family, and group-based approaches, as well as the involvement of volunteer, spiritual, or religious experts.

References

1. Palliative Care. Palliative care (who.int). Accessed 30 Sept 2023.
2. Hugar LA, Wulff-Burchfield EM, Winzelberg GS, Jacobs BL, Davies BJ. Incorporating palliative care principles to improve patient care and quality of life in urologic oncology. Nat Rev Urol. 2021;18(10):623–35.
3. Iversen K, Oechsle K, Oing C, Bokemeyer C, Seidel C. Specific characteristics of patients with advanced genitourinary cancer receiving specialized inpatient palliative care. Oncol Res Treat. 2017;40(10):609–6.
4. Hugar LA, Lopa SH, Yabes JG, Yu JA, Turner RM 2nd, Fam MM, MacLeod LC, Davies BJ, Smith AB, Jacobs BL. Palliative care use amongst patients with bladder cancer. BJU Int. 2019;123(6):968–75.
5. Tsushima T, Miura T, Hachiya T, Nakamura I, Yamato T, Kishida T, Tanaka Y, Irie S, Meguro N, Kawahara T, Nakajima N. Treatment recommendations for urological symptoms in cancer patients: clinical Guidelines from the Japanese Society for Palliative Medicine. J Palliat Med. 2019 Jan;22(1):54–61.
6. Schuler US. Early integration of palliative and oncological Care: con. Oncol Res Treat. 2019;42(1–2):19–24. https://doi.org/10.1159/000495699. Epub 2018 Dec 21. PMID: 30572330.
7. Saraiya B, Dale W, Singer EA, Cella D. Integration of palliative and supportive care into the management of genitourinary malignancies. Am Soc Clin Oncol Educ Book. 2022;42:1–10.
8. Umbehr MH, Wagg A, Habib MH, Antonelli JA, Chughtai B, Jang TL, Kaldany A, et al. Top ten tips palliative care clinicians should know about urological care. J Palliat Med. 2023;26(2):264–9.
9. Leiter RE, Bischoff KE, Carey EC, Gelfand SL, Iyer AS, Jain N, et al. Top ten tips palliative care clinicians should know about delivering specialty-aligned palliative care. J Palliat Med. 2023;26(10):1401–7.
10. Drudge-Coates L, Oh WK, Tombal B, Delacruz A, Tomlinson B, Ripley AV, Mastris K, O'Sullivan JM, Shore ND. Recognizing symptom burden in advanced prostate cancer: a global patient and caregiver survey. Clin Genitourin Cancer. 2018;16(2):e411–9.
11. Huen K, Huang C, Liu H, Kwan L, Pannell S, Laviana A, Saucedo J, Lorenz K, Bennett C, Bergman J. Outcomes of an integrated urology-palliative care clinic for patients with advanced urological cancers: maintenance of quality of life and satisfaction and high rate of hospice utilization through end of life. Am J Hosp Palliat Care. 2019;36(9):801–6.
12. de Lima MM Jr, Tobias-Machado M. Suicide in patients with genitourinary malignancies. Eur J Cancer Care (Engl). 2017;26(6) https://doi.org/10.1111/ecc.12635.
13. Andersson K-E, Wein AJ. Anatomy, physiology and pharmacology of the lower urinary tract. In: Urologic principles and practice. 2nd ed. Springer. p. 78–123.
14. Winkler D, Grohmann R, Friedrich ME, Toto S, Bleich S, Seifert J, Konstantinidis A, Shariat SF, Kasper S, Pjrek E. Urological adverse drug reactions of psychotropic medication in psychiatric inpatients – a drug surveillance report from German-speaking countries. J Psychiatr Res. 2021;144:412–20.
15. Newman DK, Wein AJ. Managing and treating urinary incontinence. 2nd ed. Baltimore: Health Professions Press.
16. Ghahestani SM, Shakhssalim N. Palliative treatment of intractable hematuria in context of advanced bladder cancer: a systematic review. Urol J. 2009;6(3):149–56.
17. Abt D, Bywater M, Engeler DS, Schmid HP. Therapeutic options for intractable hematuria in advanced bladder cancer. Int J Urol. 2013;20(7):651–60.
18. Ogita M, Kawamori J, Yamashita H, Nakagawa K. Palliative radiotherapy for gross hematuria in patients with advanced cancer. Sci Rep. 2021;11(1):9533. https://doi.org/10.1038/s41598-021-88952-.

19. Bergstra TG, Gutmanis I, Byrne J, Faulds C, Whitfield P, McCallum S, Shadd J. Urinary retention and medication utilization on a palliative Care unit: a retrospective observational study. J Pain Palliat Care Pharmacother. 2017;31(3–4):212–7.
20. Stabholz Y, Sandhu JS. Management of voiding dysfunction associated with pelvic malignancies. Int J Urol. 2021;28(1):17–24.
21. Pais R, Lee P, Cross S, Gebski V, Aggarwal R. Bladder care in palliative care inpatients: a prospective dual site cohort study. Palliat Med Rep. 2020;1(1):251–8.
22. Charach G, Greenstein A, Rabinovich P, Groskopf I, Weintraub M. Alleviating constipation in the elderly improves lower urinary tract symptoms. Gerontology. 2001;47(2):72–6.
23. Cooper FPM, Alexander CE, Sinha S, Omar MI. Policies for replacing long-term indwelling urinary catheters in adults. Cochrane Database Syst Rev. 2016;7:CD011115.
24. Pickard R, Lam T, MacLennan G, Starr K, Kilonzo M, McPherson G, et al. Antimicrobial catheters for reduction of symptomatic urinary tract infection in adults requiring short-term catheterisation in hospital: a multicentre randomised controlled trial. Lancet. 2012;380(9857):1927–35.
25. Zumstein V, Parsons BA, Dabestani S, Baranowski AP, Tidman V, Berghmans B, et al. The benefits and harms of pharmacological treatment for post-radiation pelvic pain: a systematic review by the European Association of Urology chronic pelvic pain panel with recommendations for clinical practice. Eur Urol Open Sci. 2023;56:29–38.
26. Meng E, Hsu YC, Chuang YC. Advances in intravesical therapy for bladder pain syndrome (BPS)/interstitial cystitis (IC). Low Urin Tract Symptoms. 2018;10(1):3–11.
27. De E, Gomery P, Rosenberg LB. Palliation of bladder spasms #337. J Palliat Med. 2017;20(10):1158–9.
28. Ahmed DG, Mohamed MF, Mohamed SA. Superior hypogastric plexus combined with ganglion impar neurolytic blocks for pelvic and/or perineal cancer pain relief. Pain Physician. 2015;18(1):E49–56.
29. Chiu B, Tai HC, Chung SD, et al. Botulinum toxin a for bladder pain syndrome/interstitial cystitis. Toxins (Basel). 2016;8(7):201.
30. Sinclair CT, Kalender-Rich JL, Griebling TL, Porter-Williamson K. Palliative care of urologic patients at end of life. Clin Geriatr Med. 2015;31(4):667–78.
31. Habib MH, Arnold RM. Urinary incontinence in palliative care settings: part 2: management #426. J Palliat Med. 2021;24(11):1734–5.
32. Ostaszkiewicz J, Tomlinson E, Hutchinson AM. "Dignity": a central construct in nursing home staff understandings of quality continence care. J Clin Nurs. 2018;27(11–12):2425–37.
33. Newman DK. The indwelling urinary catheter: principles for best practice. J Wound Ostomy Continence Nurs. 2007;34(6):655–61; quiz 62–63.
34. Hampson SJ, Morris SB, Gordon EM, Shearer RJ. Management of inoperable pelvic carcinomas with complex fistulas: a new approach. Ann R Coll Surg Engl. 1994;76(3):188–9.
35. Stamatakos M, Sargedi C, Stasinou T, Kontzoglou K. Vesicovaginal fistula: diagnosis and management. Indian J Surg. 2014;76(2):131–6.
36. Singh I, Strandhoy JW, Assimos DG. Pathophysiology of urinary tract obstruction. In: Wein AJ, Kavoussi LR, Novick AC, Partin AW, Peters CA, editors. Campbell-Walsh urology. 10th ed. Philadelphia: Elsevier Saunders; 2011. p. 1107–18.
37. Hsu L, Li H, Pucheril D, Hansen M, Littleton R, Peabody J, Sammon J. Use of percutaneous nephrostomy and ureteral stenting in management of ureteral obstruction. World J Nephrol. 2016;5(2):172–81.
38. Garg G, Bansal N, Singh M, Sankhwar SN. Role of percutaneous nephrostomy in bladder carcinoma with obstructive uropathy: a story revisited. Indian J Palliat Care. 2019;25(1):53–6.
39. Zhou Y, van Melle M, Lyratzopoulos G, Walter F. Factors affecting diagnostic timeliness and safety in symptomatic patients subsequently diagnosed with bladder and kidney cancer: a systematic review. J Glob Oncol. 2018;4(4_suppl_2)
40. Sountoulides P, Mykoniatis I, Dimasis N. Palliative management of malignant upper urinary tract obstruction. Hippokratia. 2014;18(4):292–7.

41. Tabib C, Nethala D, Kozel Z, Okeke Z. Management and treatment options when facing malignant ureteral obstruction. Int J Urol. 2020;27(7):591–8.
42. Liberman D, Jarosek S, Virnig BA, Chu H, Elliott SP. The patient burden of bladder outlet obstruction after prostate cancer treatment. J Urol. 2016;195(5):1459–63.
43. Yaxley JP. Urinary tract cancers: an overview for general practice. J Family Med Prim Care. 2016;5(3):533–8.
44. Aycock RD, Kass DA. Abnormal urine color. South Med J. 2012;105(1):43–7.
45. Kelemen A, Cagle J, Chung J, Groninger H. Assessing the impact of serious illness on patient intimacy and sexuality in palliative Care. J Pain Symptom Manag. 2019;58(2):282–8.
46. Bennett MR. PLISSIT interventions and sexual functioning: useful tools for social work in palliative Care? J Soc Work End Life Palliat Care. 2019;15(4):157–74.
47. Wittmann D, Bober SL. Incorporating the principles of sex therapy into urologic care. Urol Clin North Am. 2021;48(4):425–36.
48. Fabi A, Bhargava R, Fatigoni S, Guglielmo M, Horneber M, Roila F, Weis J, Jordan K, Ripamonti CI; ESMO Guidelines Committee. Electronic address: clinicalguidelines@esmo.org. Cancer-related fatigue: ESMO Clinical Practice Guidelines for diagnosis and treatment. Ann Oncol 2020;31(6):713–723.
49. Alam S, Hannon B, Zimmermann C. Palliative care for family caregivers. J Clin Oncol. 2020;38(9):926–36.
50. Oliveira C, Fonseca G, Areia NP, Sotero L, Relvas AP. Caring for people who take care: what is already done? Palliat Support Care. 2022;20(5):720–30.
51. Lim HA, Tan JY, Chua J, Yoong RK, Lim SE, Kua EH, Mahendran R. Quality of life of family caregivers of cancer patients in Singapore and globally. Singapore Med J. 2017;58(5):258–61.
52. Pannell SC, Laviana AA, Huen KHY, Shelton JB, Kwan L, Bennett CJ, Lorenz KA, Bergman J. Advance care planning and patient preferences in a feasibility pilot study to improve end-of-life communication among men with metastatic urological malignancies. Urol Pract. 2018;5(6):421–6.
53. Davis MP, Bruera E, Morganstern D. Early integration of palliative and supportive care in the cancer continuum: challenges and opportunities. Am Soc Clin Oncol Educ Book. 2013:144–50.
54. Grassi L. Bereavement in families with relatives dying of cancer. Curr Opin Support Palliat Care. 2007;1(1):43–9.
55. Chau NG, Zimmermann C, Ma C, Taback N, Krzyzanowska MK. Bereavement practices of physicians in oncology and palliative care. Arch Intern Med. 2009;169(10):963–71.